Normal and Abnormal Processes in the Basic Sciences

2nd edition

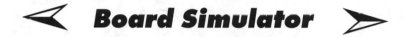

Board Simulator

Normal and Abnormal Processes in the Basic Sciences

2nd edition

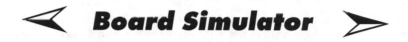

Board Simulator

DEVELOPED BY

NATIONAL MEDICAL SCHOOL REVIEW®

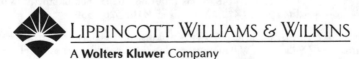

LIPPINCOTT WILLIAMS & WILKINS

A **Wolters Kluwer** Company

Philadelphia · Baltimore · New York · London
Buenos Aires · Hong Kong · Sydney · Tokyo

Editor: Elizabeth A. Nieginski
Managing Editors: Amy G. Dinkel, Darrin Kiessling
Development Editors: Melanie Cann, Beth Goldner, Carol Loyd
Manager, Development Editing: Julie Scardiglia
Editorial Assistant: Lisa Kiesel
Marketing Manager: Rebecca Himmelheber
Production Coordinator: Danielle Hagan
Text/Cover Designer: Cotter Visual Communications
Typesetter: Port City Press
Printer/Binder: Port City Press

Copyright © 1997 Lippincott Williams & Wilkins

351 West Camden Street
Baltimore, Maryland 21201-2436 USA

Rose Tree Corporate Center
1400 North Providence Road
Building II, Suite 5025
Media, Pennsylvania 19063-2043 USA

Accurate indications, adverse reactions, and dosage schedules for drugs are provided in this book, but it is possible that they may change. The reader is urged to review the package information data of the manufacturers of the medications mentioned.

Printed in the United States of America

First Edition,

Library of Congress Cataloging-in-Publication Data

Normal and abnormal processes in the basic sciences / developed by
  National Medical School Review. — 2nd ed.
      p.   cm. — (Board simulator)
  Editors and contributors, Gerald D. Barry . . . et al.
  ISBN 0-683-30297-3
  1. Medicine—Examinations, questions, etc.   2. Medical sciences—
Examinations, questions, etc.   I. Barry, Gerald D.   II. National
Medical School Review (Firm)   III. Series.
  [DNLM: 1. Medicine—examination questions.   2. Biological
Sciences—examination questions.   W 18.2 N842 1997]
  R834.5.N67   1997
  610'.76—dc21
  DNLM/DLC
  for Library of Congress   97-6602
                                                                                              CIP

The publishers have made every effort to trace the copyright holders for borrowed material. If they have inadvertently overlooked any, they will be pleased to make the necessary arrangements at the first opportunity.

To purchase additional copies of this book, call our customer service department at **(800) 638-0672** or fax orders to **(800) 447-8438**. For other book services, including chapter reprints and large-quantity sales, ask for the Special Sales department.

Canadian customers should call **(800) 665-1148**, or fax **(800) 665-0103**. For all other calls originating outside of the United States, please call **(410) 528-4223** or fax us at **(410) 528-8550**.

Visit Williams & Wilkins on the Internet: http://www.wwilkins.com or contact our customer service department at **custserv@wwilkins.com**. Williams & Wilkins customer service representatives are available from 8:30 am to 6:00 pm, EST, Monday through Friday, for telephone access.

99 00
4 5 6 7 8 9 10

DEDICATION

This book is dedicated to the loving memory of Dr. Richard Swanson: 1954–1996. Rick was an inspiration as an author, teacher, and physician. Rick led by example and his death is a loss to all of us whose lives he touched.

Rick is survived by his wife Stella, daughter Heidi, and sons Eric and Jason.

CONTENTS

EDITORS AND CONTRIBUTORS

GERALD D. BARRY, Ph.D.
Professor of Physiology and Director of the MA/MD
  Biomedical Program
Touro College School of Health Sciences

GRACE BINGHAM, Ed.D.
President and Educational Consultant
Bingham Associates, Inc.
Toms River, NJ
Coordinator of Cognitive Skills
National Medical School Review

GEORGE M. BRENNER, Ph.D.
Professor and Chairman
Department of Pharmacology
Oklahoma State University
College of Osteopathic Medicine

BARBARA FADEM, Ph.D.
Professor, Department of Psychiatry
University of Medicine and Dentistry
New Jersey Medical School

EDWARD F. GOLJAN, M.D.
Associate Professor and Chairman of Pathology
Oklahoma State University
College of Osteopathic Medicine

DAILA S. GRIDLEY, Ph.D.
Professor
Department of Microbiology and Molecular Genetics
Department of Radiation Medicine
Loma Linda University
School of Medicine

KENNETH H. IBSEN, Ph.D.
Professor, Emeritus
Department of Biochemistry
University of California at Irvine
Director of Academic Development
National Medical School Review

KIRBY L. JAROLIM, Ph.D.
Professor and Chairman
Department of Anatomy
Oklahoma State University
College of Osteopathic Medicine

KATHLEEN KEEF, Ph.D.
Professor
Department of Physiology and Cell Biology
University of Nevada
School of Medicine

JAMES KETTERING, Ph.D.
Professor and Assistant Chairman
Department of Microbiology and Molecular Genetics
Loma Linda University
School of Medicine

RICHARD M. KRIEBEL, Ph.D.
Professor
Department of Anatomy
Philadelphia College of Osteopathic Medicine

WILLIAM D. MEEK, Ph.D.
Professor
Department of Anatomy
Oklahoma State University
College of Osteopathic Medicine

STANLEY PASSO, Ph.D.
Associate Professor
Department of Physiology
New York Medical College

JAMES P. PORTER, Ph.D.
Associate Professor
Department of Physiology and Biophysics
University of Louisville
School of Medicine

VERNON REICHENBECHER, Ph.D.
Associate Professor
Department of Biochemistry and Molecular Biology
Marshall University
School of Medicine

DAVID SEIDEN, Ph.D.
Professor
Department of Neuroscience and Cell Biology
University of Medicine and Dentistry
Robert Wood Johnson Medical School

PREFACE

Since its establishment in 1988, the goal of National Medical School Review® (NMSR) has been to provide medical students and physicians with the information they need to know to pass their national licensing examinations. During this period, NMSR has developed a national reputation for high-quality programs delivered by the best teaching faculty available in United States and Canadian medical schools. Nearly 12,000 participants in NMSR programs have had access to outstanding faculty lectures as well as to diagnostic and practice examinations and high-yield notes that can be kept as learning tools. As a result, NMSR students have achieved an impressive level of success on the United States Medical Licensing Examination (USMLE) Steps 1, 2, and 3.

With the development and publication of the *Board Simulator Series* (BSS), NMSR ushered in a truly innovative new educational experience for medical students and physicians preparing for Step 1 of the USMLE. This five-volume series' unique format was designed to follow the content guidelines published by the National Board of Medical Examiners (NBME) for the USMLE, Step 1, rather than being organized strictly by isolated basic science discipline (for example, volumes dealing only with biochemistry or anatomy). Therefore, just as they appear on the real Step 1 examination, many questions in this series are preceded by a clinical vignette that often integrates two or more disciplines and can require the student to perform a multi-step reasoning process to arrive at a correct answer. Thus, students are challenged not only to recall a particular fact or principle, but to analyze and apply that information to the situation defined by the clinical vignette.

One proven way to increase the likelihood of answering these questions correctly is to practice with questions that are at a similar level of difficulty and that have a similar emphasis. The BSS series provides students with just such an experience. In fact, it is NMSR's belief that this series gives most second-year medical students attending a United States medical school the essential information and test-taking experience required to pass the USMLE, Step 1. This series could also serve as an adjunct to students who feel they would benefit from attending a structured review program.

Furthermore, the BSS series provides far more than simulated Step 1 examinations, because each question is answered with a full and detailed explanation. A student can use these explanations to clarify why the right answers are correct choices and the wrong answers are incorrect choices. In the process of doing this evaluation the student will have performed a comprehensive review of the material covered on the Step 1 examination.

To make this process even more effective, this second edition of the BSS contains 770 questions in each volume, 120 more than in the first edition. Each of the tests in each volume, with the exception of the introductory 50-question diagnostic test, contains 180 questions, which reflects the new USMLE examination booklet's length. This edition also includes a subject item index, allowing students who wish to use these books in a subject-based fashion to do so with greater ease. NMSR believes that as an educational tool this series can help maximize a student's opportunity to make reviewing for the USMLE, Step 1 both a successful and rewarding experience.

Victor Gruber, M.D.
Founder and Executive Director
National Medical School Review®

ACKNOWLEDGMENT

NMSR would like to recognize Edward F. Goljan, M.D., for his valuable contribution to the development and unique organization of topics in this series.

GUIDE TO USING THIS BOOK

During the past 10 years, a number of changes in curriculum organization have occurred in many U.S. and Canadian medical schools, particularly within the first 2 years of education. A number of meaningful innovations have been implemented, such as more self-directed learning, de-emphasis of lectures as the dominant instructional mode, earlier introduction of clinical experiences, and increases in the proportion of problem-based learning.

Today, regardless of which curriculum a medical school adopts, one trend exists even in those schools that have maintained a traditional stance: a loosening of the boundaries that organized basic science material into large territorial "subject" courses. The move is toward synthesizing domains of medical knowledge into more flexible cross-disciplinary patterns believed to approximate interactions that characterize medical practice today.

From a student's perspective, all the attention given to the number and variety of medical school curriculum reforms may have highlighted only the differences among the curricula and neglected to underscore the important similarities remaining. Regardless of the specific curriculum followed at any school, medical students are still expected to:

1. Read and understand large quantities of material. Whether the access mode is texts, handouts, specialized print materials, or computer modules, the reading demands remain significant.

2. Organize information in meaningful ways. No matter how well written a concept may appear in a text, or how well explained in a lecture, the students should *generate* the pattern of meaning that makes the most sense to them.

3. Develop relationships among experiences. All medical students are expected to engage in higher order thinking processes. New information about a topic will need to be *encoded* and *synthesized* with prior knowledge; *compared* with a lab experiment; *evaluated* through discussion with a colleague; or *solved* as a problem.

4. Store, retrieve, and remember information dependably. Historically, the demands on memory for medical personnel have been exceptional. The rapidity with which new technological advances in diagnosis and increases in treatment options are becoming available makes it more difficult than ever to learn and stay up to date in the field. Distinguishing between what needs to be mastered and recalled readily and what does not is a professional decision with which medical practitioners will struggle for the rest of their careers.

5. Demonstrate achievement through various forms of evaluation. Regardless of their curriculum model, all medical schools still require high levels of performance of their students. Evaluators can choose from a large range of methods to assess students, from the traditional instructor-designed examinations to oral evaluations, on-site observations, behavioral checklists, and product evaluations (e.g., written reports, research papers, problem solutions). Whatever the method, students will need to give evidence of competency.

6. Demonstrate competency on national standardized examinations. To qualify for licensure, students need to be successful on Steps 1, 2, and 3 of the USMLE. After further graduate training, students need to demonstrate success on specialty examinations to qualify for Board certification.

Series Design

Some of the more positive changes that characterize medical learning today are already reflected in the design of current instructional materials. One such change is the design of the five books in this series. The organization differs from the traditional subject-oriented subdivisions of basic science in that it conforms more closely to the content outline of USMLE Step 1 as presented in the *General Instructions* booklet. In Step 1, basic science material is organized along two dimensions: system (consisting of general principles and individual organ systems) and processes, which divide each organ system into normal development, abnormal processes, therapeutics, and psychosocial and other considerations.

Book I: General Principles in the Basic Sciences
Book II: Normal and Abnormal Processes in the Basic Sciences
Book III: Body Systems Review I: Hematopoietic/Lymphoreticular, Respiratory, Cardiovascular
Book IV: Body Systems Review II: Gastrointestinal, Renal, Reproductive, Endocrine
Book V: Body Systems Review III: Nervous, Skin/Connective Tissue, Musculoskeletal

Each book contains five examinations: A condensed 50-question diagnostic test; the other four tests contain 180 questions each for a total of 770 questions per book. The distribution of questions within each test in books III, IV, and V approximates subcategory percentages as follows: normal development, 10%–20%; normal processes, 20%–30%; abnormal processes, 30%–40%; principles of therapeutics, 10%–20%; psychosocial, cultural, and environmental considerations, 10%–20%. By comparing your performance on the diagnostic test in each volume, you will be able to prioritize your use of the books.

Questions in each test are presented using the two multiple-choice formats that appear in USMLE Step 1: One Best Answer (including negatively phrased items) and Matching Sets, with the largest number of questions of the One Best Answer type.

Who Can Use These Questions?

The group likely to use the questions in this series of books most frequently is students preparing for USMLE Step 1. However, other student groups who can benefit from these questions are medical students in years I, II, III, and IV. These students may turn to individual books in the series or use the entire set of books as a supplemental self-testing resource.

Students Preparing for USMLE Step 1

Students preparing for the Step 1 exam will use these books as a **diagnostic tool,** as a **guide to focus further study,** and as a **self-evaluation device.**

Specific instructions about how to use the question sets for each purpose will be described in the next section.

Students in Years I and II

Students in years I and II will use these books for **periodic self-testing.** Students in the first 2 years of medical school take a large number of examinations that evaluate their performance on material covered in their courses or other learning experiences. Those tests are usually compiled by the instructors and reflect the intructors' choice of emphasis. The questions in the five books in this series provide a sampling of the wide range of material typically taught in the first 2 years of medical school. For students who want to practice with questions that go beyond the scope of their specific school's course, these question sets will provide them with another level of testing, one that approximates more closely the expectations of the Step 1 exam. These questions also offer opportunities for practice to those students in medical school courses that use Board shelf exams as one of their required evaluations. The section How to Use These Practice Exams provides guidance on their use.

Students in Years III and IV

Students in years III and IV will use these books for **reactivating and assessing prior learning.** During their third and fourth years, students may find during clinical situations that they have forgotten some material they learned during the first 2 years. One way to stimulate, reactivate, and supplement that knowledge is by responding to questions. The content and organization of the questions in each book of the series make it possible for students in the clinical years to select and use specific segments for review.

How to Use These Practice Exams

The four sets of practice questions in this book assess knowledge of principles in ten major topics: (1) biochemistry and molecular biology, (2) biology of cells, (3) human development and genetics, (4) tissues and their responses to disease (e.g., inflammation, repair and regeneration, neoplasias), (5) psychosocial, cultural, and environmental influences on behavior, health, and disease processes, (6) multisystem processes (e.g., nutrition, temperature regulation), (7) pharmacodynamic and pharmacokinetic processes, (8) microbial biology and infection, (9) immune responses, (10) quantitative methods. Questions in this book focus on **Normal and Abnormal Processes** in reference to each of the preceding ten topics. These ten topics are cross-referenced via the subject item index to the seven traditional academic disciplines in which the topic might have been taught or may be found in other NMS or BRS review books.

Whereas the specific information to be assessed in each topic and its subtopics differs, there are certain *categories* of knowledge organization that recur regardless of differences, as can be noted in the small sampling from topics in this book:
— Abnormalities of. . . (energy metabolism; congenital origin; immunologic function)
— Adaptation to. . . (environmental extremes; chemical hazards; radiation)
— Mechanisms of. . . (antimicrobial resistance; receptors; virulence factors)
— Disease origins. . . (viral; bacterial; parasitic)
— Production and function of. . . (T lymphocytes; lymphokines; plasma cells)
— Interaction between. . . (drugs; antimicrobials and infectious agents)
— Manifestation of. . . (leukocytosis; neoplastic disorders; chronic inflammation)
— Maladaptive responses to. . . (stress and illness; lifestyle changes; death and dying)

These question sets may be used in a number of ways: (1) as a diagnostic tool (pretest), (2) as a guide and focus for further study, and (3) for self-evaluation. The least effective use of these questions is to "study" them by reading them one at at time, and then looking at the correct response. Although the questions have been compiled to be representative of the domains of information found in USMLE Step 1, simply knowing the answers to these particular 770 questions does not ensure a passing grade on the exam. The questions are intended to be an integral part of a well-planned review, rather than an isolated resource. If used appropriately, the four sets can provide self-assessment information beyond a numeric score.

As a diagnostic tool. It is possible to use each set of questions as a screening device to gather diagnostic information about relative performance across the 10 large topics presented in this book. For those who have been away from basic science study for awhile and have no other recent performance data, using a practice exam in this manner provides a form of feedback before beginning review. This method also allows students to respond to Board-type questions similar to those on the examination so they can experience the structure and complexity of such questions and acquire a sense of what the questions "feel" like.

1. Select any one of the four complete tests in this book. It does not matter which one you choose, since they are all approximately equal in terms of topics represented and question difficulty.

2. Allow yourself the same amount of time as will be allowed on the Board exam (approximately 60 seconds per question).

3. Use a separate sheet of paper for your answers (instead of writing in the book). This will make it easier for you to score, analyze, and interpret the results.

4. Score your responses (but do not read the correct answer to the question or record the correct response next to your incorrect one). Compute an accuracy level by counting the number of correct responses and dividing by the total number of questions to get the percent correct. Note your score, but be careful not to overreact to this initial score. Remember that this type of sampling provides only a rough indication of how familiar or remote this basic science material seems to you before review. Not reading the correct answer to these questions may seem a bit strange at first, but by not doing so now, you will be able to use these questions again later in your review as a posttest to check progress.

5. Know your distribution of errors across the topics. To find out, categorize each error (e.g., biochemistry, cell biology, genetics; tissue biology, pharmacokinetics, multisystem processes). If in doubt about how to categorize a particular question, check the reference listed in the answer and use that to make your decision.

6. Arrange topics in a hierarchy from relatively strong (few errors) to relatively weak (many errors). Did you do well in those topics you thought you would do well in, and vice versa, or were there some unexpected highs or lows?

To guide further study. After reviewing the material of the major areas noted previously and giving the information a complete "first pass," it is time to test yourself using another question set in this book. Your purpose is to check your estimates of which topics and subtopics have been learned well, which are still shaky, and which are quite weak. To do that:

1. Follow the first five steps described previously.

2. Analyze errors using the guidelines described in the section "Monitoring Functions for Consolidating Information."

3. Focus your follow-up study on the content areas or specific subtopics noted to still be weak. Pay particular attention to whether a pattern of errors has emerged (e.g., questions requiring understanding of genetic principles; questions requiring knowledge of repair and regenerative processes; or questions requiring knowledge of metabolic pathways and associated diseases).

There is another possible use for these questions. If you already know from experience the two or three major topics in this book that cause you the greatest concern, you can:

1. Select from *two* question sets only those questions that deal with those specific topics. (You can identify them easily because each answer is topically keyed.)

2. If the number of questions is large, you may want to divide the number in half and reserve one half for a later test.

3. Follow steps 2 to 4 from the diagnostic testing section.

4. In conducting error analysis, try to pin down more specifically your within-topic errors, so that in follow-up study you can concentrate on strengthening weaknesses that remain.

5. When you feel you have firmed up your information base, test yourself with the other half of the questions and note your progress, as well as any remaining subtopics for follow-up study. The questions not used in the first two sets of questions, as well as the two full sets, can be used as your review progresses.

For self-evaluation. As the last few weeks before the exam approach, some students begin to experience feelings of "approach/avoidance"; they would like to know if they are close to, or even beyond, the minimum needed to pass, but they also fear that if they find a large discrepancy, it may deplete their efforts during the final phase of their review. This situation is less likely to occur with students who have engaged in self-testing throughout their preparation. These students have been collecting and analyzing test data all along and adjusting their study agenda accordingly. The last level of evaluation is not likely to give them any surprises about strengths and weaknesses, but will identify areas in which they can continue to fine-tune.

There are a few different ways to handle the last round of self-testing. Some students feel less anxious if they do the final round of self-evaluation in the first few days of the last week and reserve the rest of the time for last-minute follow-up study. Other students prefer to start the week with a composite test, continue with further study, and then take another practice test 2 or 3 days before the exam.

1. If you have used one full question set as a pretest, it would now be informative to start with those questions as a posttest. Follow the steps described previously and compare performance (both total score and the score across each large basic science topic).

2. The remaining tests can be used as individual question sets, or they can be combined into one large composite set.

3. If none of the tests has been used for pretesting, you might take every other question from all five tests (385 questions) and follow up later with the remaining 385 questions.

4. If you are using other books in this series, you can select a set from each of the other four books to form a comprehensive final evaluation.

Score Interpretation

Keeping in mind that the percentage of items needed to pass the USMLE Step 1 is between 55% and 65% should help you interpret accuracy levels from your self-testing. The practice test samples suggested here (usually 180 questions) provide useful feedback to chart your progress. On your tests, percentages between 55% and 60% are minimal, but encouraging. Percentages between 60% and 75% show you are moving beyond the bare minimum needed for passing. Scores of 75% and above are indicators of substantial strength.

EXAM PREPARATION GUIDE

USMLE Step 1: What to Expect

USMLE Step 1 is the first examination of the three-step sequence required for medical licensure, so it is not surprising that its approach engenders apprehension in many students. Successful performance is particularly consequential in those medical schools that require successful passage of Step 1 before permitting students to proceed to third year. The "new" Step 1 has been in effect since 1991, and although most people are now familiar with its general contours, some "myths" still circulate.

The sources that contain the most complete and specific information about the examination are those distributed to students when they register to take Step 1: *Bulletin of Information* and *USMLE Step 1— General Instructions, Content Outline, and Sample Items.* **Both books should be read in their entirety before taking the examination.** What follows is a brief summary of what can be found in much more detail in those materials.

Description. The purpose of the Step 1 exam is to assess students' understanding and application of important concepts in the basic biomedical sciences: anatomy, behavioral science, biochemistry, microbiology, pathology, pharmacology, and physiology. Emphasis is placed on **principles and mechanisms underlying health, disease, and modes of therapy.**

A "blueprint" in the Guidelines booklet shows how basic science material is organized for the examination. Two dimensions are used: system and process. The first dimension includes a section on General Principles and ten Individual Organ Systems. The second dimension is divided into normal development; normal processes; abnormal processes; principles of therapeutics; and psychosocial, cultural, and environmental considerations. Also shown are the percentages of questions across categories of the two dimensions. The percentages are rather close between General Principles, 40%–50%, and Individual Organ Systems, 50%–60%. Of the categories in dimension 2, abnormal processes has the largest percentage (30%–40%). A more detailed breakdown of content can be found in the *Step 1 Content Outline,* but not all the topics listed are included in each test administration.

Students are expected to respond to some questions that require straightforward basic science knowledge, but the majority of questions require application of basic science principles to clinical situations. There are also questions that require interpretation of graphic and tabular data and identification of gross and microscopic specimens. There seems to be more coverage of content typically taught in the second year, but interdisciplinary topics such as Immunology, which is usually taught in the first year, receive quite a bit of attention.

Format. The 2-day examination consists of four books with approximately 180 items in each book (total, 720 questions). Two books are given on each of the days. Three hours are allowed to complete each book, or approximately 60 seconds per question.

Question types. Two types of questions are on the exam: single best answer and matching sets, which begin with a list of a certain number of response options used for all items in the set.

Scores. Passing is based on the total score. Raw scores are converted to a standard score scale with a mean of 200 and a standard deviation of 20. A score of 176, or 1.2 standard deviations below the mean, is needed to pass.

Examinees will receive a total test score, a pass/fail designation, and a graphic performance "profile" depicting strengths and weaknesses by discipline and organ system. No individual subscores are reported. A two-digit score is also reported, in which a score of 75 corresponds to the minimum passing score and 82 is equivalent to the mean of 200.

A Framework for Successful Preparation

By the time you reach medical school, you have been a student for most of your life. You have learned in a variety of settings and have achieved a number of personal goals. There is probably little that you have not observed about your own learning. Despite this, you may still approach medical studies with some degree of apprehension and have questions about the effectiveness of your study strategies, specific skills, and attitudes.

After experiencing medical courses during their first year or two, most students accommodate well and, if necessary, make whatever adjustments in their study patterns seem warranted. But, even the most competent student, given the pressure of frequent and demanding examinations, will have occasional doubts regarding the efficiency of a particular study method. For those planning to take USMLE Step 1, many questions arise about how best to proceed. "How much time is adequate for review?" "What materials should I use?" "What should I study and in what order?" In discussions with other students, you will hear about approaches they took and what worked for them. But, eventually, you will need to make important decisions for yourself about how to *initiate* and *sustain* a preparation plan that results in success on the exam.

This preparatory guide selects and summarizes, from many different areas of cognitive and educational psychology, those findings that have most applicability to a medical learning context. Strategies, skills, and functions are organized according to their potential utility for students as they move progressively from initial encounter with new learning at stage I, acquiring information, to stage II, consolidating information, and finally to the goal of self-confident achievement, stage III, reaching mastery. In the sections that follow, the conceptual framework shown in Figure 1 will be used to discuss specific suggestions and activities.

FIGURE 1. Medical learning framework.

Cognitive Learning Strategies

Stage I. Acquiring Information

Stage II. Consolidating Information

Stage III. Reaching Mastery

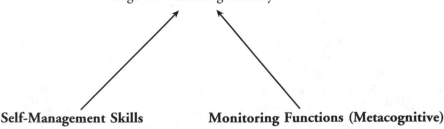

Self-Management Skills	Monitoring Functions (Metacognitive)
Time allocation	Study progress
Effort expenditure	Feelings/stress
Study resources	Self-evaluation

Three main subdivisions are represented in this Medical Learning Framework: cognitive learning strategies, self-management skills, and monitoring functions.

Cognitive learning strategies. These strategies can be used to acquire, retain, and master a massive amount of information in the basic sciences. The strategies will be arranged according to which ones are appropriate at each stage in the learning sequence.

Self-management skills. At each stage of learning noted previously, there are skills that can help students allocate time efficiently, expend effort productively, and use study resources effectively.

Monitoring functions. In addition to the cognitive dimensions, medical learning requires metacognitive functions—the ongoing self-regulation that helps students track their progress and decide whether they need to modify or fine-tune any behaviors. Students also need to monitor and try to control potentially interfering negative feelings and stress.

Cognitive Learning Strategies

Any learning experience a student engages in, whether listening to a lecture, reading a text, observing a demonstration, or viewing a video presentation can be said to move through three stages as the learner proceeds from initial encounter to eventual mastery. Many factors influence the progression from one stage to another, among them the characteristics of the student, such as ability, motivation, attitudes, and interests. Also influential are the characteristics of the material, its conceptual difficulty, its organization, and its relationships to the learner's prior knowledge. The specific study activities the student uses also will have an effect. Whether you are trying to learn medical material for the first time, or reviewing information you learned before and need to reactivate and strengthen, the three-stage concept of how learning takes place offers a handy scheme for deciding which study strategies to use when.

Strategies for Acquiring Information

In this first stage, as you read or listen to a lecture, the main task is consciously and intentionally to generate as much *meaning* (understanding) as you can. Because studies have shown that strong initial *encoding* influences to a large extent what will be stored in long-term memory, there is a payoff for being *active* at this stage. The ongoing task is to decide if what you are reading or hearing is unfamiliar information, somewhat familiar, or already part of your fund of knowledge. Rarely will you encounter something that is completely new, but some topics will seem more remote than others if your previous experience with them has been limited. As you move through the information, do so at as brisk a pace as you can without sacrificing meaning. Following are some productive strategies that can be used at this stage:

1. Preview. Before starting to read, notice how a topic or other chunk of material has been organized. Use external arrangements such as titles and subheadings to get an idea of how the topic has been segmented. One technique is to convert these subdivisions into questions. Study any pictorial material, such as figures and diagrams. Read the introduction, summary, and questions, if available. Read anything that is printed in different type, such as italic, or highlighted. Notice unfamiliar terms and look them up. Remember that the purpose of previewing is to give you a preliminary cognitive "map" that should help you extract more meaning from your subsequent reading.

2. Read actively. When reading a text, handouts, and notes, some parts will trigger recollection from your previous learning. When you encounter familiarity, try *prompting*: Pause and look away from the page, anticipate what will be coming, and try to bring forth from your memory whatever you can recall about that topic. Also, try to read as if on a *search*. Having looked at the subheading of a section and raised questions in your mind about what to expect, read to see if you can find responses to your questions.

3. Link information. Many medical students acknowledge that this is an important and useful strategy for enhancing understanding, yet few actually implement it. As you read, stop periodically and (a) summarize in your own words, (b) draw relationships to other knowledge by comparing and contrasting, (c) make an educated guess (inference), and (d) raise questions (What would happen if. . .?). If you are wondering whether you have time to think about the material given the usual pressures, remind yourself that these are the very thinking processes that are built into the questions of the Step 1 exam.

4. Construct notes. You probably have been taking notes in class since your earliest school days, and you may have developed a system for reducing and compacting lecture information that has served you well in the past. If so, continue using it. If, however, you are still trying to listen and write as much as you can, and as fast as you can, then perhaps you want to try a different method. When an instructor has provided a handout or other type of script before a lecture, preview it ahead and "cue" the sections that are obscure and need more elaboration. Then, you can limit note taking to what is essential to make sense of that script. Use whatever symbols you wish as cues (e.g., stars, circles, triangles) and assign a particular meaning to each. When you return to that handout after the lecture, you can translate your cues into further study activities (e.g., rewrite a particular section, supplement from a text, memorize a procedure).

One activity you might find helpful to institute fairly early is a last-minute study list consisting of those topics, mechanisms, procedures, and details that you find particularly problematic. Record either a brief explanation or the page and reference source where the information can be found. This list is particularly useful toward the end of your exam preparation sequence when you will want to make the most effective use of whatever time remains.

Self-Management Skills

At this early stage there are certain activities related to time, effort, and resources that are appropriate to carry out.

Time

Form a realistic study plan. Before plunging in, give some thought to how you want to organize your plan of study and which factors you need to consider. What is the amount of time you can reasonably allocate to preparation for the exam? If you are preparing for Step 1, it might be 3 or 4 months. If your experience with basic science material goes back a number of years, you will be doing more than simply activating former learning. There will be chunks of recent scientific knowledge that will require more intensive processing and more study time to reach a level of familiarity.

There are a few principles worth observing regardless of the total time actually allocated: (a) Use whatever diagnostic information you have (data-based, if possible) to assign time on the basis of relative strengths and weaknesses. Your review should be comprehensive, but some topics should be given more time than others. (b) Draft a long-range, tentative plan across the time you have available and estimate approximately how much you want to assign to each segment of content. Even a rough plan written down will reduce concern about whether you can fit everything in. You will be able to observe whether you underestimated the number of hours needed and increase them as you implement your plan. (c) Leave the last 2 weeks unscheduled so that you can return to areas that need a second pass. (d) At the end of each week, look at your plan and make changes based on your experiences during that week.

Effort

Get started. Perhaps what takes the most effort at this stage is just "lifting off" and getting into some type of study routine. You may find yourself putting off the actual start until you can finish other "essential" things, but you are probably procrastinating. It may help if you begin by studying something that you are strong in because a feeling of success will encourage you to continue. Gradually, shift to a topic that is less familiar and requires a little more intentional effort.

Select conditions conducive to study. Find a place where you can sustain a study block with few or no distractions. Put yourself in an active study posture, sitting upright, not lying on a couch or bed. Make yourself go to your study place as part of your routine. Staying in your apartment may be convenient, but it also makes it tempting to give in to other distractions.

Establish a reasonable, steady pace. If you are highly motivated, you may be tempted to work for exceptionally lengthy stretches, particularly during the early days of your review. Try, instead, to establish a reasonable routine that allows you to get a return from each study block. Know what your peak work periods are and do your most difficult studying at those times. Pay attention to whether you are getting fatigued and losing your ability to concentrate. Build in breaks that will reenergize you and help you feel refreshed when you return to studying.

Resources

Select effective study materials. Whether you are studying for a class exam or USMLE Step 1, finding just the right study material often can prove frustrating. Although quite a number of study resources are available in bookstores, each differs in purpose, format, depth, and comprehensiveness of coverage. For review, your own notes, charts, and handouts are good sources if you still have them available. They are familiar and have personal associations helpful for recalling information. To initiate review, look for publications that summarize or "compact" information, are not excessively wordy, but still provide enough narrative for you to make sense of the topic. The purpose of such books (e.g., Williams & Wilkins' *Board Review Series*) is to stimulate recall of material learned previously. Finally, have a reliable text available in each of the basic sciences so that you can use them selectively as a supplemental resource, if needed.

Monitoring Functions

Since you are just beginning to get into your study routine, this is the time to:

Initiate self-observations. These are the "informal" impressions, thoughts, and reactions that you form as you experience certain learning activities. For example, as you listen to a lecture, everything is making sense and fitting in with what you already know. Or, you feel some discomfort because the lecture is moving at too rapid a pace for you to process material meaningfully. Your reactions may be telling you that all is going well, and you should continue without change, or they may be signaling the need for some attention and possible adjustment in your study strategies.

Monitor emerging negative thoughts. If in reviewing you are reactivating without difficulty material you studied previously, you will feel productive and have a sense of accomplishment. But, there will be times when the proportion of understanding will seem relatively meager, and some discouragement will be felt. Try to confine your discouragement to the specific event that prompted the feeling without letting it generalize to *all* study activities.

Strategies for Consolidating Information

After you have listened to lectures or have read sections of material, you probably have acquired a reasonable percentage of the meaning. But, you also know that to *retain* what you understood, you will need to engage in other study activities. Of the multitude of activities from which you could choose, the following have been found to be effective to *maintain, consolidate, integrate,* and *synthesize* your knowledge.

1. Fill in gaps in your understanding. As soon after a lecture as is practical, follow up any of the "cued" sections in your notes or handouts by filling in what was unclear or incomplete. You can use another reference book, discuss the lecture with a peer, or ask for clarification from the instructor. Whatever action you take will make your learning stronger and move the information to long-term memory.

2. Reorganize for recall. Most students are familiar with the devices that can be used to reorganize information for better retrieval and recall: outlines, charts, index cards, concept maps, tree diagrams, and so forth. Following are guidelines for whether you should bother restructuring information and, if so, when it should be done.

If the material being used for study is already well organized, little if any restructuring may be needed. Sometimes, however, a different schematic format may make even well-organized material easier to recall.

If you reorganize, arrange the information so that *meaning* is emphasized. Note prototypes such as the most common and least common disease for a category, and the most frequent and least frequent treatment. In a set of diseases sharing similar symptoms, note particularly the differentiating feature(s).

If you decide to use one or more of the preceding devices, remember to do so during this stage, rather than close to the exam deadline, so you will have sufficient time to incorporate what you have restructured into your memory.

3. Synthesize from multiple sources. Avoid studying the same topic in three or four different sources. Use one substantive source as your "road map" and check other sources if you think yours is not comprehensive enough. Notice what needs to be added to make yours more complete, but end up with one dependable "script" that you can use for any subsequent study.

4. Rehearse to strengthen recall. Many students read things over and over. Rereading alone is not likely to be effective. The following habits could lead to more durable learning because they involve more active processing:

Use visual imaging. Visualize what you are trying to learn by "seeing" it in the form you will use when you want to retrieve it later (e.g., an anatomic structure as you saw it in lab, or as a schematic representation from the text, or as the instructor detailed it on a transparency).

Form analogies. Wherever possible, try to associate a new concept to a similar and simpler one that is already familiar to you.

Elaborate verbally. Talk about what you want to remember. Say it either to yourself or to others, but in your own words. "Stretch" beyond the script in the book or handout and develop inferences (make reasonable guesses about other relationships or applications).

Use mnemonics. These mental cues can be used to associate a wide range of medical information. Many can be found in student resources, or you can construct your own. Although you can be creative and even bizarre, avoid complexities that make the mnemonic harder to remember than the material itself. Using the first letter of each word to **form acronyms** is a common mnemonic device. For example, the causes of coma are AEIOU TIPS, which means *a*lcoholism, *e*ncephalopathy, *i*nsulin excess or deficiency, *o*piates, *u*remia, *t*rauma, *i*nfection, *p*sychosis, *s*yncope. **Method of loci** is one of the oldest mnemonic devices. You "place" mentally what you want to remember in certain familiar locations, such as rooms in your house, or locations within a room.

5. Establish patterns of practice. Certain "essentials" may need to be memorized and recalled almost verbatim. For such learning, **distribute the practice** so that you rehearse for a number of short periods with breaks, and other activities interspersed, rather than trying to sustain one lengthy period. Try **cumulative practice** by learning a few "chunks" at one session; then at a subsequent session, review those and add a few more. Continue the same pattern until all you want to memorize has been incorporated.

6. Study with others. This can be an effective study activity if used properly. An initial exploration of material by each student in the group will make group discussion more valuable. Discussion can then focus on clarifiying material and confirming and extending understanding. Studying with others works best if the group is small so everyone participates, and if some ground rules are established about how the sessions will be conducted.

7. Self-test periodically. The purpose of self-testing at this stage is **to guide further study.** Self-testing can help you decide which topics need more intense study, which are fairly close to being learned, and which have been learned well. Resources to use for this purpose and the sequence to follow will be described in later sections.

Applying Effective Testing Skills

Following are suggestions that will increase the likelihood that what you have learned and can recall from your study will translate into correct responses on multiple-choice examinations.

General test-taking skills

Read carefully for comprehension, not speed and respond to questions in sequence. Mark every item on your answer sheet as you go along, even if you are not completely sure of your choice. Cue the questions to which you want to return if there is time.

Be positive. Suppose the first question you see as you open the test book is a particularly difficult one, and you can feel yourself getting anxious. After giving it a try, go to the second question and respond to that one, which in all likelihood will feel more manageable.

Avoid mechanical errors. At the end of each page of questions, before going to the next page, check to make sure the **number of the question** you just finished **matches the number on your answer sheet.**

Be alert to key terms in the question stem such as "most," "least," "primarily," "frequently," "most often," and "most likely." Notice transition words that signal a change in meaning, such as "but," "although," and "however."

Let your original response stand unless you have thought of additional information.

Pace yourself. You will have approximately 60 seconds per question. Avoid dwelling on any one question, or rushing to finish. Set up checkpoints in your test booklet of where you want to be at the end of the first hour, second hour, and so on. You will know before you get close to the end whether you need to adjust your pace.

Analyzing questions

When you first read a question and look at the options, the answer may not be immediately apparent. Although you may be uncertain, don't just pick an answer arbitrarily. You can apply systematic skills of logic and deduction to narrow the five options to two or three possibilities.

Search for key information. As you read the question stem, notice key information (e.g., age, symptoms, lab results, chronic or acute condition, history). Highlight the key information by underlining or circling. **Notice particularly the request of the question** in phrases such as "the most likely diagnosis is," "the most appropriate initial step in management is," "which initial diagnostic evaluation is most appropriate." Take a quick look at the last line of the stem before reading the specific information in the remainder of the stem, especially if it is lengthy.

Analyze options. As you read each option, **try to eliminate** those that are inconsistent with the information you highlighted in the stem. For example, if a question concerns a 65-year-old woman, you would eliminate a procedure that you know applies only to children.

Cue each option. As you consider each option, mark down your initial reaction. In a "one best answer" question there are four "false" options and one "true" answer. For negative one best answer questions, the reverse applies. As you read each option, cue those you are sure of with a symbol such as "F," "N," or a minus sign. Cue true responses with a "T," "Y," or a plus sign. Cue those options you are uncertain about with the symbol you are using and a question mark.

Analyze structural clues in words. Pay attention to the meaning of prefixes, suffixes, and root words, which can sometimes help you decide whether to eliminate an option.

Approaching questions strategically. The following examples show how you might approach questions found in the books of this series.

Example: An infant who had been thriving well until 6 months of age started to develop nausea with vomiting, night sweats, and lassitude. His fasting blood glucose level was 62 mg/dl. On taking a history, the pediatrician determined that before this time the baby's diet was limited to mother's milk, and that the onset of the symptoms roughly coincided with intermittent addition of fruit juices to the diet. The pediatrician recommended the immediate return to mother's milk as the sole food in the baby's diet, with particular emphasis on the avoidance of fruit juices, fruits, and sweets. On this new regimen, the symptoms disappeared and the child continued to thrive. To obtain a definitive diagnosis of the infant's malady, the pediatrician would most likely recommend:

A. a fructose tolerance test
B. isolation and culture of fibroblasts from an innocuous source with the subsequent determination of aldolase B activity
C. determination of urinary fructose levels a week after having been placed on the restricted diet
D. liver biopsy and determination of aldolase B activity
E. determination of urinary-reducing sugar levels immediately on admission, while the infant is still showing symptoms

Analysis: The infant began to have difficulty when baby foods were introduced. Since they are sweetened with fructose, this may be a case of fructose intolerance, particularly considering that when the baby was put back on mother's milk, in which the sugar is lactose, the symptoms disappeared. As I look at the options, I can eliminate C since it is illogical—there would be no fructose after having been on a restricted diet. I can eliminate B since aldolase B is a liver enzyme and is not found in fibroblasts. I can also eliminate E since this is something that might have been done at the time of admission, but *not* when the baby is on a fructose-free diet. Option A, a fructose tolerance test, might be risky. Given the description in the case, there is the possibility that this baby would experience a severe reaction. Because the question asks about a *definitive* diagnosis, my choice is D.

Comment: This question is tapping knowledge of the biochemical cause of an inborn error of metabolism—fructose intolerance. To answer this question the student needs to know that fructose intolerance is caused by a deficiency in aldolase B activity, which results in accumulation of fructose 1-phosphate within the hepatocyte.

Example: A 2-month-old male infant is brought to the clinic with pronounced muscular flabbiness. The attending physician orders a muscle biopsy. Histologically, the muscle fibers are reported as abnormal. Other members of the family appear to be unusually weak and have an underdeveloped muscular system. Many relatives on the mother's side of the family complain of chronic fatigue and weakness. Muscle biopsy samples from these relatives show a variable histological pattern with abnormalities similar to those which predominate in the affected child. The same families also had several children who died in infancy for unidentified reasons. On the other side of the family, the father and all his relatives have normal muscular and fatigue patterns as well as normal biopsies. These findings lead the physician to consider that the proband very likely suffered from a hereditary mitochondrial myopathy with maternal transmission of the abnormal gene.

Assuming the physician's hypothesis is correct, in which of the following would an abnormality in enzymes be expected?
A. The tricarboxylic acid (citric acid or Krebs) cycle
B. Oxidative phosphorylation
C. Fatty acid degradation
D. Mitochondrial membrane structure
E. Fatty acid elongation

Analysis: I think the hypothesis is correct, since many relatives on the mother's side of the family also show similar abnormalities. This question has to do with mitochondrial

DNA, and since mtDNA is inherited only from the mother, only daughters can transmit mtDNA to their children. I think all of the choices involve mitochondrial proteins, but only those involved in oxidative phosphorylation are coded by mtDNA, so my choice is B.

Comment: To respond to this question the student needs to know the basic function of each of the biochemical mechanisms stated in the options. But the key is knowing that the proofreading mechanism for mtDNA is not as efficient as for nuclear DNA, so there is a higher mutation rate in mtDNA replication. Therefore, genetic defects involving oxidative phosphorylation are often inherited maternally.

Relying on test question cues

The ability to use the characteristics or the formats of the test itself to increase your score is sometimes referred to as "test wiseness." It is possible to make use of idiosyncrasies in the way the questions are constructed to decide on the correct choice. This technique should be used only if you are unable to answer the question based on direct knowledge or reasoning. The following are examples of the principles of test wiseness, but you may have little opportunity to use them on USMLE Step 1, because the experts who construct the questions eliminate these cues.

Length of an option. If an option is much longer or much shorter than the others, it is more likely to be correct.

Grammatical consistency. Options that are not grammatically aligned with the stem are probably false.

Specific determiners. Options that contain words such as "all," "always," and "never" overqualify an option and are likely to be false.

Overuse of the same words or expressions. Some test makers have a tendency to repeat words or phrases in the options. If you are unsure of an answer, select from the options with the repeated words or phrases. Another variation of this principle is to select an option in which a key word from the stem is repeated.

Numeric midrange. When all options can be listed in numeric order (e.g., percentages), the correct choice will most often be one of the two middle values.

Guessing

The following are "last resort" strategies, but you should be aware of them.

1. If you have eliminated one or two options, but have no idea about the remaining ones, choose the first in the list.

2. If you are unable to eliminate any options, choose A, B, or C.

3. If you have a number of questions left to do and time is running out, **do not leave blanks.** Choose A, B, or C, and fill in the same letter for all remaining questions.

Self-Management Skills

Time

Study in blocks. Assuming you plan to study 4 to 5 hours each night, you might consider dividing those hours into two study blocks. This allows you to study two areas, one that is weaker and therefore requires more time, and another that is relatively strong and can be allocated less time. The advantage of studying two sciences concurrently is that you will move through your strong science with ease and feel a sense of accomplishment, even if the weaker science does not reach the same level of confidence.

Set goals for each study block. Begin by identifying a few goals you think can be accomplished within that block of time. The goals need not be elaborately stated. Identifying what you think is important to study increases the chances that you will study *actively* (with heightened awareness) since you are controlling the purpose, direction, and rate of the studying.

Set realistic deadlines. Although your accuracy in estimating how long it takes you to complete a study agenda will vary, observe whether you habitually overestimate. Arbitrary deadlines are self-defeating if you have little or no chance of meeting them. Set more realistic targets and attempt to meet them most of the time.

Use record-keeping devices. Calendars and appointment books will help you schedule your study agenda and permit you to look ahead and adjust plans to meet deadlines.

Control distractions. There are many kinds of distractions, some of which are self-imposed. Others, such as telephone calls, can interrupt concentration and make it harder to get back to work. If a call is not urgent, decide on a response within the first 30 seconds (e.g., "I'll call you back later. I'm in the middle of something important."). When you do call later, use it as a reward for having worked well, and enjoy It. Also, learn to say "No" to requests that take time and distract you from your schedule.

Effort

Avoid activities that dissipate effort. Be aware of whether there are things you do each day that reduce your total energy, and particularly the energy you want to give to studying. Think about which of the "nonessential" tasks you can delegate to other family members, or to friends who want to be helpful. Give them some direction about what kind of help you would appreciate most.

Try to anticipate crises. There are disruptive life events that happen to all of us that we cannot anticipate but must deal with as best we can. But, there are other events of a less traumatic nature that, if they occur, can interrrupt the flow of a study plan and throw you off course (e.g., the car breaking down and needing immediate repair, a relative who wants to come and stay with you, or a friend who needs your advice on a troublesome problem). Anticipate crises that may happen during the span of your preparation and have alternative plans ready that permit you to be a part of what is going on but do not derail you completely.

Reward yourself for good effort. After having sustained a stretch of "heavy duty" studying, reward yourself by doing something that for you is pleasurable. A phone call to or from a friend that might be a distraction if it happens when you are trying to study can be a source of pleasure if you can defer it until you have completed your agenda for that day.

Resources

The following testing materials are appropriate for self-testing to guide further study. Their use is described in the next section.

Instructor content tests. These tests consist of questions prepared by the instructor who taught a particular segment of content. Some medical schools retain former course exams on file for student practice. Although the questions may not be structured as they appear on the Step 1 exam, they are good for pinpointing specific gaps or confusions in your knowledge base. Keep records of each practice test result and note relative performance across sciences and across topics in each science. For example, in pathology, note if one system (e.g., respiratory, cardiovascular, endocrine) is notably weaker than another. Cue topics that will need more sustained study. Take advantage of the instructor's presence to seek help, if needed.

Published books of practice questions. The books in this series arrange basic science content into "principles" (one book), "normal and abnormal processes" (one book), and "body systems" (three books).

Monitoring Functions

Monitor study progress
During this phase, when you are strengthening your learning, you will want to get **data-based feedback** using numeric scores to chart your progress.

Use questions to monitor progress

The pattern that works best is study, test, follow-up. Although there are times when it is appropriate to use questions before study to stimulate motivation or trigger recall, at this stage the best use of questions is after preliminary study. When you believe you have learned a segment of material, try a batch of questions. If time permits, you might want to test yourself on each major topic after completing its study, and before testing yourself on a mixed batch of topics in a science. However, if time is limited, select those topics about which you feel the most uncertainty, and use the feedback to guide additional study.

Select a representative sample of questions and complete them using the same time limits as will be used on your class exam or Board exam (approximately 60 seconds per question). Record your answers on a sheet of paper rather than in the question book or on the class practice exam. A separate sheet will allow you to do error analysis (described later) and keeps the book "clean" for future question retakes. **Do not do questions one at a time and then read the answer.** The purpose is not to learn a particular question, but to find out which topics require follow-up.

Score your responses, but do not read answers immediately since you may want to give some questions a second try. After performing error analysis, decide which topics need further study and the type of study needed.

Compute an accuracy percentage by dividing the number correct by the total number of questions. Keep a record of your scores and note whether your accuracy level is approaching the percentage required for passing (for Board exams, between 55% and 65%). For class exams, the percentage may be higher.

Analyze for errors. It is important to analyze more specific aspects of your study and test-taking behavior to direct further study and make it more focused and productive.

1. Were patterns of errors noted (e.g., questions related to DNA principles, or questions about immune responses, or questions regarding quantitative methods)?
2. Did you misread or misinterpret the question?
3. Were questions missed because, although you understood the concept, you forgot important details?
4. Did you note errors in addressing the *decision* required by the question? For example, although you knew much about the disease process described, you could not differentiate a likely diagnosis, or you were unable to form a judgment about a mechanism involved, draw an inference about the appropriate next step in management, or make a prediction about which drug would cause an adverse effect. In other words, you were unable to transform your conceptual and factual knowledge to meet the request of the question.

Monitor test anxiety

One aspect of self-testing that you should be monitoring is whether you are experiencing *inordinate* anxiety when dealing with test questions. It is not unusual to feel some elevation in anxiety when facing a comprehensive and consequential examination such as Step 1. But, if the amount of worry and the physiologic aspects (rapid breathing, sweaty palms, increased heartbeat) become so preoccupying that they interfere with productive studying, then some professional attention may be needed. If, however, test anxiety is of reasonable proportion, then remember what many studies have found. The best defense against test anxiety is a combination of strong review of subject matter, practice on tests similar to the target test, and positive self-reinforcement throughout the preparation process.

Combat negative self-statements

Part of your monitoring should include awareness of your moods and general state of being. Be sensitive to when you are about to give yourself a negative self-evaluation and combat it with an accurate, but positive one. "What if I don't. . ." statements will intrude periodically and, if permitted, can change your mood and distract you from your study. Start practicing self-talk by having a positive statement ready to use to redirect yourself back to your agenda ("I've been studying well and my scores show I'm making progress. . . I just need to keep going!" or "I can't afford the time to worry now; maybe late tonight; back to the topic now").

Strategies for Reaching Mastery

By the time you reach this stage you should feel more confident that your knowledge is firmer and that you can retrieve information dependably. The tasks of this stage deal with refining, or fine-tuning, for increased accuracy.

1. Focus on follow-up study. Your study agenda at this stage should be based on findings from your error analysis of questions you practiced, as well as any behavioral observations you noted from monitoring your performance.

If there are topics you need to reinforce, check your resources to note if those explanations are adequate, or if confusions still remain that may need to be clarified through use of another text or discussion with a peer.

If details are eluding you, engage in some of the memory strengthening activities noted in the previous stage, particularly use of mnemonics, and cumulative practice.

If you misread information in questions, remember to highlight pertinent cues as you read, to focus on comprehension and avoid regressions, and to vary your rate to emphasize meaning.

If one of the patterns you noted is that errors were made on questions with very long stems, practice by first reading the "request" at the end of the question stem. You may then be able to interpret the direction and relevance of the information in the question more quickly and accurately.

If you found that you were unable to translate your knowledge to the specific *thinking* requirement of the question (form a judgment, integrate information to form a conclusion, draw an inference), first check to make sure you know the principles or mechanisms the question assumes you know (e.g., biosynthesis and degradation, dose–effect relationships, alterations in immunologic function). Then, analyze the question through a "think aloud" procedure, with a peer if possible, and try to identify why your thinking is inaccurate.

2. Engage in comprehensive self-evaluation. If you have practiced questions topically, and through a systems approach, as in this series, and followed up with focused review, you should be ready to test yourself with comprehensive question sets. These sets will contain questions that sample most of the domains of information represented on the target exam. The procedure in using those questions, scoring them, and analyzing errors is the same as described previously. Since the question sets are likely to be longer (approximately 150–200 questions), schedule them during the last 2 or 3 weeks, with time between each to benefit from the feedback. Some students end self-evaluation before the last week because further testing too close to the exam date heightens their anxiety.

3. Deal with interfering test-taking behaviors and attitudes. If your self-observations have noted any test-taking behaviors that need improvement, this is the time to correct them.

Impulsive responding. Do you find yourself getting annoyed if the answer to a question is not immediately apparent, and simply choose an option impulsively? Try to curb your impatience, and remind yourself that some questions are designed to engage you in an internal dialogue before deciding on a response.

Inability to move on. Are you unable to disengage from a particularly troublesome question and move on to the next one? This is especially bothersome when you have that tip-of-the tongue feeling that the answer is something you know, but seems just a little out of reach. Difficult as it seems, try not to allow yourself to become irritated and get "stuck" to that question. Choose an answer and move on. It is likely that if you return to it later on, something may trigger recall.

Carrying over previous unsuccessful testing experiences. If comprehensive multiple-choice exams have been problematic for you in the past, and particularly if a recent attempt has not been successful, you may be tempted to see yourself as a "poor test-taker" and allow a defeatist attitude to permeate your self-testing activities. It would be better to start by asking yourself,

"Why do I not do as well as I would like on multiple-choice exams?" Then, through your self-observations and data-based assessments, note any interfering behaviors you would like to change and implement activities that are more effective and can lead to success on such exams.

Self-Management Skills

Time

Set and maintain study priorities. One of the biggest problems experienced by some medical students at any level of training is approaching an exam deadline realizing that there is still so much to learn that they will not reach the stage of "mastery." After some last-minute cramming they may even "pass," but the feeling of personal accomplishment eludes them. Although this has happened to all of us at one time or another, if it occurs as an ongoing pattern, then some change is needed. Make a list at the beginning of the week of all the study activities you want to accomplish and rank them in order of *importance* and *urgency*. At the beginning of the next week look at any low-priority items left undone and decide where to arrange them in that week's list. Make a record of each time you procrastinated or gave in to other distractions. Also note how often you kept to your schedule—it can motivate and encourage you to stay with it.

Schedule time for self-testing. Avoid deferring your first self-testing until just before an exam deadline. Build it into your schedule as part of your ongoing study activities and benefit from the feedback. You can then do "last-minute" testing to aim for greater accuracy.

Effort

Avoid excessive fatigue. It is expected that you will work hard to be ready for an exam, but allowing yourself to get excessively tired and sleep deprived sabotages your goal. Respond to your body's need for rest instead of pushing for another hour's study with little to show for it. Try to pace yourself so that you have energy left to think clearly when you take the exam.

Keep motivation high. One of the possible pitfalls toward the end of your review is a reduction in your level of attention and concentration, because of either fatigue or emerging apprehension about the imminence of the exam. If you have done some record keeping during the preparation sequence, it is now helpful to look back and acknowledge how far you have come from the point where you started. Reward yourself for progress by planning a pleasurable activity following a block of concentrated study, and enjoy it without guilt.

Resources

Comprehensive question sets. For USMLE Step 1, materials such as Williams & Wilkins' *Review for USMLE Step 1* (NMS series), which provides five practice exams with approximately 200 questions in each exam, will be useful for comprehensive evaluation.

Monitoring Functions

As the exam deadline approaches, you may find that you are experiencing frequent mood shifts. When things are going well, your spirits may be high, but after a disappointing day you may feel blue, gloomy, or even angry. Recent research has found that some techniques work better than others to escape from a bad mood:

1. Take some action. If possible, do something to solve the problem that is causing the bad mood.
2. Spend time with other people, particularly to shake sadness. Focus on something other than what is getting you down.
3. Exercise. The biggest boost comes to people who are usually sedentary, rather than the already aerobically fit.
4. Pick a sensual pleasure, such as taking a hot bath or listening to a favorite piece of music. Be careful of using eating for this purpose; it may work in the short run, but may backfire, leaving you feeling guilty. Drinking and drugs are to be avoided for obvious reasons.

5. Try a mental maneuver such as reminding yourself of previous successes to help bolster your self-esteem.

6. Take a walk. Cool down before confronting whatever gave rise to your negative feelings.

7. Try to see the situation from the other person's point of view—why someone might have done whatever provoked your anger.

8. Lend a helping hand to someone in need. If you are studying, offer to help someone understand a science topic in which you feel very competent.

9. Use stress reduction techniques. Among the most effective are progressive relaxation, which uses tension and tension release in the body's muscle groups; mental imagery, which is putting yourself mentally in a location that evokes feelings of calm and peacefulness; and meditation, which aims for a state of relaxed alertness.

Grace Bingham, Ed.D.

◄ Diagnostic Test ►

QUESTIONS

DIRECTIONS:

Each of the numbered items or incomplete statements in this section is followed by answers or by completions of the statement. Select the ONE lettered answer or completion that is BEST in each case.

1. As an adult ages, his or her need for sleep

(A) increases
(B) decreases
(C) remains the same
(D) shows a significant gender difference
(E) shows a significant ethnic difference

2. When pyruvate is utilized as a substrate for gluconeogenesis

(A) the pyruvate carboxylase reaction is blocked by acetyl CoA
(B) the pyruvate carboxylase reaction is reversed
(C) oxaloacetate combines with acetyl CoA to form citrate
(D) the pyruvate dehydrogenase complex is inhibited by acetyl CoA
(E) the pyruvate is converted into oxaloacetate, which diffuses from the mitochondria into the cytosol, where it is converted into phosphoenolpyruvate

3. Which of the following items has the highest point value in the Holmes and Rahe social readjustment rating scale?

(A) Marital separation
(B) Divorce
(C) Death of a spouse
(D) Legal violation
(E) High mortgage

4. Studies of maternal (nurturing) behavior in rats indicate that

(A) female rats begin to show maternal behavior approximately 24 hours after their pups are born
(B) male rats show maternal behavior after repeated exposure to pups
(C) pheromones produced by pups increase estrogen levels in virgin female rats
(D) hormones are unrelated to the display of maternal behavior in rats
(E) virgin female rats will only show maternal behavior toward offspring that are genetically related to them

5. The most effective pain management technique after a surgical procedure is to administer pain medication in a relatively

(A) low dose only when the patient requests it
(B) high dose only when the patient requests it
(C) low dose before the pain starts
(D) high dose before the pain starts
(E) moderate dose only when the patient requests it

6. What is the general adaptation syndrome described by Hans Selye?

(A) A model of the doctor–patient relationship
(B) A syndrome of self-induced modification of cortisone release
(C) A model of compliance
(D) A posthypnotic side effect
(E) The stages the body goes through in response to stress

7. A 35-year-old man is to be treated for tension headaches using a biofeedback technique. What would be the most specific and effective biofeedback technique for this patient?

(A) Breathing using the upper chest
(B) Increasing skin perspiration
(C) Relaxing the frontalis muscle
(D) Warming the hands
(E) Warming the feet

8. Pharyngeal infection may lead to postinfectious, acute rheumatic heart disease or glomerulonephritis. Which of the following organisms is directly responsible for these complications?

(A) *Streptococcus mutans*
(B) *Streptococcus faecalis*
(C) *Streptococcus pyogenes*
(D) *Streptococcus pneumoniae*
(E) *Streptococcus agalactiae*

Questions 9-10

A consumer group would like to evaluate the success of three different medications for hypertension. To obtain this information, blood pressure readings are obtained from three groups of 25 patients (total number of patients = 75) who are then put on three different medications. At the end of 6 weeks, blood pressure readings are obtained from all subjects.

9. Which test can determine whether the difference in blood pressure between the three groups is significantly different at the end of the 6 weeks?

(A) Independent *t*-test
(B) Dependent *t*-test
(C) Analysis of variance
(D) Correlation
(E) Chi-squared test

10. Which test is used to determine whether blood pressures of all subjects at the start of the study are significantly different than blood pressures of all subjects at the end of the 6-week study?

(A) Independent *t*-test
(B) Dependent *t*-test
(C) Analysis of variance
(D) Correlation
(E) Chi-squared test

Questions 11-12

Seven weeks after visiting the "red light" district in New Orleans, a 24-year-old man develops a nonpruritic, maculopapular rash. The rash is generalized and includes the hands, feet, and mucous membranes of the oral and anogenital areas. The rapid plasma reagin (RPR) test is negative at the standard dilution.

11. Which of the following organisms is the most likely cause of his infection?

(A) *Haemophilus ducreyi*
(B) *Treponema pallidum*
(C) *Treponema carateum*
(D) *Chlamydia trachomatis*
(E) *Neisseria gonorrhea*

12. The gold standard test for the diagnosis of this patient's condition is

(A) *Treponema pallidum* immobilization test
(B) fluorescent treponemal antibody test
(C) darkfield microscopy
(D) Wasserman test
(E) Venereal Disease Research Laboratory (VDRL) test

13. Two hundred children go to the museum on a school outing. One hundred children eat hamburgers at the museum restaurant, and 100 eat a lunch that they had brought. Fifty of the children who ate at the restaurant developed hepatitis A. The attack rate for hepatitis A among those who ate at the restaurant is

(A) 5%
(B) 15%
(C) 25%
(D) 50%
(E) 75%

Questions 14-15

A cell-free extract prepared from type S pneumococcus is incubated with type R cells. Some cells in the culture become converted to type S.

14. What is the name of the process by which type R cells become converted to type S?

(A) Transduction
(B) Conjugation
(C) Transformation
(D) Transposition
(E) Differentiation

15. When incubated with the cell-free extract, which of the following enzymes would prevent the formation of type S cells?

(A) DNAase
(B) RNAase
(C) Protease
(D) Phosphatase
(E) Reverse transcriptase

16. The following table shows the prevalence and incidence of diseases Q,R,S,T and V per a population of 100,000 people.

Disease	Prevalence	Incidence
Q	150	25
R	300	20
S	75	15
T	50	1
V	6	2

Which one of these diseases has the longest duration?

(A) Disease Q
(B) Disease R
(C) Disease S
(D) Disease T
(E) Disease V

Questions 17-18

A 23-year-old man, who recently returned from a camping trip, complains of headache, nausea, and sore throat. He has a convulsive seizure while at home. His wife is concerned because the campground had signs warning of rabies, and her husband was bitten by a raccoon that was acting strangely.

17. Of the following, the most reliable method by which to make a rapid definitive diagnosis of rabies is to

(A) detect Negri bodies in corneal or brain tissue
(B) inoculate a blood sample into cell culture and identify cytopathic effects
(C) determine if there is a fourfold rise in antibody titer over a 2-week period
(D) capture the raccoon and perform a necropsy
(E) do nothing until the symptoms become more specific for rabies

18. Which of the following is most likely to be injected partly around the bite wound and partly intramuscularly in this patient?

(A) Antirabies serum
(B) Nerve tissue vaccine
(C) Rabies immune globulin
(D) Live attenuated vaccine
(E) Interferon-α

19. In city Z, there are 1000 HIV-positive people, out of whom 10 people died within one year. The case fatality rate, expressed as a percent, is

(A) 1%
(B) 2%
(C) 5%
(D) 10%
(E) Cannot be determined from the data given

20. Which of the following best exemplifies the mode of action of oxidizing agents?

(A) Damage to DNA
(B) Protein denaturation
(C) Disruption of cell membrane or wall
(D) Removal of free sulfhydral groups
(E) Chemical antagonism

21. A telephone survey is conducted to determine whether bronchial asthma is more common in employed or unemployed adults. This study design is a

(A) cross-sectional study
(B) case-control study
(C) historical cohort study
(D) concurrent cohort study
(E) randomized controlled trial

22. Investigators identified 200 women with breast cancer seen at two hospitals in New York City from 1987–1992. On the basis of interviews with the women, it was determined that they were more likely to report a history of smoking than 500 women admitted to the surgical service of the same hospitals for disorders not involving the breast. The study design is an example of a

(A) cross-sectional study
(B) case-control study
(C) historical cohort study
(D) concurrent cohort study
(E) randomized controlled trial

23. The wife of a 70-year-old man has just died. How long does normal bereavement most commonly last?

(A) 1 month
(B) 2 months
(C) 4 months
(D) 1 year
(E) 3 years

24. The periplasm in gram-negative bacteria is significant in the colonization of tissues and metabolism because

(A) it contains a variety of genes for antibiotic resistance
(B) it mediates adherence of bacteria to cell surface
(C) it contains many hydrolytic enzymes, including β-lactamases
(D) it is the site of oxidative and transport enzymes
(E) it protects the bacteria against phagocytosis

25. During a routine tubal ligation, a surgeon discovers that a 40-year-old woman has a malignant ovarian tumor. The surgeon should

(A) remove the tumor immediately while the patient is still under anesthesia
(B) discuss the patient's options with her after she recovers from the anesthesia
(C) ask the husband for consent to remove the tumor while the patient is still under anesthesia
(D) ask the hospital administration for permission to remove the tumor while the patient is still under anesthesia
(E) call in a gynecologic oncologist to remove the tumor while the patient is still under anesthesia

26. *Staphylococcus aureus* produces a superantigen that contributes to massive disease caused by cytokines that are released from polyclonal T-cell activation. Which one of the following best fits this description of a superantigen?

(A) Exfoliative toxin
(B) Protein A
(C) Coagulase
(D) Toxic shock syndrome toxin
(E) Beta hemolytic hemolysin

27. Which one of the following brain wave patterns is most likely to be seen on an electroencephalogram (EEG) of an awake, relaxed, and calm 34-year-old female patient with her eyes closed?

(A) Alpha
(B) Beta
(C) Delta
(D) Theta
(E) Sawtooth

28. In von Gierke's disease, glycogen accumulation is limited to the liver and kidneys because these two organs have

(A) more glycogen than other organs
(B) gluconeogenic enzymes
(C) glycogen synthetase
(D) a greater concentration of uridine diphosphate (UDP)-glucose than other organs
(E) a greater concentration of glucose 1-phosphate than other organs

DIRECTIONS:

Each of the numbered items or incomplete statements in this section is negatively phrased, as indicated by a capitalized word such as NOT, LEAST, or EXCEPT. Select the ONE lettered answer or completion that is BEST in each case.

29. Which of the following statements does NOT apply to hepatitis C virus (HCV)?

(A) HCV can be identified by a specific serologic test for anti-HCV antibodies
(B) HCV is the leading cause of posttransfusion hepatitis
(C) Chronic, asymptomatic carriers for HCV have not been documented
(D) HCV causes chronic hepatitis that usually is less severe than that caused by hepatitis B virus (HBV)
(E) HCV was previously referred to as non-A, non-B (NANB) hepatitis virus

30. Five people attempt suicide using five different methods. Which method is LEAST likely to result in death?

(A) Hanging
(B) Shooting
(C) Jumping from a high place
(D) Drug overdose
(E) Crashing an automobile

31. Which of the following organisms is LEAST likely to be associated with a disease involving type III hypersensitivity?

(A) *Treponema pallidum*
(B) Hepatitis B virus
(C) Group A streptococcus
(D) *Plasmodium malariae*
(E) *Streptococcus pneumoniae*

32. Which one of the following is MOST likely to commit suicide?

(A) A 60-year-old black woman
(B) A 60-year-old black man
(C) A 60-year-old white woman
(D) A 60-year-old white man
(E) A 60-year-old Hispanic woman

33. Some microorganisms produce pigments, giving their colonies characteristic colors that may be useful in identification and diagnosis. Which of the following organism–colony color associations is NOT correct?

(A) *Staphylococcus aureus*—yellow
(B) *Staphylococcus epidermidis*—white
(C) *Pseudomonas aeruginosa*—blue-green
(D) *Serratia marcesens*—red
(E) *Mycobacterium kansasii*—white

34. Which one of the following completions of the statement is LEAST likely to be true? In general, pain in children is

(A) undertreated
(B) overtreated
(C) underreported
(D) misunderstood
(E) as common as in adults

35. Which one of the following cytokine relationships is INCORRECT?

(A) Interleukin-1: stimulates the synthesis of acute phase reactants

(B) Tumor necrosis factor-α: mediates cachexia in cancer patients

(C) Interleukin-2: downregulates CD8 cytotoxic T cells

(D) Interleukin-3: enhances hematopoiesis

(E) Interleukin-6: induces B cell differentiation and synthesis of acute phase reactants

36. A 25-year-old man has just been diagnosed with AIDS. Which one of the following actions is LEAST appropriate?

(A) The physician should quickly tell the patient all of the facts at once

(B) The physician should find out how much the patient wants to know about the illness

(C) The physician should find out how much the patient already knows about the illness

(D) The physician should sit down when speaking with the patient

(E) The physician should explain that he will not abandon the patient, no matter how ill he becomes

37. All of the following associations between anatomic locations and normal flora are correct EXCEPT

(A) Nasopharyngeal—*Streptococcus aureus*
(B) Skin—*Staphylococcus epidermidis*
(C) Colon—group D streptococci
(D) Vagina—group D streptococci
(E) Trigeminal ganglia—herpex simplex virus I

38. Which one of the following is NOT normally seen in a 75-year-old man?

(A) Neurofibrillary tangles
(B) Senile plaques
(C) Loss of cortical neurons
(D) Severe memory loss
(E) Increased ventricular size

DIRECTIONS:

Each set of matching questions in this section consist of a list of four to twenty-six lettered options (some of which may be in figures) followed by several numbered items. For each numbered item, select the ONE lettered option that is most closely associated with it. To avoid spending too much time on matching sets with large numbers of options, it is generally advisable to begin each set by reading the list of options. Then for each item in the set, try to generate the correct answer and locate it in the option list, rather than evaluating each option individually. Each lettered option may be selected once, more than once, or not at all.

Questions 39-41

For each of the following functions, select the appropriate lipase.

(A) Gastric lipase
(B) Pancreatic lipase
(C) Capillary lipoprotein lipase
(D) Hormone-sensitive lipase
(E) Acid lipase

39. It is the primary digestive lipase

40. It is responsible for removal of lipids from very–low-density lipoproteins (VLDL) and chylomicrons for use in tissues

41. It is responsible for liberating free fatty acids from adipocytes in the fasting state

Questions 42-44

Match each description with the appropriate term.

(A) Psychic causality
(B) Preconscious
(C) Primary process
(D) Libido
(E) Parapraxis

42. A colleague who is pleased about a recent promotion says, "That promotion will be a land mine for me."

43. A student taking an exam is able to recall the correct answer to a question.

44. A woman complains to her doctor of an increased desire for sexual gratification.

Questions 45-47

For each description of clinical findings, select the appropriate disorder.

(A) α-L-Iduronidase deficiency
(B) Galactokinase deficiency
(C) Fructokinase deficiency
(D) M-Lactate dehydrogenase deficiency
(E) Vitamin B_6 deficiency
(F) Aldolase B deficiency
(G) Fructose 1,6-bisphosphatase deficiency
(H) Biotin deficiency
(I) Thiamine deficiency

45. Decreased ability to catabolize fatty acids to carbon dioxide and water

46. Decreased ability to synthesize ribose 5-phosphate from fructose 6-phosphate and glyceraldehyde 3-phosphate

47. Corneal clouding, dwarfism, mental retardation, and gargoylism

Questions 48-50

Use the following data to answer the questions.

	A	B	C	D	E
Plasma (glucose)	↓	↑	↓	↑	↓
Plasma (insulin)	↑	↓	↓	↑	↑
Plasma (C peptide)	↑	↓	↓	↑	↓

↑ = increased compared with normal
↓ = decreased compared with normal

48. Which column is most consistent with an insulinoma?

49. Which column is most consistent with 24 hours of fasting?

50. Which column is most consistent with untreated type II diabetes?

ANSWER KEY

1. C	10. B	19. A	27. A	35. C	43. B
2. D	11. B	20. D	28. B	36. A	44. D
3. C	12. C	21. A	29. C	37. D	45. H
4. B	13. D	22. B	30. D	38. D	46. I
5. D	14. C	23. D	31. E	39. B	47. A
6. E	15. A	24. C	32. D	40. C	48. A
7. C	16. D	25. B	33. E	41. D	49. C
8. C	17. A	26. D	34. B	42. E	50. D
9. C	18. C				

ANSWERS AND EXPLANATIONS

1. The answer is C. *(Behavioral science)*
As an adult ages, his or her need for sleep remains the same. While the need for sleep remains the same in the elderly as in younger people, sleep in the elderly is of poorer quality than in young people and is characterized by decreased rapid eye movement (REM) sleep and slow-wave sleep. There are no significant gender or ethnic differences in the need for sleep at any age.

2. The answer is D. *(Biochemistry)*
Acetyl CoA and other products generated from the beta oxidation of even-chained fatty acids inactivate the pyruvate dehydrogenase complex, so that pyruvate preferentially forms oxaloacetate via pyruvate carboxylase in an irreversible reaction. Acetyl CoA also activates pyruvate carboxylase and phosphoenolpyruvate carboxykinase. Oxaloacetate is unable to diffuse out of the mitochondria, so it is first converted into malate, which is transported from the mitochondria into the cytoplasm, where it is reoxidized back into oxaloacetate. Oxaloacetate is then converted into phosphoenolpyruvate via phosphoenolpyruvate carboxykinase using guanosine-5'-triphosphate (GTP), thus completing the first step in the gluconeogenic process, namely forming phosphoenolpyruvate from pyruvate.

3. The answer is C. *(Behavioral science)*
Death of a spouse has the highest point value in the Holmes and Rahe social readjustment scale. After death of a spouse, in descending order on the scale are divorce, trouble with the law, marital separation, and high mortgage.

4. The answer is B. *(Behavioral science)*
Studies of maternal behavior in rats indicate that hormones are associated with the display of this behavior because female rats show maternal behavior immediately after their pups are born. While hormones are associated with the initiation of maternal behavior in parturient rats, exposure to pups alone can induce maternal behavior in virgin female rats and in male rats without alteration of hormone levels. Having a genetic relationship to the pups is not important for stimulating maternal behavior in rats. Results of these

and other animal studies are one reason that parents are now encouraged to touch their newborn infants as much as possible, even if they are premature.

5. The answer is D. *(Behavioral science)*
The most effective technique for managing postoperative pain is to administer pain medication in a relatively high dose before the pain starts, so that pain does not become associated with receipt of pain medication. In the United States, pain patients have generally been undermedicated because of fears of addiction. However, such fears have proven to be unfounded because pain patients do not become addicted to opiates the way that addicts do (i.e., they no longer need the medication when the pain remits).

6. The answer is E. *(Behavioral science)*
The general adaptation syndrome, described by Hans Selye, refers to the stages the body goes through in response to stress. These stages include the alarm reaction, followed by adaptation in the form of psychosomatic illness, and finally, exhaustion.

7. The answer is C. *(Behavioral science)*
Relaxing the frontalis muscle is the most specific and effective biofeedback technique for treating tension headaches. Warming the hands and feet is a specific and effective biofeedback technique for the treatment of migraine headaches. Lower (not upper) chest breathing and decreasing (not increasing) skin perspiration are general relaxation techniques.

8. The answer is C. *(Microbiology)*
Streptococcus pyogenes, the type of organism of Lancefield's group A streptococci, produces most human infections. It is beta hemolytic. It routinely causes streptococcal sore throat and may spread to other body locations to cause disease (e.g., erysipelas, septicemia, pyoderma, and endocarditis). It also causes postacute group A infection complications, such as acute glomerulonephritis and rheumatic heart disease. The kidney infections are usually self-limited, whereas progressive damage in the heart may cause life-threatening situations.

Streptococcus mutans is alpha hemolytic and involved in production of caries. Alpha-hemolytic streptococci are the main organisms involved in subacute bacterial endocarditis. *Streptococcus* (or *Enterococcus*) *faecalis* is normally in the intestine and is a tremendous opportunist outside of that location. *Streptococcus pneumoniae* is the most significant cause of bacterial pneumonia, whereas *Streptococcus agalactiae* is part of the normal vaginal flora and is significant in neonatal infections.

9-10. The answers are: 9-C, 10-B. *(Behavioral science)*

Differences in means among more than two groups are tested using analysis of variance. Differences between means of two samples are tested using independent and dependent (paired) *t*-tests. Correlation examines the mutual relationship between two continuous variables, while the chi-squared test is used to test differences between frequencies in a sample.

Differences in mean blood pressure values for the same people sampled on two occasions are tested using a dependent *t*-test. An independent *t*-test would be used to test the difference between the mean blood pressure of two different, unrelated groups of people.

11-12. The answers are: 11-B, 12-C. *(Microbiology)*

This patient most likely has secondary syphilis caused by *Treponema pallidum*, given the description of the rash, its distribution, and the time of its appearance. The rapid plasma reagin (RPR) test is negative because of the prozone phenomenon. In the case of secondary syphilis, a high antibody level may interfere with antigen–antibody complex formation and may be interpreted as negative. The RPR test is widely used for screening reagin in serum from patients infected with the organism.

Humans are the only natural hosts of *T. pallidum*. Transmission is usually through direct sexual contact. Transmission can also occur from mother to fetus or through blood transfusion, although this mode of transmission is rare. Usually the organisms enter through mucous membranes or through abrasions in the skin.

The gold standard test for this patient's condition is darkfield microscopy. Spirochetes, with the exception of *Borrelia* species, are too thin to be seen through a regular light microscope. A drop of fluid or exudate from a primary or secondary lesion is placed on a slide, covered with a coverslip, and examined under oil emersion. The characteristic spiral shape and motility are seen in positive specimens.

The illumination for darkfield microscopy is passed through a special condenser that blocks direct light rays and deflects light off a mirror on the side of the condenser at an oblique angle. The reflected rays are deflected from the edge of the organisms up to the objective, making the spirochetes appear larger than they are. They appear white against a dark background. Special stains (e.g., silver stains) and direct labeling of treponemes with fluorescent antibodies can also be performed to view the organisms in a specimen.

13. The answer is D. *(Behavioral science)*

The attack rate is the number of people who get sick in the time period divided by the number of people at risk in the time period. It is generally used for conditions in which the population is at risk for a short time (e.g., food-borne illness). Among the 100 children who ate at the restaurant (i.e., those at risk), 50 developed hepatitis A. The attack rate is 50 divided by 100, or 50%.

14-15. The answers are: 14-C, 15-A. *(Biochemistry)*

This is an example of the process of transformation, in which genetic information is transmitted from one bacterium to another by means of a naked DNA molecule. In this case, type R cells take up DNA from the type S extract. This DNA becomes incorporated into the type R chromosomes and transforms the cells to type S. The process of transduction is similar, except that a bacteriophage vector is used to transmit the DNA from donor to recipient. In conjugation, direct contact between the two bacteria is required to transmit genetic information. Transposition involves the movement of mobile genetic elements called transposons. Differentiation involves the specialization of cell types during development.

Because the component of the cell extract causing transformation is DNA, an enzyme that degrades DNA would prevent the cell conversion from occurring. DNAase is a nuclease that degrades DNA molecules to its deoxynucleotide building blocks.

Enzymes such as RNAase, which destroys RNA, or proteases, which destroy proteins, have no effect on transformation. Other ineffective enzymes include phosphatases, which only remove exposed phosphate groups from various compounds, and reverse transcriptase, which has the ability to synthesize DNA using an RNA template.

16. The answer is D. *(Behavioral science)*

Disease T has the longest duration. Prevalence is the number of existing cases of an illness divided by the total population over a period of time (usually 1 year). Incidence is the number of new cases occurring in a given year. And, prevalence equals incidence multiplied by the duration of the disease (or $P = I \times D$). Therefore:

1. Disease Q : $150 = 25 \times D$, and $D = 6$
2. Disease R: $300 = 20 \times D$, and $D = 15$
3. Disease S: $75 = 15 \times D$, and $D = 5$
4. Disease T: $50 = 1 \times D$, and $D = 50$
5. Disease V: $6 = 2 \times D$, and $D = 3$

17-18. The answers are: 17-A, 18-C. *(Microbiology)*

The testing of tissues (i.e., impression preparations of cornea or brain) for Negri bodies by direct immunofluorescence using antirabies serum is currently the most rapid and reliable method of diagnosis. Negri bodies are spherical viral inclusions with a characteristic internal structure containing basophilic granules. The cytoplasm of one infected neuron may have several Negri bodies. Detection of Negri bodies is diagnostic for rabies.

Virus isolation by intracerebral injection into suckling mice results in flaccid paralysis of the legs, encephalitis, and death. Virus identification can also be done with neutralization tests after culturing available tissue in hamster and mouse cell lines. However, these assays are relatively slow (several days).

Viremia does not occur at any time during the progression of rabies; thus, a culture of blood from the patient would not be useful. The virus first multiplies locally in muscle or connective tissues at the site of the bite and spreads along peripheral nerves to the central nervous system. It multiplies in the brain and continues to spread through nerves to other parts of the body including the salivary glands.

Antibodies against the rabies virus generally do not appear until relatively late in the disease (i.e., after it has already reached the brain and started to spread to other tissues). Waiting for a fourfold rise in antibody titer would not be appropriate, since death usually occurs in 3 to 5 days after onset of symptoms.

With regard to performing a necropsy on the raccoon, it is highly unlikely that the animal responsible for the bite could be found and captured.

One should not wait for symptoms to appear in a human bitten by a wild animal suspected of being rabid. Rabies is an acute, fulminating encephalitis. A prodrome of malaise, headache, nausea, vomiting, and other nonspecific symptoms is followed by increasing nervousness, hyperventilation, salivation, and confusion. Violent spasms of the throat muscles upon offer of a glass of water (hydrophobia) is virtually diagnostic for rabies; however, hydrophobia is not present in all infected individuals. The disease is nearly 100% fatal once symptoms appear, if untreated. Respiratory paralysis is the major cause of death.

It is most likely that rabies immune globulin will be administered (passive immunization). The preparation contains high levels of neutralizing immunoglobulin G antibody against the rabies virus. It is prepared from the plasma of hyperimmunized human volunteers. Standard procedure involves injecting one half of the preparation around the bite wound and the other half intramuscularly. There is only one antigenic type of rabies virus. The patient will also be vaccinated with human diploid cell vaccine (active immunization).

Antirabies serum is obtained from hyperimmunized horses. Because this is a heterologous preparation, it has a shorter half-life after administration, and there is an increased risk for hypersensitivity reactions compared with preparations made from human immunoglobulins. For these reasons, rabies immune globulin is always preferred over antirabies serum.

Nerve tissue vaccine is made from virus grown in brain tissues from sheep, goats, or mice. Postvaccinal encephalitis occurs with considerable frequency. It is no longer used in the United States.

A live attenuated vaccine (Flury strain) is available for dogs and cats. Attenuation is accomplished by serial passage in embryonated chicken eggs. Genetically engineered oral vaccines for wild animal populations are currently being tested.

Genetically engineered interferon-α, as well as the other interferons, are being tested for a variety of viral infections (e.g., rabies, herpes encephalitis, cytomegalovirus, hemorrhagic fever, hepatitis B and C, influenza). Nervous system and gastrointestinal side effects, however, are common at the dosages used.

19. The answer is A. *(Behavioral science)*
The case fatality rate is the number of deaths due to a specific disease divided by the number of people who have the disease. The case fatality rate for these data is 10 per 1000, or 1%.

20. The answer is D. *(Microbiology)*
Oxidizing agents, including hydrogen peroxide, iodine, and chlorine, are capable of causing widespread damage. They inactivate cells by oxidizing, or removing, free sulfhydral groups.

Compounds containing alkyl groups are toxic to cells at relatively high concentrations. Seventy percent of ethanol and isopropyl alcohol act as mild protein denaturants.

Detergents are surface-active agents. They collect at lipid-containing membrane-aqueous medium interfaces and disrupt cell membranes or walls. Detergents are either anionic (negative charge) or cationic (positive charge).

Chemotherapeutic agents (e.g., antibiotics) have the ability to directly damage DNA (actinomycin D) or produce chemical antagonism (as with sulfa drugs).

21. The answer is A. *(Behavioral science)*
Random telephone surveys are often used in epidemiologic research. Because data are being collected at one point in time and the population is chosen at random, this is a cross-sectional study. A cohort study starts with a group of well people and either follows them to see who becomes ill (concurrent approach) or looks at their records (historical approach) to determine who was and was not exposed to a risk factor and who did and did not become ill. In a case-control study, individuals who are ill and those who are well are chosen, and their previous exposure to a risk factor is assessed. A randomized controlled trial is a type of cohort study that includes a clinical intervention.

22. The answer is B. *(Behavioral science)*
In this case-control study, individuals who had an illness (breast cancer) and those who did not have the illness were chosen and their prior exposure to a risk factor (smoking) was assessed. In cross-sectional studies, data are collected at one point in time and the population is chosen at random. A cohort study starts with a group of well people and either follows them ahead in time to see who becomes ill or looks at their records to determine who was and who was not exposed to a risk factor and who did and who did not become ill. The former cohort approach is known as a concurrent cohort study; the latter is a historical cohort study. A randomized controlled trial is a type of cohort study that includes some type of clinical intervention.

23. The answer is D. *(Behavioral science)*
The period of normal bereavement most commonly lasts about 1 year.

24. The answer is C. *(Microbiology)*
The periplasm, or periplasmic space, is the space between the cytoplasmic membrane and the outer membrane of the gram-negative bacterial cell wall. This space contains many hydrolytic enzymes, including β-lactamases. The availability of these enzymes allows the organisms to utilize a variety of complex chemicals as food nutrients and to inactivate β-lactam antibiotics (e.g., penicillin, cephalosporins). These products also allow efficient colonization of tissue sites.

Plasmids, small circles of DNA, are located in the cytoplasm and contain a variety of genes associated with antibiotic resistance, enzymes, and toxins. Pili, or fimbriae, mediate close adherence of bacteria to cell surfaces. Phagocytosis would be indirectly inhibited by the close, tight attachment of the bacteria. The cytoplasmic, or plasma, membrane is the site of significant oxidative and transport enzymes. Capsules, composed of a thick polysaccharide layer around the bacteria, directly interfere with white blood cell phagocytic ability.

25. The answer is B. *(Behavioral science)*
Prior to performing any surgical procedure, the surgeon must receive informed consent from the patient. This patient has not consented to removal of an ovarian tumor; therefore, the surgeon should discuss the finding and treatment options with the patient after she recovers from the anesthesia. In order to obtain informed consent, the surgeon must inform the patient of the risks and benefits of the procedure and explain what will happen if the procedure is not performed. Asking either the husband or the hospital administration for permission, or calling in another doctor to remove the tumor is inappropriate because the patient is competent and therefore capable of giving her own consent. Ignoring the presence of the tumor is criminal.

26. The answer is D. *(Microbiology)*
Superantigens can bind to major histocompatibility (MHC) class II molecules outside the peptide-bonding cleft, as well as to the T-cell receptor. Superantigen binding stimulates the release of large amounts of cytokines, including interleukin I and tumor necrosis factor. This mechanism is caused by stimulation of a high percentage of the pool of T lymphocytes (polyclonal activation) and explains to a large extent the pathogenesis of diseases caused by organisms with superantigens. *Staphylococcus aureus* produces both toxic shock syndrome toxin and enterotoxins (food poisoning), which exhibit the superantigen characteristics.

Although toxic and harmful, exfoliative toxin, protein A, coagulase, and beta hemolytic hemolysin respond as regular antigens in the immune response and are specific in their destructive action in the body. Exfoliative toxin includes at least two proteins that cause the generalized desquamation seen in the scalded skin syndrome. Protein A nonspecifically binds to the Fc portion of immunoglobulin G molecules and prevents complement attachment and activation. Coagulase clots citrated plasma, with the help of a serum factor, and probably assists in the development of the abscess lesion. *S. aureus* produces several hemolysis, or exotoxins. They damage erythrocytes, platelets, and other cells in the body.

27. The answer is A. *(Behavioral science)*
Alpha waves are associated with an awake state of relaxation and calm with the eyes closed. Beta waves are associated with awake, alert, active mental concentration. Delta and theta waves are associated primarily with stage 4 and stage 1 of sleep, respectively. Sawtooth waves are associated with REM sleep.

28. The answer is B. *(Biochemistry)*
In von Gierke's disease, an autosomal recessive glycogen storage disease, the absence of glucose 6-phosphatase causes glucose-6-phosphate to build up. This compound is converted to glucose 1-phosphate and then into uridine diphosphate (UDP)-glucose. Glucose 6-phosphate also enhances glycogen synthetase activity and the UDP-glucose is used to generate glycogen. The liver and kidneys do not have a greater concentration of glycogen synthetase, glucose 1-phosphate, or UDP-glucose. The liver and muscle contain the greatest amounts of glycogen.

29. The answer is C. *(Microbiology)*
Both asymptomatic carriers and individuals with chronic hepatitis have been documented in people infected with hepatitis C virus (HCV). The frequency of chronic HCV hepatitis is high, but its course is considered less severe than that of hepatitis B virus (HBV). Complete resolution occurs in almost all cases of HCV infection.

Up to 25% of sporadic hepatitis may be caused by HCV, and 90% of the transfusion-associated hepatitis cases. Serologic markers associated with active hepatitis A virus (HAV), HBV, and other viral agents are absent, but anti-HCV antibodies can be detected. HCV was referred to as non-A, non-B (NANB) transfusion-associated hepatitis, until a specific serologic test became available in recent years. Interestingly, HCV is classified as an RNA-containing Flavivirus. The virus has not been definitely seen by electron microscopy, yet its entire genome has been sequenced and translated. Proteins from the translation serve as antigens in the serologic test.

30. The answer is D. *(Behavioral science)*
Attempting suicide by overdosing on drugs is less likely to result in death than a violent method, such as hanging, shooting, jumping from a high place, or crashing an automobile. Most people do not understand how much or what type of medication is needed to cause death. Furthermore, "effective" medications

for committing suicide (e.g., barbiturates) are not easily available.

31. The answer is E.   *(Pathology)*
Streptococcus pneumoniae, a gram-positive diplococcus, is the most common cause of community acquired pneumonia. It is not associated with any immune complex disease, unlike its relative, group A streptococcus, which is involved in producing immune complex poststreptococcal glomerulonephritis. Damage in immune complex disease is associated with activation of the complement system and the chemotaxis of neutrophils to the area of deposition.

Treponema pallidum (etiologic agent in syphilis), hepatitis B virus, and *Plasmodium malariae* are all associated with an immune complex, membranous type of glomerulonephritis that produces a nephrotic syndrome.

32. The answer is D.   *(Behavioral science)*
Male sex and white race are associated with the highest rate of successful suicide attempts. Therefore, a white man would be the most likely of the five people listed to commit suicide.

33. The answer is E.   *(Microbiology)*
Mycobacterium kansasii is one of four well-defined photochromogenic mycobacteria that display a pigment following exposure to light. If cultures are grown in the dark, the colonies are cream-color, but they become a bright lemon-yellow if exposed to light. Crystals of beta carotene form on the surface of colonies, especially when growth is heavy. *M. kansasii* is the best recognized member of this group and is responsible for pulmonary disease in humans. The disease is indistinguishable from that caused by *Mycobacterium tuberculosis*, but follows a more chronic course.

Staphylococcus aureus produces yellow colonies (*aures* means golden); however, color may vary according to culture conditions.

Staphylococcus epidermidis (former name was *albus*, which means white) has white colonies.

Pseudomonas aeruginosa produces a blue-green color because of the production of pigments (pyoverdin = green and pyocyanin = blue); a sweet or grape-like odor is another characteristic.

Serratia marcesens routinely produces red-pigmented colonies.

34. The answer is B.   *(Behavioral science)*
In general, pain in children is not overtreated. Rather, pain in children is undertreated, underreported, misunderstood, and as commonly seen as in adults.

35. The answer is C.   *(Microbiology)*
Interleukin-2, produced by activated CD4 T helper cells, is an activator of T cells in that it increases production and differentiation of CD8 cytotoxic T cells and induces the synthesis of T cell cytokines. It increases the cytotoxicity of natural killer (NK) cells and is a cofactor for B cell proliferation and immunoglobulin secretion. Interleukin-1, produced by macrophages, stimulates the synthesis of acute phase reactants in the liver during inflammation, activates T cells, enhances hematopoiesis, increases adhesion molecule synthesis, causes the release of the postmitotic neutrophil pool from the bone marrow, and is responsible for fever in inflammation. Tumor necrosis factor-α, produced by macrophages, NK cells, and T lymphocytes, is a mediator of cachexia in cancer patients, has antiviral and antitumor properties, increases adhesion molecule synthesis, increases B cell proliferation and secretion of immunoglobulins, increases the synthesis of acute phase reactants in the liver, and stimulates the production of fever. Interleukin-3, produced by T lymphocytes, enhances hematopoiesis by stimulating the pluripotential stem cell. Interleukin-6, produced by T lymphocytes, induces B cell differentiation and synthesis of acute phase reactants.

36. The answer is A.   *(Behavioral science)*
When delivering a bad medical diagnosis to a patient, it is appropriate to tell him the news slowly, giving him the facts one at a time so that he can become adjusted to them. It is not appropriate to tell the patient all of the facts at once because he may become overwhelmed and anxious. It is appropriate to find out how much the patient already knows about the illness as well as how much he wants to know. Physicians should always sit down with their patients; standing gives the impression that the physician is in a hurry. Finally, the physician should explain that he

will not abandon the patient no matter how ill he becomes.

37. The answer is D.   *(Microbiology)*
Group B streptococci (e.g., *Streptococcus agalactiae*) are members of the normal flora of the female genital tract and are an important cause of neonatal sepsis and meningitis. They are beta hemolytic. Group D streptococci are normally found in the intestinal tract and are opportunists outside of this area.

Staphylococcus aureus* normally implants itself in the nasopharyngeal area, and thus prevention of nosocomial transmission is important. This type of colonization may be transient or permanent and may be detected by culture. The normal flora member, *Staphylococcus epidermidis*, is routinely found on the skin or also in the nasal area. Herpes simplex virus I resides in the trigeminal ganglia in latent infection and may reoccur periodically.

38. The answer is D.   *(Behavioral science)*
Although neurofibrillary tangles, senile plaques, loss of cortical neurons, and increased ventricular size are seen in Alzheimer's disease, these findings also occur to a lesser extent as part of the normal aging process. Whereas some mild memory impairment occurs with normal aging, severe memory loss that interferes with a normal life (e.g., leaving the stove on, starting a fire) is a sign of dementia in an elderly patient.

39-41. The answers are: 39-B, 40-C, 41-D.   *(Biochemistry)*
Pancreatic lipase hydrolyzes triacylglycerides, which pass essentially unaltered to the small intestine where they are emulsified with the aid of bile salts. The emulsification process increases the surface area of the lipid droplets so that the digestive enzymes can act effectively. Colipase, a protein also secreted by the pancreas, aids in this process by anchoring and stabilizing pancreatic lipase.

Insulin-enhanced capillary lipoprotein lipase binds to the luminal surface of the endothelial cells lining the capillaries, where it is activated by apolipoprotein C-II to degrade triacylglycerol in circulating chylomicrons and very–low-density lipoproteins (VLDLs). The free fatty acids released from this reaction are then taken up by tissues, where they are used as fuel

or, in the case of the adipocyte, for storage as triacylglycerides.

Hormone-sensitive lipase is activated by a catecholamine-mediated phosphorylation when glucose levels are low (as in the fasting state), or when an individual is under stress. This results in the release of free fatty acids, which associate with serum albumin and are then transported to tissues to use as fuel via β-oxidation. Insulin, which is the key hormone in the fed state, inhibits hormone-sensitive lipase, so the triacylglyceride remains in storage.

Gastric lipase plays a minor role in digestion, except in infants, in whom it may help digest the triacylglycerides containing short- and medium-chain fatty acids, which are typically found in milk.

Acid lipase, also known as acid-stable lipase or lingual lipase, originates from glands at the back of the tongue. This lipase is active at the acid pH of the stomach, but it contributes little to digestion because the triacylglycerol molecules are not emulsified. Emulsification only occurs in the small intestine after the lipid is mixed with bile. Except for the role of gastric lipase in infants, dietary lipids are minimally, if at all, degraded in the mouth or stomach.

42-44. The answers are: 42-E, 43-B, 44-D.   *(Behavioral science)*
In the first example, the colleague really meant to say "That promotion will be a gold mine for me," but his underlying repressed fears about possible negative consequences of the promotion have prompted this slip of the tongue or parapraxis.

Memories that can be recalled, such as the answers to exam questions, reside in the preconscious mind; those that cannot be recalled to the conscious mind reside in the unconscious mind.

Libido is the force that represents sexual drive in the mind.

45-47. The answers are: 45-H, 46-I, 47-A.   *(Biochemistry)*
Vitamin B, thiamine, is used as the cofactor for four reactions: pyruvate dehydrogenase, α-ketoglutarate dehydrogenase, branched-chain ketoacid decarboxylase, and transketolase. It is the latter reaction that permits ribose-phosphate to be formed from glycolytic reactants.

Biotin is required for the carboxylation of pyruvate to form oxaloacetic acid (OAA); it is a cofactor for pyruvate carboxylase. This anaplerotic (replenishing) reaction is important in the citric acid (Krebs) cycle, supplying the OAA that is required to condense with acetyl-CoA formed from fatty acid catabolism. Biochemists have summarized the importance of this reaction in the phrase, "Fat burns in the flame of carbohydrate." This reaction also supplies the cycle with carbons used for synthetic processes, including heme synthesis and glutamic acid and aspartic acid formation.

Lack of the lysosomal enzyme, α-L-iduronidase, results in the accumulation of dermatan sulfate and heparan sulfate in lysosomes. Children who are homozygous for this autosomal recessive deficiency are seemingly normal at birth, but their status gradually deteriorates as these glycosaminoglycans (formerly called mucopolysaccharides) accumulate in the brain and other tissues. A deficiency of α-L-iduronidase is known as Hurler syndrome. Hunter disease is a similar, slightly milder, sex-linked recessive disease. Vitamin B_6, as the cofactor pyridoxal phosphate, plays a central role in amino acid, not fatty acid, metabolism.

48-50. The answers are: 48-A, 49-C, 50-D.   (*Pathology*)

An insulinoma is a functional tumor (micro- or macroadenoma) of the islet of Langerhans that secretes insulin and C peptide. The increased plasma insulin produces hypoglycemia by increasing delivery of glucose to muscle and adipose tissue.

During a fast, blood glucose levels decrease. The hypoglycemia inhibits insulin and C peptide secretion and stimulates glucagon secretion.

Type II diabetes mellitus is characterized by insulin resistance. Hence, blood glucose is elevated and stimulates the β cells to secrete insulin and C peptide.

Column E could result from injection of insulin. Commercial insulin, which is devoid of C peptide, produces hypoglycemia and suppresses endogenous secretion of insulin and C peptide. The reported increase in plasma insulin is from the injected insulin.

Test 1

QUESTIONS

DIRECTIONS:

Each of the numbered items or incomplete statements in this section is followed by answers or by completions of the statement. Select the ONE lettered answer or completion that is BEST in each case.

1.   In the United States, most elderly people reside in

(A) a skilled nursing care facility
(B) an intermediate nursing care facility
(C) a residential nursing care facility
(D) the home of relatives
(E) their own residence

2.   Organisms that can use only molecular oxygen as the final hydrogen acceptor are known as

(A) obligate anaerobes
(B) strict anaerobes
(C) facultative anaerobes
(D) obligate aerobes
(E) aerotolerant anaerobes

Questions 3-5

The following figure represents biochemical pathways in the liver. Letters *A* through *G* represent key substrates. Numbers *1* through *8* represent enzymes.

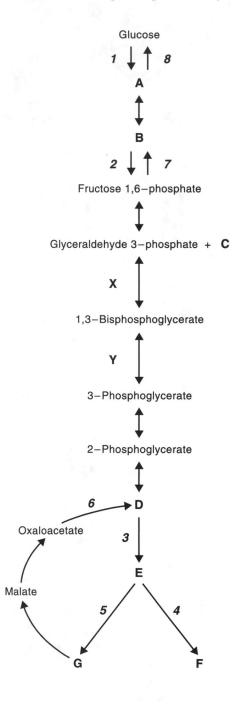

3.   Which one of the following enzyme relationships is correct?

(A)   Enzymes 1 and 2 are activated by fructose 2,6-bisphosphate in the fed state

(B)   Enzyme 3 is inactivated by protein kinase A action in the fasting state

(C)   Enzyme 4 catalyzes a reversible reaction-forming oxaloacetate and uses thiamine as a cofactor

(D)   Enzyme 5 catalyzes a reversible reaction-forming acetyl CoA and uses biotin as a cofactor

(E)   Enzymes 6, 7, and 8 are predominantly operative in the fed state

4.   Which one of the following relationships is correct?

(A)   Substrate A is an intermediate that is used in forming ribose 5-phosphate, glycogen, and reduced nicotinamide adenine dinucleotide phosphate (NADPH)

(B)   Substrate C is an intermediate formed during the metabolism of galactose

(C)   Substrate D is the primary substrate for gluconeogenesis

(D)   Substrates F and G combine to form oxaloacetate

(E)   Substrate A is produced via the action of fructokinase

5.   Which one of the following groups of substrates is used as intermediates for the synthesis of glycogen, glycerol-phosphate, and fatty acids, respectively?

(A)   Substrates A, B, and F

(B)   Substrates B, C, and G

(C)   Substrates A, C, and F

(D)   Substrates B, D, and G

(E)   Substrates B, C, and F

6. Which of the following growth alterations has the greatest risk for malignant transformation?

(A) Actinic keratosis
(B) Peutz-Jeghers polyp
(C) Duodenal ulcer
(D) Bronchial hamartoma
(E) Prostatic hyperplasia

7. Which of the following is a transversion mutation?

(A) The substitution of a GC base pair for an AT base pair
(B) The substitution of a CG base pair for a GC base pair
(C) The deletion of three base pairs
(D) The insertion of two base pairs
(E) All point mutations

8. A 30-year-old male known to have type I hypersensitivity undergoes hyposensitization. Which of the following statements best describes this procedure?

(A) Antibodies that compete with histamine for H1 and H2 receptors are induced
(B) T-suppressor cells are activated in order to reduce immunoglobulin E (IgE) production
(C) A substance that relaxes smooth muscle and decreases vascular permeability is induced
(D) Mast cells and basophils are slowly degranulated over a period of several hours
(E) Blocking immunoglobulin G (IgG) is induced so that the allergen will be intercepted

9. Genes containing a homeobox are most likely involved in

(A) causing cancer
(B) coding for glycolytic enzymes
(C) causing homocystinuria
(D) controlling development
(E) coding for hemoglobin

10. Which of the following descriptions best characterizes the growth alteration referred to as a malignant process?

(A) A tumor in the parotid gland that recurs after being previously removed, without a margin of normal tissue around the mass
(B) A mass compressing the cerebral cortex with swirls of meningothelial cells surrounding a psammoma body
(C) An encapsulated follicular tumor of the thyroid with absence of capsular and vessel invasion
(D) A solitary nodular mass in the liver with nests of mucin secreting glands and focal areas of necrosis
(E) A smooth muscle tumor in the myometrium with one normal mitotic spindle in ten high-powered fields

11. The only codon for tryptophan is UGG. The anticodon portion of the transfer RNA (tRNA) that carries tryptophan is most likely to be

(A) ACC
(B) UGG
(C) TCC
(D) CCA
(E) GGU

12. Which of the following statements concerning chemical carcinogenesis is correct?

(A) Promotion must precede the initiation of a transformation cell before malignancy transformation can occur
(B) Initiation produces a permanent mutational change in the cell's DNA
(C) Promotion is mutagenic and activates oncogenes by inducing point mutations in nucleotides
(D) Estrogen is primarily an initiator in chemical carcinogenesis
(E) Once the mutational change has occurred in the DNA, no further cell division is necessary

Questions 13-14

The following pedigree shows a family in which the father (I-1) and mother (I-2) are both carriers of the autosomal recessive disease phenylketonuria (PKU). Their firstborn son (II-1) is affected by the disease. The figure also shows Southern blots of a restriction fragment length polymorphism (RFLP) marker located close to the phenylalanine hydroxylase gene for each family member.

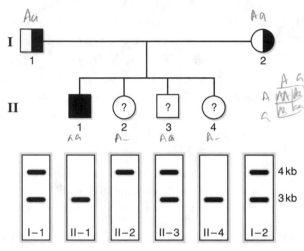

13. What is the status of the firstborn daughter (II-2) and secondborn son (II-3), respectively?

(A) Carrier; homozygous normal
(B) Affected; carrier
(C) Affected; homozygous normal
(D) Homozygous normal; carrier
(E) Homozygous normal; affected

14. If these parents have another child, what is the probability that it will have PKU?

(A) 0%
(B) 25%
(C) 50%
(D) 75%
(E) 100%

15. An all-day family reunion was held on a summer day when the temperature soared to 103°F. The picnic food included potato salad, chicken, and hamburgers. The next morning, five family members experienced diarrhea, fever, and abdominal pain, which lasted for several days. One person was eventually hospitalized, and gram-negative H_2S-producing rods were isolated from the stool. Which of the following bacteria was most likely the cause?

(A) *Shigella dysenteriae*
(B) *Shigella sonnei*
(C) *Shigella flexneri*
(D) *Salmonella typhimurium*
(E) *Salmonella typhi*

Questions 16-17

The following pedigree shows a family in which the firstborn son (II-1) is affected by the X-linked disease hemophilia A. The figure also shows Southern blots of a restriction fragment length polymorphism (RFLP) marker in an intron of the factor VIII gene for each family member.

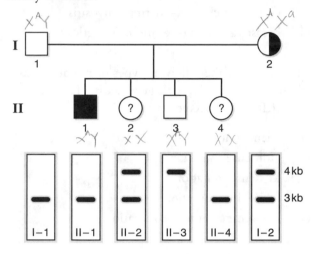

16. What is the status of the first- and second-born daughters (II-2 and II-4), respectively?

(A) Carrier; homozygous normal
(B) Carrier; affected
(C) Affected; homozygous normal
(D) Homozygous normal; carrier
(E) Homozygous normal; affected

17. If these parents have another son, what is the probability that he will be affected by hemophilia A?

(A) 0%
(B) 25%
(C) 50%
(D) 75%
(E) 100%

18. Which of the following cancer–oncogene relationships is correct?

(A) Breast cancer—ras oncogene
(B) Burkitt lymphoma—c-myc oncogene
(C) Neuroblastoma—abl oncogene
(D) Chronic myelogenous leukemia—N-myc oncogene
(E) Colon cancer—erb-B3 oncogene

19. Which of the following sugars is an anomer of α-D-glucose?

(A) α-D-Fructose
(B) β-D-Glucose
(C) α-D-Galactose
(D) α-L-Glucose
(E) β-L-Glucose

20. Which of the following is the most important factor that determines the prognosis of a patient with breast cancer?

(A) Estrogen receptor and progesterone receptor assay results
(B) DNA ploidy studies
(C) S-phase studies
(D) Grade of the cancer
(E) Stage of the cancer

21. The following figure shows results of DNA typing performed in two cases of disputed paternity. The *lanes* show Southern blots for a polymorphic marker derived from each of the involved individuals. Which of the following statements about these cases is correct?

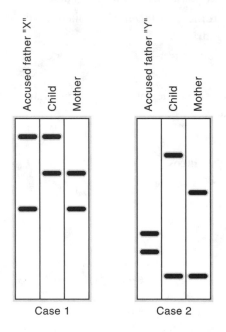

(A) Individual X is the father in case 1, whereas individual Y is not the father in case 2

(B) Individual X is not the father in case 1, whereas individual Y may be the father in case 2

(C) Individual X may be the father in case 1, whereas individual Y is definitely the father in case 2

(D) Individual X is not the father in case 1, whereas individual Y is the father in case 2

(E) Individual X may be the father in case 1, whereas individual Y is definitely not the father in case 2

22. Which of the following organisms are found only in humans?

(A) *Salmonella typhimurium*
(B) *Salmonella typhi*
(C) *Salmonella choleraesuis*
(D) *Yersinia enterocolitica*
(E) *Pasteurella multocida*

23. Which of the following cancer–paraneoplastic syndrome relationships is correctly matched?

(A) Small cell carcinoma of the lung—hypercalcemia
(B) Pancreatic carcinoma—hypertrophic osteoarthropathy
(C) Thymoma—pure red blood cell aplasia
(D) Gastric carcinoma—dermatomyositis
(E) Breast carcinoma—acanthosis nigricans

24. Which of the following types of mutations usually involves mutation of a gene coding for a transfer RNA (tRNA) molecule?

(A) Silent mutation
(B) Nonsense mutation
(C) Missense mutation
(D) Frameshift mutation
(E) Nonsense suppressor mutation

25. Which of the following screening tests has contributed most to the decline in the incidence of a specific cancer in the United States?

(A) Mammography
(B) Stool guaiac
(C) Cervical Papanicolau (PAP) smear
(D) Rectal exam
(E) Prostate-specific antigen

26. During a trip to the desert, a 14-year-old boy is bitten by a rattlesnake. He is treated with serum made in hyperimmunized horses, which contains antibodies against the snake venom. Approximately 9 days later, the boy develops a generalized rash. Which of the following diagnoses is most likely?

(A) Serum sickness
(B) Arthus reaction
(C) Type II hypersensitivity
(D) Disseminated intravascular coagulation
(E) Type IV hypersensitivity

27. The rooting reflex characteristic of newborn infants usually disappears by the age of

(A) 1 month
(B) 3 months
(C) 8 months
(D) 10 months
(E) 12 months

28. A characteristic response to infection with *Mycobacterium tuberculosis* is granuloma formation. Which of the following cell types are important in mediating this type of reaction?

(A) Neutrophils and other granulocytes
(B) T-helper cells and macrophages
(C) B lymphocytes and basophils
(D) Mast cells and eosinophils
(E) Neutrophils and basophils

29. The rate of DNA synthesis in a cell could be determined most specifically by measuring the incorporation of radioactive

(A) leucine
(B) thymidine
(C) uridine
(D) phosphate
(E) ribose

30. Use of certain antibiotics (e.g., tetracycline) may result in a disturbance of the normal flora of the mouth and subsequent predominance of which one of the following organisms?

(A) *Haemophilus influenzae*
(B) *Nocardia asteroides*
(C) *Candida albicans*
(D) *Treponema pallidum*
(E) *Cryptococcus neoformans*

31. Myoglobin has a hyperbolic oxygen dissociation curve, while hemoglobin has a sigmoidal curve. This is a reflection of the fact that

(A) myoglobin is a monomer, while hemoglobin consists of four subunits
(B) myoglobin has quaternary structure
(C) the iron in myoglobin is in the Fe^{2+} form, while it is in the Fe^{3+} form in hemoglobin
(D) myoglobin binds protons more efficiently than does hemoglobin
(E) myoglobin binds carbon dioxide more efficiently than does hemoglobin

32. A 9-year-old boy goes on a camping trip with his parents. Upon arrival, he eagerly jumps out of the car and runs into the bushes to play. The next day he complains of intense itching and blistering of the hands, arms, and legs. Which of the following conditions is he most likely to have?

(A) Serum sickness
(B) Hay fever
(C) Arthus reaction
(D) Contact dermatitis
(E) Farmer's lung disease

33. A 5-year-old boy with normal motor skills has severe language delay, shows no interest in interacting with other children or with adults, and spends a lot of time spinning around. The most likely diagnosis for this child is

(A) attention deficit hyperactivity disorder (ADHD)
(B) Rett syndrome
(C) conduct disorder
(D) mental retardation
(E) infantile autism

Questions 34-35

A 45-year-old male with end-stage renal disease is prepared to receive a kidney from his wife. Assays for HLA antigens indicate that the donor and recipient are not 100% compatible. The patient is given an immunosuppresive drug regimen. Three months after transplantation, laboratory tests indicate that the patient's kidney function is declining. There is a rapid decrease in urine output and the urine contains blood cells and a high level of protein. The engrafted kidney is enlarged and tender. After treatment with antilymphocyte serum (ALS), the patient's critical condition is reversed.

34. The type of graft this patient has received is a(n)

(A) isograft

(B) syngraft

(C) allograft

(D) autograft

(E) xenograft

35. During the crisis period, the patient was most likely experiencing

(A) acute rejection

(B) chronic rejection

(C) graft-versus-host disease

(D) hyperacute rejection

(E) toxicity to the drugs

36. Patients with diabetes mellitus often show an increase in the type of hemoglobin known as

(A) HbA

(B) HbA_{1c}

(C) HbA_2

(D) HbF

(E) Hb Gower 1

37. A 4-year-old child attending a day care center developed abdominal pain, a low-grade fever, and watery diarrhea. The next day his condition became worse and the mother took him to a pediatrician. Microscopic examination of the stool revealed the presence of numerous red and white blood cells and mucus. Blood cultures were negative, but a lactose negative, nonmotile gram-negative rod was isolated from the stool. Which of the following is the most likely causative organism?

(A) *Escherichia coli*

(B) *Enterobacter* species

(C) *Klebsiella* species

(D) *Salmonella typhi*

(E) *Shigella sonnei*

38. Which of the following amino acids is most likely to be located in the interior of a soluble protein molecule, not in contact with water molecules of the solvent?

(A) Aspartic acid

(B) Arginine

(C) Lysine

(D) Valine

(E) Serine

39. In which of the following organisms is mycolic acid present and responsible for identification in clinical material?

(A) *Nocardia*

(B) *Actinomyces*

(C) Corynebacteria

(D) Mycobacteria

(E) Actinobacillus

40. A crisis in a patient with sickle cell disease is most likely to be caused by

(A) alkalosis
(B) acidosis
(C) increased oxygen concentration
(D) decreased CO_2 concentration
(E) decreased 2,3-bisphosphoglycerate concentration

41. A 57-year-old male with acute lymphocytic leukemia (ALL) fails all standard chemotherapies. Preparative chemoradiotherapy and broad-spectrum antibiotics are administered before proceeding with a bone marrow transplant from an HLA-nonidentical donor. Within 2 to 4 weeks, engraftment of the cells is confirmed by rising lymphocyte and granulocyte numbers. Approximately 2 months after the transplant, the patient develops a skin rash, severe diarrhea, and jaundice. Which of the following reactions is most likely occurring?

(A) Cyclosporin A toxicity
(B) Host-versus-graft rejection
(C) *Staphylococcus* infection
(D) Recurrence of ALL
(E) Graft-versus-host disease

42. A 5-year-old boy told his mother that he had an accident with his bicycle because he was thinking of taking some money from his brother. This type of reasoning is known as

(A) adaptive reasoning
(B) magical thinking
(C) concrete operations
(D) abstract reasoning
(E) preoperational thinking

43. Meningitis caused by *Cryptococcus neoformans* is most often acquired by

(A) head trauma
(B) primary gastrointestinal infection
(C) hematogenous spread of fungus from the lung
(D) orthopedic surgery
(E) ingesting pigeon droppings

44. A father and daughter have a close relationship with each other, but neither one gets along well with the mother. In the family system, this is an example of

(A) an executive subsystem
(B) a triangle
(C) an emotional cutoff
(D) mutual accommodation
(E) multigenerational transmission process

45. A microscopic examination of a 10% potassium hydroxide preparation of a skin scraping is most useful in the diagnosis of

(A) tinea versicolor
(B) histoplasmosis
(C) coccidioidomycosis
(D) blastomycosis
(E) chromoblastomycosis

46. A 6-year-old child develops abdominal pain early every Monday morning. A comprehensive medical workup fails to reveal a physiologic problem. This symptom is most likely caused by

(A) genetic factors
(B) a learning disability
(C) developmental immaturity
(D) separation anxiety
(E) mental retardation

Questions 47-48

A 30-year-old homeless, alcoholic man, who has recently lost 15% of his body weight, develops night sweats, fever, and a productive cough. His sputum is greenish and flecked with blood. A radiograph shows a cavitary lesion in the apex of his left lung. He has had a positive tuberculin skin test for approximately 10 years.

47. Which of the following bacteria is the most likely causal organism?

(A) *Mycobacterium scrofulaceum*
(B) *Mycobacterium marinum*
(C) *Mycobacterium tuberculosis*
(D) *Mycobacterium ulcerans*
(E) *Mycobacterium fortuitum-chelonae*

48. Which of the following statements regarding the tuberculin skin test is true?

(A) A positive result may indicate past or present infection with *Mycobacterium tuberculosis*
(B) Live, attenuated *Mycobacterium tuberculosis* is injected intradermally
(C) A positive reaction establishes a diagnosis of active tuberculosis
(D) A positive reaction is caused by antibodies against *Mycobacterium tuberculosis*
(E) Positive reactivity usually disappears a few months after infection

49. Which of the following conditions is consistent with increased 24-hour urinary excretion of calcium and phosphate?

(A) Dietary calcium deficiency
(B) Dietary vitamin D deficiency
(C) Primary hyperparathyroidism
(D) Primary hypoparathyroidism
(E) Pseudohypoparathyroidism

50. An avid gardener developed a painless nodule in the finger that, over the ensuing weeks, spread up the arm, leaving a series of subcutaneous nodules. Some of these were draining pus. The most likely diagnosis in this patient is

(A) mucormycosis
(B) mycetoma
(C) *Trichophyton rubrum* infection
(D) favus, caused by *Trichophyton schoenleinii*
(E) sporotrichosis

51. Helping a 25-year-old male schizophrenic patient learn self-care is an example of

(A) primary prevention
(B) secondary prevention
(C) tertiary prevention
(D) active prevention
(E) retroactive prevention

52. A mycosis caused by a dimorphic fungus that is characterized by yeast found intracellularly in reticuloendothelial cells is

(A) coccidioidomycosis
(B) histoplasmosis
(C) cryptococcosis
(D) blastomycosis
(E) mucormycosis

53. A patient with xeroderma pigmentosum is most likely to be defective in the process of

(A) purine degradation
(B) pyrimidine biosynthesis
(C) DNA repair
(D) antibody production
(E) collagen production

54. Observation of yeast cells with multiple budding in tissue in the form of a "ship's wheel" is highly suggestive of

(A) blastomycosis
(B) coccidioidomycosis
(C) paracoccidioidomycosis
(D) histoplasmosis
(E) sporotrichosis

55. Training of an expectant couple in the principles of child development is an example of

(A) primary prevention
(B) secondary prevention
(C) tertiary prevention
(D) active prevention
(E) retroactive prevention

56. The cord factor is a virulence factor for a/an

(A) gram-positive rod
(B) gram-negative rod
(C) gram-positive filamentous bacteria
(D) acid-fast bacteria
(E) gram-positive diplococcus

57. Livingston is a town of 100,000 people. During 1960, there were 1000 deaths from all causes. All cases of tuberculosis were found and totaled 300, 200 male cases and 100 female cases. Also during 1960, there were 60 deaths from tuberculosis; 50 of them were male. The sex-specific mortality rate for tuberculosis in males is

(A) 5 per 100,000
(B) 50 per 200 × 1000
(C) 60 per 300 × 1000
(D) 60 per 100,000 × 1000
(E) not calculable from the data given

58. The following drugs are frequently associated with sideroblastic anemia. Which would most likely be used to treat active tuberculosis?

(A) Kanamycin
(B) Isoniazid
(C) Amikacin
(D) Dapsone
(E) Streptomycin

59. A man is suffering from acute intestinal pains, hair loss, nausea, and anemia. The physician suspects arsenic poisoning. The recommended treatment for this suspected arsenic poisoning is

(A) parenteral administration of ethylenediaminctet-raacetate (EDTA, edetate)
(B) peritoneal dialysis or hemodialysis
(C) parenteral administration of 2,3-dimercaptol-1-propanol (dimercaprol)
(D) parenteral administration of penicillamine
(E) parenteral administration of deferoxamine

60. Which of the following statements applies to both *Mycobacterium tuberculosis* and *Mycobacterium leprae*?

(A) Disease progresses rapidly compared with most other pathogens
(B) The incidence of drug-resistant strains is decreasing
(C) Delayed-type hypersensitivity is usually not detectable after infection
(D) Biochemical tests need to be performed after in vitro culture
(E) There are no serologic tests that are useful in diagnosis

61. Which of the following examples best illustrates prevalence rate?

(A) Number of new cases of multiple sclerosis per 100,000 population per year

(E) Number of men who die per year per 100,000 population per year

(B) Number of new cases of cancer of the prostate per 100,000 men per year

(C) Number of 10-year-old children who die of leukemia per 100,000 population per year

(D) Number of multiple sclerosis patients per 100,000 population per year

(E) Number of men who die per 100,000 population per year

62. Which of the following symptoms would most likely be found in a patient with lepromatous leprosy?

(A) No bacteremia

(B) Macrophages with a foamy appearance in the dermis

(C) A positive lepromin reaction

(D) A high cell-mediated response against *Mycobacterium leprae*

(E) Skin infiltration with T-helper lymphocytes

63. A Poly A base sequence would be most likely found at the

(A) 5′ end of a prokaryotic messenger RNA (mRNA)

(B) 3′ end of a prokaryotic mRNA

(C) 5′ end of a eukaryotic mRNA

(D) 3′ end of a eukaryotic mRNA

(E) 3′ end of both prokaryotic and eukaryotic mRNA

64. Dysphonia in a 2-year-old child with a grayish exudate in the posterior pharynx and massive, tender cervical lymphadenitis is most likely caused by

(A) *Corynebacterium diphteriae*

(B) *Corynebacterium pseudodiphtheriticum*

(C) group A *Streptococcus*

(D) *Propionibacterium* species

(E) *Erysipelothrix rhusiopathiae*

65. The percentage of the gross domestic product spent on health care in 1992 was approximately

(A) 4%

(B) 6%

(C) 13%

(D) 22%

(E) 35%

66. Which of the following statements applies to the diphtheria toxin?

(A) All *Corynebacterium diphtheriae* produce it

(B) It inhibits protein synthesis in mammalian cells

(C) Its effects cannot be prevented

(D) It increases the intracellular level of cyclic adenosine monophosphate (cAMP)

(E) It is an endotoxin

67. The standardized mortality ratio (SMR) for office workers is 0.95. This suggests that when compared with the general population in a given year, office workers are

(A) more likely to die

(B) less likely to die

(C) equally likely to die

(D) at the highest risk for dying

(E) at the lowest risk for dying

68. A bacteria with tumbling end-over-end motility is isolated from the cerebrospinal fluid of a 2-day-old infant with meningitis. This organism is likely to be

(A) *Escherichia coli*

(B) β-hemolytic *Streptococcus*

(C) *Listeria monocytogenes*

(D) *Haemophilus influenzae*

(E) *Neisseria meningitidis*

69. A young woman is homozygous for an unusual form of succinate thiokinase that has a very high Michaelis-Menten constant (K_m) for succinate. Because of this aberration, this enzyme can only catalyze the forward reaction, which is the formation of succinate, guanosine triphosphate (GTP), and coenzyme A (CoA) from succinyl CoA and guanosine diphosphate (GDP). In a normal individual, the reverse reaction is used to form succinyl CoA from oxaloacetate (OAA) via fumarate and succinate under high-energy charge conditions, which inhibit isocitrate dehydrogenase and the other early reactions in the citric acid (Krebs) cycle. Consequently, the young woman cannot synthesize more succinyl CoA than is required to maintain the energy needs of her cells. A physician expects this young woman would be prone to develop

(A) a lower than normal red blood cell adenosine triphosphate (ATP) level
(B) hemolytic anemia
(C) microcytic anemia associated with a defect in heme synthesis
(D) megaloblastic anemia associated with a functional folate deficiency
(E) pernicious anemia

70. A gold miner in the Southwest who contracts plague most likely had contact with a/an

(A) arthropod
(B) rodent
(C) wild dog
(D) dead bird
(E) human

71. To assess the strength of association between two variables that are hypothesized to be linearly related, which of the following tests is the most appropriate?

(A) Fisher exact test
(B) t-Test
(C) Analysis of variance (ANOVA)
(D) Correlation
(E) Chi-square test

72. A 5-year-old boy has just recovered from a rotavirus infection. When given milk, he develops watery diarrhea. Which of the following conversion problems is described by these symptoms? The conversion of

(A) starch to limit dextrins and milk albumin to polypeptides
(B) lactose to galactose plus glucose and small peptides to free amino acids
(C) lactose to galactose plus glucose and milk albumin to polypeptides
(D) starch to limit dextrins and small peptides to free amino acids
(E) maltose to glucose and milk albumin to polypeptides

73. The average life expectancy for all Americans at birth is approximately

(A) 71 years
(B) 76 years
(C) 78 years
(D) 80 years
(E) 82 years

74. A nutritionist is working on the problem of feeding starving populations in Africa and Asia. The American Dairy Association, because of a large surplus, offers to supply the nutritionist with all the milk products she wants. Her problem is that both populations live in remote tropical areas with no refrigeration. The nutritionist decides to accept the offer with the condition that the supplied milk is in the form of

(A) a desiccated powder
(B) cheese
(C) yogurt
(D) butter
(E) cream

75. Which of the following disorders is consistent with ketoacidosis?

(A) Type II diabetes
(B) Positive nitrogen balance   anabolic.
(C) Low plasma [C peptide]
(D) Increased lipogenesis
(E) Expanded blood volume

76. Women are more likely than men to

(A) suffer from hypochondriasis
(B) show aggression
(C) seek medical attention
(D) suffer from spinal cord injuries
(E) have a homosexual orientation

77. Medicaid is financed by

(A) the federal government
(B) state governments
(C) municipal governments
(D) federal and state governments
(E) federal, state, and municipal governments

78. What happens during the process of DNA replication in *Escherichia coli*?

(A) Newly synthesized strands are made in the 3′ → 5′ direction
(B) A newly synthesized strand has an identical sequence to that of its template
(C) Okazaki fragment synthesis is initiated by synthesis of an RNA primer
(D) A "proofreading" activity is provided by the 5′ → 3′ exonuclease activity of DNA polymerase III
(E) DNA ligase provides a "swivel"

79. When compared with a 55-year-old African-American woman, a 55-year-old white woman is more likely to show which of these conditions?

(A) Obesity
(B) Schizophrenia
(C) Diabetes
(D) Suicidal tendencies
(E) Hypertension

80. Fluoroquinolones such as ciprofloxacin are usually avoided in children because of the potential for

(A) damage to growing cartilage
(B) hyperpyrexia
(C) macrocytic anemia
(D) ototoxicity
(E) permanent staining of the teeth

81. Improving the nutrition of an 18-year-old pregnant woman is an example of

(A) primary prevention
(B) secondary prevention
(C) tertiary prevention
(D) active prevention
(E) retroactive prevention

82. Which antiviral agent most often causes anemia, leukopenia, or thrombocytopenia?

(A) Ribavirin
(B) Zidovudine
(C) Amantadine
(D) Acyclovir
(E) Didanosine

83. A drug has a 10% rate of side effects. If a physician puts two patients on this drug, what is the probability that both will develop side effects?

(A) 1%
(B) 2%
(C) 5%
(D) 10%
(E) 15%

84. The component of the extracellular matrix that is responsible for tracking adhesion of embryonic cells and is lost from the cell surface of cancer cells is

(A) laminin
(B) integrin
(C) glycocalyx
(D) fibronectin
(E) hyaluronic acid

85. A persistent or chronic infection of hepatitis B virus (HBV) is usually detected by measuring

(A) hepatitis B surface antigen (HBsAg) for less than 3 months
(B) HBsAg for more than 6 months
(C) HBsAg antibody for more than 6 months
(D) hepatitis B coreantigen (HBcAg) antibody for less than 3 months
(E) hepatitis Be antigen (HBeAg) anytime

86. Specific cell surface proteins, such as alkaline phosphatase, acetylcholine esterase, and lipoprotein lipase, are anchored to the cell membrane. This anchoring is accomplished by covalent binding through an oligosaccharide bridge to a component of the cell membrane. This component is

(A) sphingomyelin
(B) phosphatidic acid
(C) phosphatidylserine
(D) phosphatidylinositol
(E) phosphatidylethanolamine

87. A 2-year-old girl is 33 inches tall. Which of the following measurements is the best estimate of her adult height?

(A) 60 inches
(B) 62 inches
(C) 66 inches
(D) 70 inches
(E) 72 inches

88. For the following data, the attributable risk of smoking to bladder cancer in men is

Bladder cancer per 100,000 men per year	
Smokers	48.0
Non smokers	25.4

(A) 48.0/25.4 = 1.89
(B) 48.0 - 25.4 = 22.6/100,000
(C) 48.0
(D) 48.0/100,000 = 0.00048
(E) not calculable from these data

89. A 78-year-old man whose wife died six months ago has lost 15 pounds, cries most of the time, and refuses to leave his apartment. He tells you that it is his fault that his wife died because he did not appreciate her. You should

(A) increase the number of appointments with the patient
(B) give him a trial of antidepressant medication and see him weekly
(C) tell him to get out more and to see friends
(D) reassure him that he will be feeling better in another few weeks
(E) contact his children and tell them to call him more often

Questions 90-91

A previously healthy, 53-year-old sheep farmer is admitted to the hospital. Two months prior to admission, he developed swollen lymph nodes and myalgia. Approximately one week prior, he began having daily fevers, chills, and night sweats. Blood cultures were positive for a bacterium after prolonged incubation. Histologic examination of a liver biopsy revealed the presence of noncaseating granulomatous lesions.

90. Which of the following microorganisms is the most likely cause?

(A) *Francisella tularensis*
(B) *Salmonella typhi*
(C) *Brucella melitensis*
(D) *Brucella canis*
(E) *Mycobacterium bovis*

91. Of the following factors, the most important in the outcome of this disease is the

(A) activation of T-suppressor lymphocytes
(B) production of complement-activating antibodies
(C) action of lysozyme
(D) ability of macrophages to kill the organisms
(E) environment of the patient

92. A 54-year-old physician with undiagnosed pancreatic cancer is suffering severe pain and appears jaundiced. Upon learning about his symptoms, his close friend and colleague, also a physician, tells him that his symptoms are probably caused by an infection. The reason for the colleague's misdiagnosis is most likely

(A) transference
(B) countertransference
(C) rationalization
(D) displacement
(E) projection

93. N-linked glycosylation of a protein is most likely to begin in the

(A) cytoplasm
(B) Golgi apparatus
(C) lysosomes
(D) nucleus
(E) endoplasmic reticulum

94. A 20-year-old male college student develops a sore throat, fever, generalized lymphadenopathy, and splenomegaly. Serologic tests reveal that he has heterophile antibodies and nucleic acid hybridization performed on immortalized B lymphocytes from the patient reveals viral infection. Which of the following viruses is most likely to be the etiologic agent?

(A) Human immunodeficiency virus type-1
(B) Human T leukemia virus type-I
(C) Human herpes virus type 6
(D) Epstein-Barr virus (EBV)
(E) Cytomegalovirus (CMV)

95. Which of the following statements describes the grade rather than the stage of a cancer?

(A) The tumor measures 2 x 2 x 2 cm and extends to the serosal surface of the colon
(B) Sections through the tumor reveal sheets of malignant cells with focal areas of gland formation and mucin production.
(C) Three out of 20 lymph nodes are involved with metastatic disease.
(D) The proximal and distal margins of the colon resection are free of tumor
(E) Sections of a liver biopsy reveal malignant cells similar to those seen in the primary site in the colon

96. The single most important risk factor that contributes to mortality in the Unites States is

(A) diet
(B) alcohol
(C) smoking
(D) accidents
(E) lack of exercise

97. In which of the following sites is the most likely primary cancer an adenocarcinoma?

(A) Cervix
(B) Lung
(C) Esophagus
(D) True vocal cord
(E) Bladder

98. Which of the following tumor–chromosome relationships is correctly matched?

(A) Neuroblastoma—chromosome 1
(B) Wilm's tumor—chromosome 7
(C) Osteogenic sarcoma—chromosome 8
(D) Retinoblastoma (Rb)—chromosome 11
(E) Neurofibromas—chromosome 13

99. A pathology report on a dilatation and curettage specimen from a 62-year-old woman with vaginal bleeding reads as follows: "Sections of tissue labelled 'endometrial tissue' reveal numerous tightly packed glands lined by columnar cells with enlarged, irregular nuclei and prominent irregular nucleoli. Atypical mitotic spindles are frequently present. Multiple foci of necrosis are noted within the gland lumens. There is no intervening stroma between many of the glands. One of the tissue fragments exhibits a focus of bland squamous epithelium with focal areas of keratinization blending imperceptibly into one of the glands. It makes up less than 1% of the specimen submitted. No myometrial tissue is readily identified in the tissue submitted." Which of the following statements best describes this specimen? It is a/an

(A) atypical endometrial hyperplasia with focal areas of squamous metaplasia
(B) high-grade cancer of the endometrial glands with focal invasion into the cervix
(C) well-differentiated squamous cancer infiltrating into the endometrial cavity
(D) low-grade endometrial adenocarcinoma with focal areas of benign squamous epithelium
(E) anaplastic endometrial cancer with squamous cell carcinoma (adenosquamous carcinoma)

100. An increased insulin–glucagon ratio most likely

(A) increases protein kinase A activity
(B) inactivates dephosphorylated phosphofructokinase-2
(C) activates fructose bisphosphate phosphatase-2
(D) increases the concentration of fructose 2,6-bisphosphate
(E) activates adenylate cyclase

101. In which stage of bacterial growth is there a slow loss of cells through death that is balanced by the formation of new cells through binary fission?

(A) Lag stage
(B) Acceleration
(C) Exponential (or logarithmic) stage
(D) Stationary
(E) Deceleration

DIRECTIONS:

Each of the numbered items or incomplete statements in this section is negatively phrased, as indicated by a capitalized word such as NOT, LEAST, or EXCEPT. Select the ONE lettered answer or completion that is BEST in each case.

102. Which of the following patients is LEAST likely to visit the office of a private physician?

(A) An affluent 45-year-old man
(B) An affluent 45-year-old woman
(C) A low-income 45-year-old woman
(D) A low-income 45-year-old man
(E) A middle-income 45-year-old woman

103. Which one of the following is NOT a fuel for gluconeogenesis?

(A) Acetyl CoA
(B) Glycerol
(C) Lactate
(D) Oxaloacetate
(E) Propionyl CoA

104. Which of the following is LEAST likely to be involved in oncogenesis?

(A) Inactivation of suppressor genes
(B) Activation of growth-promoting oncogenes
(C) Chromosomal translocations
(D) Point mutations
(E) Shortening of the cell cycle

105. Which one of the following statements is NOT applicable to pyruvate?

(A) It is operative in the Cori cycle
(B) It is the gateway to the tricarboxylic acid cycle
(C) It is transaminated into aspartate
(D) It is converted into lactate during anaerobic glycolysis
(E) It is an α-ketoacid

106. Which of the following statements is NOT true of fungi?

(A) Fungi contain 80S ribosomes
(B) Fungal nuclei are surrounded by nuclear membranes
(C) Fungal cytoplasmic membrane contains sterol
(D) Some fungi produce sexual spores
(E) Fungal cell walls are made of peptidoglycan

107. Which of the following statements is NOT a characteristic of the genetic code?

(A) Each codon consists of three bases
(B) A single amino acid can have more than one codon
(C) A single codon can correspond to more than one amino acid
(D) Codons are nonoverlapping
(E) *Escherichia coli* and humans have the same genetic code

108. Of the following disorders, age is the LEAST important risk factor for

(A) breast cancer
(B) coronary artery disease
(C) prostate cancer
(D) colon cancer
(E) lung cancer

109. Which of the following actions is LEAST characteristic of a normal 3-year-old boy?

(A) Putting on shoes without tying the laces
(B) Knowing that he is a boy
(C) Following a three-step command
(D) Drawing a detailed figure of a person
(E) Riding a tricycle

110. All of the following statements regarding the role of macrophages in AIDS patients are correct EXCEPT

(A) they can be infected with HIV-1
(B) they exhibit defective chemotaxis
(C) they produce an inhibitor of interleukin-1
(D) they present antigen normally
(E) they are reservoir cells for the virus

111. A drug is discovered that is very effective in curing a form of cancer that was previously rapidly fatal. Which of the following factors would be LEAST affected by this drug discovery for this form of cancer?

(A) Crude mortality rate
(B) Cause-specific mortality rate
(C) Point prevalence rate
(D) Incidence rate
(E) Period prevalence rate

112. All of the following statements regarding a typical HIV-1 infection are correct EXCEPT

(A) T-cell response to mitogens declines
(B) the first antibody class to appear is immunoglobulin M (IgM)
(C) p24 antigen titer is high early after infection
(D) p24 antigen titer is high at the terminal stage of AIDS
(E) anti-p24 antibody titer is high at the terminal stage of AIDS

113. Which specialty is LEAST likely to have a surplus of physicians by the end of the century?

(A) Obstetrics and gynecology
(B) Internal medicine
(C) Ophthalmology
(D) Neurosurgery
(E) Emergency medicine

Questions 114-116

A 25-year-old male is physically fit and healthy until stung on the cheek by a wasp. He has been previously stung on several occasions and has experienced some respiratory discomfort. The last time this occurred was approximately 3 weeks ago. Within 5 minutes he feels faint, develops edema of the face and neck, makes gasping sounds, and collapses. He is treated promptly in the emergency room and the symptoms resolve within several hours.

114. The most likely diagnosis is

(A) type I hypersensitivity
(B) type II hypersensitivity
(C) type III hypersensitivity
(D) type IV hypersensitivity
(E) C1 esterase inhibitor deficiency

115. The mechanism of the reaction directly involves all of the following EXCEPT

(A) immunoglobulin E (IgE)
(B) mast cells
(C) complement
(D) FcεRI receptors
(E) histamine

116. Which of the following is most likely to be given first in the treatment of this patient?

(A) Topical corticosteroids
(B) Cyclosporin A
(C) Methotrexate
(D) Cromolyn sodium
(E) Epinephrine

117. Target-tissue insensitivity to parathyroid hormone produces all of the following EXCEPT

(A) decreased plasma levels of parathyroid hormone
(B) hypocalcemia
(C) hyperphosphatemia
(D) decreased activity of 1α-hydroxylase
(E) decreased bone resorption

118. When compared with white Americans, Native Americans are less likely to

(A) be alcoholic
(B) commit suicide
(C) have high incomes
(D) have an infant that dies in its first year of life
(E) have emotional problems

119. All of the following actions occur in mitosis EXCEPT

(A) cytokinesis
(B) chromatids separate
(C) DNA replication
(D) the kinetochore becomes evident
(E) the nuclear membrane and nucleolus disappear

120. All of the following physiologic changes are associated with aging EXCEPT

(A) impaired immune responses
(B) decreased fat relative to muscle
(C) decreased brain weight
(D) enlarged brain ventricles
(E) decreased blood flow to the gastrointestinal system

121. Which of the following fungi is LEAST likely to cause pulmonary disease?

(A) *Aspergillus fumigatus*
(B) *Blastomyces dermatitidis*
(C) *Coccidioides immitis*
(D) *Epidermophyton floccosum*
(E) *Histoplasma capsulatum*

122. Which of the following patients is LEAST likely to experience erectile dysfunction?

(A) A 65-year-old man who is alcoholic and taking disulfiram (Antabuse)
(B) A 65-year-old male with Parkinson disease who is taking L-dopa
(C) A 65-year-old man who is taking guanethidine
(D) A 65-year-old man who has just had a myocardial infarction
(E) A 65-year-old diabetic man

123. Which of the following enzymes is NOT involved in the digestion of starch?

(A) α-Amylase
(B) Maltase
(C) Isomaltase
(D) Glucoamylase
(E) Trehalase

124. By 2 weeks of age, infants normally show all of the following signs EXCEPT

(A) copying facial expressions
(B) stepping
(C) palmar grasp
(D) the rooting reflex
(E) a negative Babinski reflex

125. Which of the following choices is NOT a metabolite involved in regulating glycolysis?

(A) Glucose 1-phosphate
(B) Fructose 6-phosphate
(C) Fructose 2,6-bisphosphate
(D) Citrate
(E) Adenosine triphosphate (ATP)

126. All of the following characteristics describe temperament EXCEPT

(A) level of motor activity
(B) emotional intensity
(C) adaptability to change
(D) intelligence
(E) biological predictability

127. Which of the following statements does NOT apply to *Mycobacterium tuberculosis*, or to the disease it causes?

(A) Tubercle bacilli can grow in virtually all parts of the body.
(B) Inflammation often results in containment of the organisms.
(C) Tubercle bacilli may be disseminated via the blood and lymphatics.
(D) The organisms can remain viable for years within the host.
(E) Most individuals exhibit little or no resistance to the organisms.

128. Which of the following characteristics is LEAST typical of a 9-year-old child?

(A) Engaging in risky behavior
(B) Interest in artistic projects
(C) Industriousness and hard work
(D) Telling riddles and jokes
(E) Understanding the concept of conservation

129. All of the following processes occur in the eukaryotic cell nucleus EXCEPT

(A) transcription
(B) translation
(C) removal of introns
(D) DNA replication
(E) capping of messenger RNA (mRNA)

130. Which of the following statements concerning the immunoglobulin G (IgG) molecule is NOT correct?

(A) The two heavy chains are identical to each other
(B) The two light chains are identical to each other
(C) The two antigen-binding sites are identical to each other
(D) The antigen-binding sites are located near the carboxy termini of the chains
(E) Each individual plasma cell produces just one type of antibody

131. Which of the following growth alterations is NOT considered a precursor lesion for cancer?

(A) Koilocytic atypia with human papilloma virus types 16, 18, 31
(B) Barrett's esophagus
(C) Lichen sclerosis et atrophicus
(D) Vaginal adenosis
(E) Intestinal metaplasia in chronic atrophic gastritis

132. Which of the following inherited diseases is LEAST likely to predispose a patient to lymphoid malignancies or leukemia?

(A) Xeroderma pigmentosum
(B) Fanconi syndrome
(C) Ataxia telangiectasia
(D) Bloom syndrome
(E) Bruton agammaglobulinemia

133. Which of the following cancer–putative viral associations is NOT correctly matched?

(A) Anal carcinoma in homosexuals—HIV
(B) Hepatocellular carcinoma—hepatitis B and hepatitis C
(C) Nasopharyngeal carcinoma—Epstein-Barr virus
(D) Adult T-cell leukemia—human T-cell leukemia virus, type I
(E) Cervical carcinoma—human papilloma virus types 16, 18, 31

134. Glycerol is the backbone of all of the following phospholipids EXCEPT

(A) Phosphotidylethanolamine
(B) Cardiolipin
(C) Phosphotidylcholine
(D) Sphingomyelin
(E) Phosphotidylinositol

DIRECTIONS:

Each set of matching questions in this section consists of a list of four to twenty-six lettered options (some of which may be in figures) followed by several numbered items. For each numbered item, select the ONE lettered option that is most closely associated with it. To avoid spending too much time on matching sets with large numbers of options, it is generally advisable to begin each set by reading the list of options. Then for each item in the set, try to generate the correct answer and locate it in the option list, rather than evaluating each option individually. Each lettered option may be selected once, more than once, or not at all.

Questions 135-138

Match each description with the appropriate cause of amenorrhea.

(A) Pregnancy
(B) Menopause
(C) Prolactinoma
(D) Sheehan syndrome

135. Can be treated with bromocriptine

136. Associated with high circulating levels of follicle-stimulating hormone (FSH) and luteinizing hormone (LH)

137. Associated with high circulating levels of estrogen and progesterone

138. Associated with anterior pituitary infarction

Questions 139-143

For each effect, pick the pair of drugs in which the first would promote the effect, and the second would counteract it.

(A) Pancuronium—acetylcholine
(B) Isoproterenol—propranolol
(C) Acetylcholine—atropine
(D) Pancuronium—isoproterenol
(E) Phenylephrine—prazosin
(F) Atropine—histamine
(G) Propranolol—dopamine
(H) Histamine—diphenhydramine

139. Increased heart rate

140. Skeletal muscle relaxation

141. Vasoconstriction

142. Increased capillary permeability

143. Pupillary constriction

Questions 144-149

Match the terms to the correct description.

(A) Phosphatidic acid
(B) Phosphatidylserine
(C) Phosphatidylethanolamine
(D) Phosphatidylcholine
(E) Phosphatidylinositol
(F) Phosphatidylglycerol
(G) Cardiolipin
(H) Phosphatidalethanolamine
(I) Sphingomyelin

144. A phosphorylated derivative is acted upon by phospholipase C as part of a second messenger system.

145. Acted upon by phospholipase A_2 to produce arachidonic acid, leading to the synthesis of prostaglandins

146. An example of a plasmalogen

147. Major lipid component of lung surfactant

148. Has two phosphate groups and is the only human phospholipid that is antigenic

149. Requires S-adenosylmethionine (SAM) for its de novo synthesis

Questions 150-154

Select the drug that best matches the following descriptions.

(A) Ribavirin (Virazole)
(B) Acyclovir (Zovirax)
(C) Zidovudine (Retrovir)
(D) Amantadine (Symmetrel)
(E) Ganciclovir (Cytovene)

150. Preferred drug for genital herpes infections

151. Prevents penetration/uncoating of influenza A virus

152. Inhibits RNA-dependent DNA polymerase

153. Blocks guanosine monophosphate formation

154. Most active drug for cytomegalovirus infections

Questions 155-160

The figure below illustrates part of the cascade that regulates glycogen synthesis and breakdown in the liver. Match each phrase with the appropriate location on the diagram.

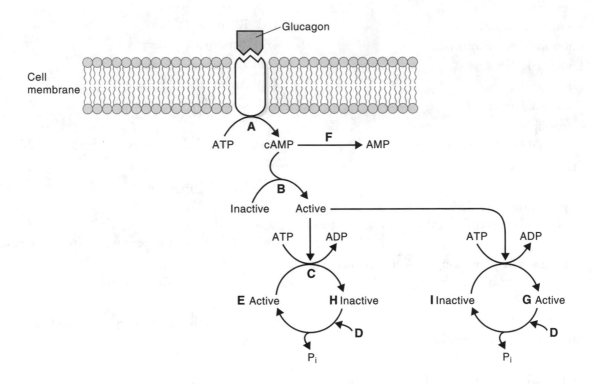

155. Phosphorylates phosphorylase

156. Activated by a G_s protein

157. Glycogen synthetase A

158. Protein phosphatase 1

159. Protein kinase A

160. Inhibited by caffeine

Questions 161-165

Select the antibiotic(s) that inhibits the designated step of bacterial protein synthesis.

(A) Chloramphenicol and erythromycin
(B) Tetracyclines and chloramphenicol
(C) Streptomycin (aminoglycosides)
(D) Erythromycin and clindamycin

161. Formation of the initiation complex of 30S and 50S subunits, messenger RNA (mRNA), and formyl methionine transfer RNA (tRNA)

162. Binding of aminoacyl tRNA to mRNA codon

163. Peptide bond formation catalyzed by peptidyl transferase

164. Normal reading of the genetic code of mRNA

165. Translocation of the peptide chain from the aminoacyl site to the peptidyl site

Questions 166-168

Use the following data to answer the questions.

	A	B	C	D	E
Plasma (ACTH)	↑	↑	↑	↓	↓
Plasma (cortisol)	↓	↑	↑	↓	↓
Plasma (aldosterone)	↓	↑	↔	↓	↔

↑ = increased compared with normal
↓ = decreased compared with normal
↔ = within normal range

166. Which column is consistent with an adrenocorticotropic hormone (ACTH)-secreting tumor?

167. Which column is consistent with secondary adrenal insufficiency?

168. Which column is consistent with Addison disease?

Questions 169-172

Match the lipoproteins to the functions they perform.

(A) Apolipoprotein B-100
(B) Apolipoprotein B-48
(C) Apolipoprotein C-II
(D) Apolipoprotein E
(E) Apolipoprotein A-1

169. Absence of this lipoprotein is responsible for the genetic disorder, familial type III hyperlipoproteinemia (also known as familial dysbetalipoproteinemia, or remnant disease)

170. Absence of this lipoprotein is a cause of the childhood genetic disorder, familial type I hyperlipoproteinemia

171. This lipoprotein is required for the normal endocytosis of low-density lipoprotein (LDL)

172. Carried on high-density lipoprotein (HDL), this lipoprotein serves to activate phosphatidylcholine: cholesterol acyltransferase (PCAT)

Questions 173-177

Select the receptor–second-messenger pair that mediates each physiologic effect.

(A) Cholinergic muscarinic—increased cyclic guanosine monophosphate (cGMP)

(B) α_1-Adrenergic—formation of inositol triphosphate (IP_3)

(C) α_2-Adrenergic—decreased cyclic adenosine monophosphate (cAMP)

(D) β_1-Adrenergic—increased cAMP

(E) β_2-Adrenergic—increased cAMP

(F) β_2-Adrenergic—formation of diacylglycerol (DAG)

(G) Cholinergic muscarinic—formation of IP_3

173. Feedback inhibition of neurotransmitter release

174. Vasoconstriction

175. Bronchoconstriction

176. Cardiac stimulation

177. Vasodilation

Questions 178-180

For each statement, select the appropriate cell structure.

(A) Cytosol

(B) Endoplasmic reticulum

(C) Golgi apparatus

(D) Mitochondrion

(E) Nucleus

178. Proteins containing a homeodomain are active here

179. Carbamoylphosphate synthetase I is found here

180. Terminal glycosylation of proteins occurs here

ANSWER KEY

1. E	31. A	61. D	91. D	121. D	151. D
2. D	32. D	62. B	92. B	122. B	152. C
3. B	33. E	63. D	93. E	123. E	153. A
4. A	34. C	64. A	94. D	124. E	154. E
5. C	35. A	65. C	95. B	125. A	155. G
6. A	36. B	66. B	96. C	126. D	156. A
7. B	37. E	67. B	97. B	127. E	157. E
8. E	38. D	68. C	98. A	128. A	158. D
9. D	39. D	69. C	99. D	129. B	159. B
10. D	40. B	70. B	100. D	130. D	160. F
11. D	41. E	71. D	101. D	131. C	161. C
12. B	42. B	72. B	102. D	132. A	162. B
13. D	43. C	73. B	103. A	133. A	163. A
14. B	44. B	74. B	104. E	134. D	164. C
15. D	45. A	75. C	105. C	135. C	165. D
16. D	46. D	76. C	106. E	136. B	166. C
17. C	47. C	77. D	107. C	137. A	167. E
18. B	48. A	78. C	108. E	138. D	168. A
19. B	49. C	79. D	109. D	139. B	169. D
20. E	50. E	80. A	110. D	140. A	170. C
21. E	51. C	81. A	111. D	141. E	171. A
22. B	52. B	82. B	112. E	142. H	172. E
23. C	53. C	83. A	113. E	143. C	173. C
24. E	54. C	84. D	114. A	144. E	174. B
25. C	55. A	85. B	115. C	145. E	175. G
26. A	56. D	86. D	116. E	146. H	176. D
27. B	57. E	87. C	117. A	147. D	177. E
28. B	58. B	88. B	118. C	148. G	178. E
29. B	59. C	89. B	119. C	149. D	179. D
30. C	60. E	90. C	120. B	150. B	180. C

ANSWERS AND EXPLANATIONS

1. The answer is E.   *(Behavioral science)*
In the United States, most elderly people live in their own residence. The elderly are expected to be independent and not require their relatives' care. Only 5% of the elderly reside in nursing care facilities (i.e., nursing homes).

2. The answer is D.   *(Microbiology)*
Obligate aerobes specifically require oxygen and lack the capacity for substantial fermentation. Some of these aerobes are facultative, able to live aerobically or anaerobically; others are obligate anaerobes, requiring a substance other than oxygen as the hydrogen acceptor, and are sensitive to oxygen inhibition.

The toxicity of oxygen is a result of its reduction by enzymes (flavoproteins) in the cell to hydrogen peroxide (H_2O_2) and the even more toxic-free radical, superoxide (O_2^-). Aerobes and aerotolerant anaerobes are protected from these products by superoxide dismutase (SOD) and catalase. Lactic acid bacteria depend on peroxidases.

Bacteroides fragilis, for example, lacks SOD, but contains small amounts of catalase. This organism, if collected in a clinical specimen, cannot grow but is viable until a true anaerobic atmosphere is provided.

3-5. The answers are: 3-B, 4-A, 5-C. *(Biochemistry)*
To understand the glycolytic sequence, the following figure identifies all of the enzymes and substrates.

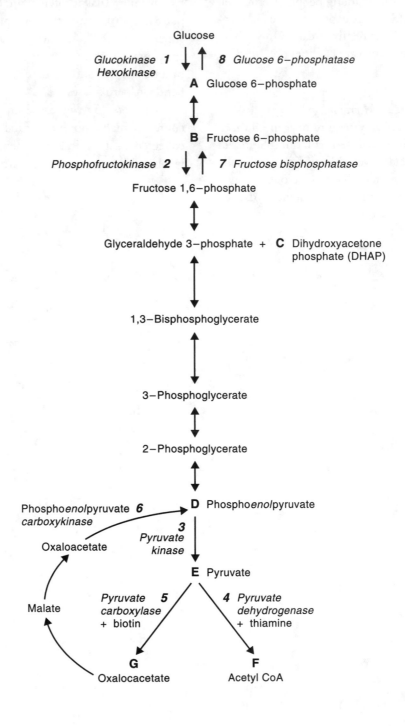

Substrate A is used to synthesize glycogen; substrate C is used to form glycerol 3-phosphate; and substrate F is used for fatty acid synthesis.

Enzyme 3 (liver-pyruvate kinase) is inactivated by phosphorylation using protein kinase A in the fasting state and effectively prevents glycolysis when gluconeogenesis is required.

Only enzyme 2 (phosphofructokinase-1) is activated by fructose 2,6-bisphosphate in the fed state.

Enzyme 4 does not catalyze a reversible reaction-forming oxaloacetate. This is an enzyme complex called pyruvate dehydrogenase, which catalyzes an irreversible reaction that converts pyruvate into acetyl CoA, using thiamine as a cofactor. Two nicotinamide adenine dinucleotides (NADH) are also generated per glucose used. This provides six adenosine triphosphates via oxidative phosphorylation.

Enzyme 5 (pyruvate carboxylase) does not catalyze a reversible reaction-forming acetyl CoA. It catalyzes an irreversible reaction in which pyruvate is converted into oxaloacetate, using biotin as a cofactor.

Enzymes 6, 7, and 8 are predominantly operative in the fasting, not the fed, state.

Substrate A (glucose-6-phosphate) is the intermediate used by the pentose phosphate shunt to generate reduced nicotinamide adenine dinucleotide phosphate (NADPH) for reducing equivalents and ribose-5-phosphate for DNA synthesis. It is also the intermediate for glycogen synthesis, the first metabolite in the glycolytic sequence and the last phosphorylate reactant in the gluconeogenic sequence.

Substrate C [dihydroxyacetone phosphate (DHAP)] and glyceraldehyde 3-phosphate are three-carbon intermediates derived from fructose 1,6-bisphosphate. DHAP can be converted into glycerol 3-phosphate, the carbohydrate backbone of triacylglycerol, which is packaged in the liver forming very-low-density lipoproteins.

Substrate D (phosphoenolpyruvate) is not the primary substrate for gluconeogenesis; substrate E (pyruvate) is.

Substrates F (acetyl CoA) and G (oxaloacetate) combine to form citrate, not oxaloacetate.

Fructokinase catalyzes the formation of fructose 1-phosphate, not substrate A (glucose 6-phosphate).

6. The answer is A. *(Pathology)*
An actinic keratosis has the greatest risk for malignant transformation, most commonly into a squamous cell carcinoma on sun-damaged skin.

A Peutz-Jeghers polyp is a hamartoma, or non-neoplastic polyp, with an overgrowth of tissue that is normally present in the gastrointestinal tract. This is an autosomal dominant hereditary polyposis, which is rarely associated with malignant transformation, unlike most of the other hereditary polyposis syndromes.

It is a maxim of gastrointestinal pathology that duodenal ulcers never transform into adenocarcinoma. This underscores why they are rarely biopsied during endoscopy. Gastric ulcers have a small risk for malignant transformation.

Bronchial hamartomas, by definition, are non-neoplastic and would not be expected to have a malignant potential.

Unlike ductal hyperplasia in the breast, which can progress to ductal cancer, prostatic hyperplasia does not progress into prostatic cancer, even though the two may be together in the prostate at the same time.

7. The answer is B. *(Biochemistry)*
A mutation is a permanent change in a DNA molecule, and single base pair changes are referred to as point mutations. A transversion is a point mutation in which a purine base is substituted for a pyrimidine base, and a pyrimidine is substituted for a purine (e.g., CG changed to GC or AT). A transition is a point mutation in which a purine is substituted for the other purine, and a pyrimidine is substituted for the other pyrimidine (e.g., GC changed to AT or AT changed to GC). Insertions and deletions can involve any number of base pairs.

8. The answer is E. *(Microbiology)*
Hyposensitization is done by administering, once or twice each week, subcutaneous injections of the allergen at increasing doses until a small area of inflammation is produced at the injection site. The purpose of this immunotherapy is to induce immunoglobulin G (IgG) specific for the allergen. The IgG is thought to intercept the allergen during natural exposure to agents implicated in type I hypersensitivity. For this reason, the IgG is often referred to as "blocking" antibody.

The procedure tends to work well for Hymenoptera insect venoms and seasonal pollens; however, its effectiveness begins to wane after treatment is stopped.

The antibodies that are generated do not compete with histamine for its receptors on target organs. Antihistamines, however, do compete with histamine for H1 and H2 receptors.

There is little or no evidence that the procedure activates T-suppressor cells specific for IgE-producing B lymphocytes.

It is believed that the procedure does not induce production of a substance that relaxes smooth muscle or decreases vascular permeability. Epinephrine (adrenalin), however, does have this effect on target tissues.

Hyposensitization is done over a period of weeks. Occasionally, slow degranulation of mast cells and basophils (over a period of several hours) is done by serial injections of a substance that the patient is known to be allergic to, but needs for treatment. An example would be therapeutic antibodies against snake venom made in an animal species.

9. The answer is D.   *(Biochemistry)*
The homeobox is a portion of certain genes that codes for the homeodomain of the corresponding protein products. The homeodomain binds to specific sequences of DNA and controls development in all eukaryotes. Homeotic, or HOX, genes were first discovered in *Drosophila*, where mutation of these genes converts one body part to another.

Cancer-causing genes are called oncogenes. Homocystinuria is caused by mutation of the enzyme cystathionine synthetase.

10. The answer is D.   *(Pathology)*
Adenocarcinoma, most likely in the colon or pancreas, can be described as a solitary nodular mass in the liver with nests of mucin-secreting glands and focal areas of necrosis. A primary hepatocellular carcinoma is not mucin secreting, nor are any benign liver tumors (hepatic adenoma).

A tumor in the parotid gland that recurs after being previously removed, without a margin of normal tissue around the mass, is a classic benign mixed tumor. These tumors are the most common overall in the salivary glands. Because of an incomplete capsule and extension of the tumor beyond the capsule, removal of the tumor without taking a margin of normal tissue usually results in recurrence. This is not an example of malignancy, because it is not invasion through the capsule as much as a problem with an incomplete capsule.

A mass compressing the cerebral cortex with swirls of meningothelial cells surrounding a psammoma body is a benign meningioma. These tumors derive from the arachnoid granulations. As a rule, psammoma bodies (calcium concretions) are associated with malignant tumors (e.g., papillary adenocarcinoma of the thyroid and serous cystadeno-carcinoma of the ovary).

An encapsulated follicular tumor of the thyroid with absence of capsular and vessel invasion is a classic description of a benign follicular adenoma. These account for 25% of all "cold nodules" on radioactive scans.

A smooth muscle tumor in the myometrium with one normal mitotic spindle in ten high-powered fields is consistent with a benign leiomyoma of the uterus, which is the most common overall benign tumor in women. Normal mitotic spindles are important in excluding malignancy; however, the presence of more than ten mitotic spindles in one high-powered field is highly suggestive of a leiomyosarcoma, which is the most common sarcoma of the uterus. It rarely derives from a leiomyoma.

11. The answer is D.   *(Biochemistry)*
The anticodon on the transfer RNA (tRNA) molecule binds to the codon on the message because the two are complementary to each other. Complementary base sequences are of opposite polarities, or directions. By convention, nucleic acid sequences are written in the 5′ → 3′ direction. The anticodon complementary to the codon 5′ UGG 3′ would be 3′ ACC 5′, or, by convention, 5′ CCA 3′.

12. The answer is B.   *(Pathology)*
In chemical carcinogenesis, the transformation of a cell into a malignant cell is caused by the process of initiation followed by promotion. Initiation is the first step in the transformation of a cell, in which the proto-oncogene (normally functioning oncogene) becomes activated into a c-onc (e.g., ras oncogene has a point mutation and becomes c-ras). Initiation is rapid, prefers rapidly dividing cells, has memory, is additive, and produces a permanent mutational change in the cell's DNA.

Promotion must always follow initiation. It is slow, reversible in the early stages, nonadditive, and causes the initiated cells to replicate via a growth promoter (e.g., estrogen); therefore, the mutational event is passed on to future generations of cells.

Repeated mitoses can lead to additional mutations, which ultimately transform the cell. Most carcinogens are complete carcinogens, meaning that they both initiate and promote a cell (e.g., asbestos is both an initiator and promoter).

Chemicals are either indirect-acting (transformed by the microsomal P-450 system of the liver into carcinogens) or direct-acting carcinogens (e.g., alkylating chemotherapy agents). The mutagenicity of chemical carcinogens is evaluated with the Ames test. In this test, Salmonella that is not able to synthesize histidine is mixed with the chemical in question and liver microsomes (the latter is necessary to convert chemicals into mutagens). They are cultured on histidine-free media. If Salmonella does not grow, the chemical is not a mutagen, whereas growth of the organism indicates that the chemical is a mutagen.

13-14. The answers are: 13-D, 14-B. (Biochemistry)
Phenylketonuria (PKU) is caused by mutation of the phenylalanine hydroxylase gene. Because this is an autosomal recessive disease, affected individuals carry two mutant alleles, whereas carriers carry one mutant and one normal allele. The restriction fragment length polymorphism (RFLP) marker in this example lies close to the gene in question, so the inheritance of particular alleles is observed by following inheritance of their tightly linked RFLPs.

Both the father and mother exhibit two bands, 4kb and 3kb. Because they are both carriers, one of the bands in each of them is linked to the normal allele and the other to the mutant allele. Because the affected son (II-1) has only the 3kb band, he must have inherited a 3kb band linked to a mutant allele from each parent; therefore, the 4kb band in each parent is linked to a normal allele. The firstborn daughter (II-2) exhibits only the 4kb band. She inherited a normal allele linked to the 4kb band from each parent, and she is homozygous normal. The secondborn son (II-3) shows both a 4kb and a 3kb band. He is a carrier, because he inherited the 3kb band linked to the mutant allele from one parent, and the 4kb band linked to the normal allele from the other. The secondborn daughter (II-4) has only the 3kb band and is affected by the disease.

A child has a 50% chance of inheriting the mutant allele from the father and a 50% chance of inheriting the mutant allele from the mother, which gives them a 25% chance (multiplying 50% by 50%) that the child will inherit two mutant alleles and be affected. Similarly, there is a 25% chance that the child will inherit two normal alleles and be homozygous normal. There is a 50% chance that the child will inherit one normal and one mutant allele and be a carrier.

15. The answer is D. (Microbiology)
Salmonella typhimurium is the most common cause of enterocolitis (formerly known as gastroenteritis) in the United States. S. enteritidis and many other of the 1500 to 2000 serotypes have also been implicated in the disease. It is estimated that approximately two million episodes of enterocolitis are caused by these organisms each year. Many salmonellae, but not shigellae, produce H_2S in media containing an inorganic sulfur source (e.g., triple sugar iron agar). The symptoms and the course of the disease described in the case history are typical for enterocolitis, but not for enteric fever, which is caused by Salmonella typhi.

Enterocolitis caused by Salmonella is an infection of the colon that usually begins approximately 18 to 24 hours after ingestion of the organisms. Diarrhea, fever, and abdominal pain are typical for the disease. Most cases are thought to go unreported, because the infection is usually not severe and is self-limiting within approximately 2 to 3 days. Dehydration and electrolyte imbalance are the major threats.

The Salmonella organisms can be shed for several weeks after recovery from enterocolitis, but chronic carriers are rare. Treatment with antibiotics may prolong the length of time that the organisms are shed. This reaction is opposite to that of Shigella.

The salmonella organisms associated with enterocolitis have been recovered from milk (including ice cream and cheeses), shellfish, dried or frozen eggs, poultry, beef, and water contaminated with feces. Meat products can be contaminated by animal fecal material during slaughter. Undercooking and improper storage at warm temperatures allow the organisms to proliferate to large numbers. Temperatures above 140°F will kill the organisms. The source of the Salmonella at the picnic could have been the potato salad, the chicken, or the hamburgers.

Ingestion of a relatively large number of Salmonella is required in order for symptoms to appear.

Dogs, pet turtles, and other cold-blooded animals can carry the organisms for extended periods of time. There are now restrictions on the import and sale of turtles in pet shops.

Salmonella infections cause three distinct diseases: enterocolitis, enteric fever (typhoid fever), and septicemia.

16-17. The answers are: 16-D, 17-C. *(Biochemistry)*

In X-linked genetic diseases, affected males inherit mutant alleles on chromosome X from their mothers. Females are carriers but are rarely affected by the disease because they have two X chromosomes, and the normal allele is usually dominant over the recessive mutant allele. In this example, the restriction fragment length polymorphism (RFLP) marker is tightly linked to the factor VIII gene associated with hemophilia A. Southern blots from each member of the family determine which band is linked to the normal allele and which is linked to the mutant allele. The father (I-1) is normal and exhibits a 3kb band, thus in the father the 3kb band is linked to the normal allele. The mother (I-2) is a carrier and demonstrates both a 3kb and 4kb band. However, we do not yet know which of her bands is linked to the mutant allele. The firstborn son (II-1) is affected. He shows only the 3kb band, which must be linked to the mutant allele. Because this allele was inherited from his mother, the mother's 3kb band is linked to the mutant allele. The secondborn son (II-3) is unaffected and exhibits a 4kb band, which he inherited from his mother. Therefore, the mother's 4kb band must be linked to the normal allele. The firstborn daughter (II-2) shows both a 3kb and 4kb band. The 3kb band with its linked normal allele must have come from the father, and the 4kb band with its linked normal allele must have come from the mother; she is homozygous normal for this trait. The secondborn daughter (II-4) exhibits only a 3kb band. She inherited a 3kb band with its linked normal allele from the father, and a 3kb band with its linked mutant allele from the mother; she is a carrier of the disease.

Each son inherits his single X chromosome from his mother. Because the mother in this family is a carrier, she has a 50% chance of passing the mutant allele to her son. In this family (normal father and carrier mother) 50% of the sons will be normal and 50% will be affected. Likewise, 50% of the daughters will be homozygous normal, and 50% will be carriers.

18. The answer is B. *(Pathology)*

Burkitt lymphoma is associated with c-myc oncogene, which is involved in the synthesis of nuclear regulatory proteins necessary for the growth process of B lymphocytes.

Some breast cancers (e.g., comedocarcinomas) are associated with overexpression of the erb-B-3 oncogene. The presence of this oncogene imposes a poor prognosis for the patient.

Neuroblastomas have an abnormality in the N-myc oncogene, which is normally involved in the generation of nuclear regulatory proteins.

Chronic myelogenous leukemia is associated with the c-abl oncogene, which is normally involved in nonreceptor tyrosine kinase activity for generation of second messengers.

Colon cancer is associated with the ras oncogene, which is normally involved in guanosine 5′-triphosphate (GTP) binding and the generation of second messengers.

19. The answer is B. *(Biochemistry)*

Less than 1% of the monosaccharides with five or more carbons exist in an open-chain form. They prefer a ringed structure, in which the aldehyde (or ketone) group has reacted with an alcohol on the same sugar molecule in a hemiacetal (or hemiketal) bond, forming a six (pyranose) or five (furanose) membered ring. These rings involve the aldehydic group on carbon 1 of the aldohexoses and carbon 2 of the ketohexoses and the hydroxyl on carbon 6 of all the hexoses. This reaction has made carbon atom 1 asymmetric, and two different structures, called α or β, are formed depending on the configuration of the ring. Therefore, there are two forms of D-glucose: α-D-glucose and β-D-glucose.

20. The answer is E. *(Pathology)*

The stage of cancer is the most important factor determining the prognosis, not only in breast cancer, but other cancers at well. Lymph-node status is the single most important factor that determines the prognosis in women with breast cancer.

The grade of a tumor is based primarily on the degree of differentiation of the tumor (how much it resembles its parent tissue) and on the amount of mitotic activity, which indirectly indicates its growth rate. Grading terms include low grade, or well differentiated, intermediate grade, or high grade (poorly differentiated, or anaplastic).

21. The answer is E. *(Biochemistry)*
DNA typing can rule out a man being the father of a child, but it cannot establish with absolute certainty that a man is the father of a child. Each child carries two alleles for the marker, one inherited from each parent. In case 1, the child has one band that matches a band from the mother's DNA. The child's second band matches one from accused father X. This indicates that individual X may be the father of this child. In case 2, one of the child's bands matches one of the mother's bands. However, neither of the child's bands matches any band from the DNA of the accused father, indicating that individual Y is not the father of this child.

22. The answer is B. *(Microbiology)*
Humans are the only natural hosts of *Salmonella typhi*. All other salmonellae, *Yersinia enterocolitica*, and *Pasteurella multocida* can be found in a wide variety of other animals (e.g., poultry, pigs, cattle, rodents, dogs).

Salmonella typhi (and to a lesser extent *Salmonella paratyphi* A and B) is the cause of enteric fever (typhoid fever). After ingestion of contaminated food or drink, the organisms multiply in macrophages in the Peyer patches (small collections of lymphoid tissue) of the small intestine, reach the lymphatics, and enter the blood circulation (septicemic phase of septicemia).

The disease begins slowly with fever and constipation (rather than diarrhea). High fever, delerium, tender abdomen, and splenomegaly occur after the first week. "Rose spots" (small pinkish macules that look like a rose) may be briefly present on the abdomen and chest, but occur rarely. Blood cultures are positive during the first week, whereas stool specimens should be tested during the second and third weeks. The illness is usually over by the third week. Complications such as intestinal hemorrhages or perforations may occur. The triad of sinus bradycardia, splenomegaly, and neutropenia is characteristic.

Approximately 3% of patients, especially women with previous gallbladder disease, become chronic carriers of *Salmonella typhi*. Presence of the organisms in duodenal drainage establishes the biliary tract as the site of importance in carriers. Cholecystectomy combined with antimicrobial therapy is used to eradicate the carrier state. In rare instances, the organisms may be chronically carried in the urinary tract or intestinal tract.

Sepsis can be caused by a variety of salmonellae serotypes, especially *Salmonella choleraesuis*. Fever, but little or no enterocolitis, followed by symptoms associated with involved organs are typical for this clinical entity. The bones, lungs, and meninges are most often affected. Blood cultures are positive.

Antimicrobial therapy is important for individuals with enteric fever or sepsis, whereas it is generally not needed in the majority of enterocolitis cases (which are mostly mild and self-limiting).

Antibodies against salmonellae are often detected by a tube dilution agglutination test (Widal test). At least two specimens, taken approximately 10 days apart, are needed to show a 4-fold rise in the antibody titer. A rapid slide agglutination test is useful for preliminary identification of culture isolates.

23. The answer is C. *(Pathology)*
Thymomas are often associated with pure red blood cell aplasia, the latter possibly leading to the discovery of the thymoma. Paraneoplastic syndromes often indicate the presence of an underlying neoplasm before it has progressed into an advanced stage. Unfortunately, they only occur in 10% to 15% of cases. To qualify as a paraneoplastic syndrome, the syndrome must not be caused by the direct effects of tumor invasion or metastasis. For example, hypercalcemia caused by lysis of bone by metastatic tumor does not qualify, but secretion of a parathormone-like peptide producing the hypercalcemia does qualify.

Small-cell carcinoma of the lung is associated with an increase in ADH or ACTH. Pancreatic carcinoma is associated with Trousseau superficial migratory thrombophlebitis. Gastric carcinoma is associated with acanthosis nigricans. Breast carcinoma is associated with dermatomyositis.

24. The answer is E. *(Biochemistry)*
A nonsense suppressor mutation is a secondary mutation that reverses the effect of a primary nonsense or chain-termination mutation. Ordinarily, no transfer RNA (tRNA) molecule can recognize a nonsense codon; therefore, protein synthesis terminates when the ribosome reaches such a codon. A nonsense suppressor mutation usually involves the mutation of a tRNA gene, so that the anticodon of the tRNA is altered to a sequence that is complementary to a nonsense codon. The altered tRNA can then bind to the nonsense codon and insert an amino acid at that point in the protein sequence. Thus, protein synthesis is allowed to continue, and the nonsense mutation is suppressed.

A silent mutation is one that causes no change in the amino acid sequence of a protein. A missense mutation causes a single amino acid change. A frameshift mutation is the result of an insertion or deletion that alters the reading frame of the ribosome, leading to the production of a garbled amino acid sequence.

25. The answer is C. *(Pathology)*
Cervical Papanicolau (Pap) smears have contributed most to the decline of cervical cancer. This is related to the 80% sensitivity of Pap smears in detecting cervical dysplasia, which can be treated, thus preventing squamous cancer.

Mammography is actually responsible for an increase in the incidence of breast cancer, because it detects nonpalpable masses in the breast.

Yearly stool guaiac testing in patients 50 years of age and older, who are asymptomatic and have no risk factors, has reduced the incidence of colon cancer, but not to the same degree as a cervical Pap smear for cervical cancer.

Rectal examination (gold standard) and prostate-specific antigen are recommended for prostate cancer screening in patients 50 years of age and older.

26. The answer is A. *(Microbiology)*
Serum sickness, a type III hypersensitivity reaction, occurs in a relatively high percentage of individuals approximately 1 to 2 weeks after the administration of foreign protein (e.g., horse antibodies). A later injection of the same foreign protein can produce a more severe response and even death.

In type III hypersensitivity, immunoglobulin G or immunoglobulin M (IgG or IgM), which are produced by the recipient of the foreign protein, bind to circulating antigen and form soluble, intermediate-size complexes. An intermediate-size complex usually consists of only a few molecules of antibody and antigen (e.g., Ag_2Ab, Ag_3Ab_2). The complexes lodge in the walls of the blood vessels and activate complement. The subsequent generation of C3a, C4a, and C5a (anaphylatoxins) increases vascular permeability. C5a also attracts neutrophils to the site of action. The neutrophils, in an unsuccessful attempt to phagocytize the lodged complexes, release the contents of their granules (proteases, collagenases, and vasoactive substances) into the surrounding microenvironment. These cells, as well as platelets, pile up at the reaction site and form microthrombi, which can block the blood vessels and produce hemorrhaging and necrosis.

The Arthus reaction is the classic example of a type III hypersensitivity reaction. Its mechanism of action is virtually identical to that seen in serum sickness; however, it is a localized reaction and occurs when a small amount of antigen is injected intradermally into an immune individual who already has a relatively large amount of antibody against the antigen. It is characterized by erythema and edema at the injection site.

Microbial and viral agents and soluble self-proteins are sometimes implicated as the antigens in type III hypersensitivities.

In type II hypersensitivity, IgG or IgM bind directly to antigen present on cells or tissues (i.e., form insoluble antigen–antibody complexes). Activation of complement leads to cell lysis and tissue destruction. In addition, effector cells with receptors for the Fc region of IgG can mediate the lysis. Examples of type II reactions include: hemolytic disease of the newborn (Rh⁻ mother, Rh⁺ fetus), hemolytic anemias, transfusion reactions caused by ABO incompatibility, some drug-induced hypersensitivities, and Goodpasture syndrome.

Disseminated intravascular coagulation would present as a bleeding problem, rather than as a diffuse rash.

Type IV hypersensitivity is a cell-mediated response that is most effectively induced by live whole cells.

27. The answer is B. *(Behavioral science)*
The rooting reflex is the tendency of a newborn to turn her head in the direction of a stroke on her cheek and helps the infant find the nipple. This characteristic of newborn infants usually disappears by the age of 3 months.

28. The answer is B. *(Microbiology)*
This is a typical type IV hypersensitivity reaction. The response is delayed because it generally begins hours to days after exposure to antigen (later than what is typical for type I, II, and III hypersensitivity). Granuloma formation is a common result of infection with persistent microbial agents such as *M. tuberculosis.* The reaction is initiated when antigen-presenting cells (APCs) present processed antigen to CD4$^+$ T-helper lymphocytes in the context of major histocompatibility complex (MHC) class II molecules. The T helpers become activated upon exposure to interleukin-1 (IL-1, derived from the APC), which provides a second signal, and begin secreting lymphokines. Some of the lymphokines chemotactically call in and activate macrophages. Interferon-γ (IFN-γ) is now thought to be the major factor responsible for many of the effects on macrophages. Activated macrophages have greater phagocytic ability, contain more lytic enzymes, and express greater numbers of MHC class II molecules (thereby making them more efficient in antigen presentation); however, if the antigen is not readily destroyed, the response becomes prolonged and destructive to the host. Macrophages continue to accumulate, fuse into giant cells, and form granulomas.

Granuloma formation is not seen in type I, II, or III hypersensitivity reactions.

In nearly all respects, a type IV hypersensitivity reaction is identical to a normal cell-mediated response. The key difference is that in hypersensitivity, the antigen is protected in some way, or is very persistent.

A positive tuberculin (PPD) skin test is a good example of delayed-type hypersensitivity.

Other infectious diseases in which a type IV reaction may be seen include leprosy, brucellosis, listeriosis, blastomycosis, coccidioidomycosis, leishmaniasis, and schistosomiasis.

Neutrophils are important in mediating the tissue damage seen in type III hypersensitivity.

Eosinophils accumulate at and down-regulate type I hypersensitivity.

Mast cells and basophils degranulate and release pharmacologically active mediators during type I hypersensitivity.

29. The answer is B. *(Biochemistry)*
Of the compounds listed, the incorporation of radioactive thymidine provides the best measure of the rate of DNA synthesis because thymidine is specifically found in DNA, and not RNA protein or other macromolecules. Leucine is an amino acid that could be used to measure protein synthesis. Uridine is a nucleoside found specifically in RNA and would be useful for measuring RNA synthesis. Phosphate and ribose could be incorporated into several different types of macromolecules and would not be very useful because of their lack of specificity.

30. The answer is C. *(Microbiology)*
Opportunistic fungi fail to induce disease in most normal persons but may do so in those with impaired host defenses. *Candida albicans* causes thrush, vaginitis, and chronic mucocutaneous candidiasis. Considered to be part of the normal flora, candida infections are considered to be endogenous. Relative numbers of *C. albicans* are naturally kept to a low level by the overriding effort of normal bacterial flora being able to grow more quickly and compete more successfully for available nutrition. *C. albicans* is relatively resistant to broad-spectrum antibiotics (e.g., tetracycline) and may become the predominant organism after such use.

Nocardia asteroides, Treponema pallidum, and *Cryptococcus neoformans* are not considered to be part of the normal flora.

31. The answer is A. *(Biochemistry)*
The oxygen dissociation curve for myoglobin is hyperbolic, because myoglobin consists of a single subunit and binds a single molecule of oxygen. The oxygen dissociation curve for hemoglobin is sigmoidal, because hemoglobin consists of four subunits, which show cooperative binding of oxygen. The first molecule of oxygen binds to hemoglobin with difficulty. Subsequent molecules of oxygen bind with higher affinity. The heme in both myoglobin and hemoglobin

contains iron in the ferrous (Fe^{2+}) form. Oxygen binding by myoglobin is not influenced by pH or carbon dioxide concentration.

32. The answer is D. *(Microbiology)*
It is likely that the boy has contact dermatitis (contact hypersensitivity). At the campground he may have encountered poison ivy, a plant that produces urushiols (small molecular weight oils on the underside of its leaves). Contact dermatitis is a cell-mediated, type IV hypersensitivity reaction. It occurs upon contact with small molecular weight lipid-soluble substances, which penetrate the skin and act as haptens after binding to large carrier proteins. Langerhans cells in the skin act as the antigen-presenting cells.

Itching, erythema, fluid-filled vesicles, and sometimes necrosis are typical clinical manifestations that are generally seen within 12 to 48 hours after contact. Topically applied steroid creams or systemic corticosteroids may be used in treatment. Patch testing can be used for identification of the agent responsible in contact dermatitis.

Other agents that may induce contact hypersensitivity include: poison oak, dyes, cosmetics, metals (e.g., nickel, gold), and black rubber mix.

Serum sickness and the Arthus reaction are examples of type III hypersensitivity.

Hay fever (allergic rhinitis) is the result of type I hypersensitivity.

Farmer's lung disease is the result of inhalation of spores from Actinomycetes species, a frequent resident of moldy hay. Early lesions are thought to be an immune complex hypersensitivity (type III), followed by granulomatous interstitial inflammation of the lungs, a characteristic feature of type IV cell-mediated responses. Farmer's lung disease is the prototype and most frequently reported hypersensitivity pneumonitis. Hundreds of other inhaled allergens (often associated with the workplace) have been implicated in the etiology of hypersensitivity pneumonitis.

33. The answer is E. *(Behavioral science)*
The most likely diagnosis for this 5-year-old boy with normal motor skills, severe language delay, and stereotypical spinning movements who shows no interest in interacting with others is infantile autism, a pervasive developmental disorder of childhood. In contrast, children with attention deficit hyperactivity disorder (ADHD) show problems paying attention or with excessive activity but not language delay. Children with conduct disorder show behaviors like stealing, truancy, and setting fires. Mentally retarded children may have language delay but interact with others in a relatively normal fashion. Rett syndrome, which involves some behavioral features of infantile autism such as stereotypical movements, is seen only in girls.

34–35. The answers are: 34-C, 35-A. *(Microbiology)*
This type of graft is an allograft (i.e., the graft is transferred between two members of the same species). Because the donor and recipient are histoincompatible (genetic differences exist in the human leukocyte antigen system or HLA; genetic differences are also likely in minor histocompatibility loci), rejection of the graft is likely, but could be controlled with immunosuppressive therapy (e.g., cyclosporin).

Isograft and syngraft are synonymous terms. They refer to a graft transferred between genetically identical individuals (identical twins) or highly inbred laboratory animals. The donor and recipient are histocompatible. Rejection will not occur.

An autograft is performed by transferring cells or tissues from one part of the body to another part of the same individual. Autografting of skin and bone is frequently done. Rejection will not occur.

A xenograft is transferred from a member of one species to a member of another species (i.e., baboon to human). The donor and recipient are histoincompatible. Rejection is highly likely without immunosuppressive therapy.

The patient was most likely experiencing acute rejection. This type of rejection is primarily a cell-mediated attack against the grafted organ. Antigen presentation may occur in at least two different ways. In the direct path, blood-borne cells within the graft (i.e., "passenger" dendritic cells and monocytes expressing class I and class II major histocompatibility complex [MHC] molecules) act as the antigen-presenting cells. In the indirect path, the host's antigen-presenting cells may present allogeneic class I and class II molecules that have been shed by the graft. Peptides presented in the context of MHC class I will activate CD8-positive T-cytotoxic lymphocytes, which can directly attack the graft. Peptides presented in the context of

MHC class II molecules can activate CD4 positive T-helper cells, resulting in secretion of helper factors. This intensifies the rejection by expansion of antigen-specific cytotoxic T-cell clones and accumulation and activation of macrophages. Antilymphocyte serum (anti–T-cell antibodies made in an animal) is among the agents used to reverse acute rejection episodes. Without immunosuppression of the recipient, allograft rejection usually takes place in approximately 11 to 14 days.

Chronic rejection is a slow, smoldering phenomenon that is poorly understood. The mechanisms responsible may include monocyte secretion of interleukin-1 (IL-1) and release of platelet-derived growth factor (PDGF) from platelets and endothelial cells. If it is going to occur, it generally begins several months to years after the transplantation is performed. It is characterized by proliferation of endothelial cells of blood vessels feeding the graft and fibrotic changes within the vessel wall. Blockage of the vessels results in necrosis and demise of the graft. It is not reversed by antilymphocyte serum.

In a graft-versus-host reaction, the cells of the graft attack the recipient, either directly or indirectly, by recruiting the recipient's cells to attack the host. This type of reaction is seen primarily in recipients of bone marrow grafts.

Hyperacute (accelerated or second-set) rejection is mediated by pre-existing antibodies in the recipient, which can bind to the graft and activate complement (type II hypersensitivity). These antibodies may be present as the result of sensitization by human antigens during pregnancy, previous blood transfusions, or previous transplants. This type of rejection occurs within minutes to hours. It is virtually impossible to reverse. Organ recipients are screened for antibodies against donor HLA antigens prior to transplantation.

The case history does not mention reduction in drug dosage. Administration of anti-lymphocyte serum will not reverse immunosuppressive drug toxicity.

36. The answer is B. (Biochemistry)

HbA ($\alpha_2\beta_2$) is the major normal adult hemoglobin. HbA$_2$ ($\alpha_2\delta_2$) is the minor normal adult hemoglobin. HbF ($\alpha_2\gamma_2$) is fetal hemoglobin, and Hb Gower 1 ($\zeta_2\epsilon_2$) is embryonic hemoglobin. HbA$_{1c}$ is HbA that has been modified by the nonenzymic addition of glucose. Patients with diabetes mellitus show increased levels of HbA$_{1c}$, because the hemoglobin in these patients has been exposed to higher levels of glucose during the lifetime of their red blood cells.

37. The answer is E. (Microbiology)

The most likely causative organism is *Shigella sonnei*. *Shigella* should be suspected when a nonmotile, gram-negative rod that does not ferment lactose is isolated from a case of diarrhea. An important additional clue in the case history is the presence of blood in the stool. Shigellosis is a bacillary dysentery typified by the presence of blood and mucus in stool. The organisms are capable of local invasion. They infect epithelial cells lining the intestinal tract, multiply within their cytoplasm, and spread to adjacent cells. Microabscesses form in the large intestine and terminal ileum, leading to necrosis, ulceration, and bleeding. Granulation and scar tissue may form at the ulcerative sites as the infection subsides.

Shigellae almost never invades the blood circulation, unlike *Salmonella typhi* (a motile, lactose-negative rod), which does so routinely.

Escherichia coli, *Enterobacter*, and *Klebsiella* are lactose positive.

Shigella is transmitted from person-to-person via the "four Fs": food, fingers, feces, and flies. There are no known animal reservoirs. The organisms are highly contagious and outbreaks have been reported in substandard day care centers, nursing homes, inner-city apartment dwellings, and even luxury cruise ships. Approximately one-half of all *Shigella*-positive stool cultures are from children under the age of 10 years. The incubation period is short (i.e., only 1 to 2 days).

There are four species of shigellae: *S. dysenteriae*, *S. flexneri*, *S. boydii*, and *S. sonnei*. The species can be differentiated on the basis of whether or not they ferment mannitol and produce ornithine decarboxylase.

Shigella dysenteriae generally produces the most severe disease. It can produce a heat-labile exotoxin that acts as a neurotoxin, as well as an enterotoxin. Its mechanism of action on the intestinal tract is not entirely clear, but it is thought to be similar to that of verotoxin, which is secreted by *Escherichia coli*. Its action as a neurotoxin is associated with rectal spasms, pain and excitation in the meningocortical region of the brain, and coma. *Shigella dysenteriae* is not prevalent in the United States. It is found in individuals returning from countries where the organisms are more common.

38. The answer is D.   *(Biochemistry)*
As a general rule, amino acids with nonpolar side chains tend to be located in the interior of soluble protein molecules. These nonpolar side chains can participate in hydrophobic interactions. Of the amino acids listed, valine is the only one with a nonpolar side chain. Aspartic acid has an acidic side chain, arginine and lysine have basic side chains, and serine has an uncharged polar side chain.

39. The answer is D.   *(Microbiology)*
By convention, mycobacteria are the only organisms that are referred to as "acid-fast" (i.e., it is a hallmark characteristic). They are unusual because they contain waxes or lipids (fatty acids or long-chain hydrocarbons that can be up to 90 carbons in length) that give them the ability to retain dyes during treatment with acid solutions. Mycolic acid (a β-hydroxy fatty acid) is the major wax. Muramyl dipeptide bound to mycolic acids can induce granuloma formation.

Because of their lipid layers, mycobacteria are relatively impermeable. For example, they do not take up the gram stain (or other conventional laboratory stains) and therefore are not referred to as gram-positive or gram-negative.

The Ziehl-Neelsen technique is a universally accepted acid-fast stain. A slide with the mycobacteria is flooded with basic fuchsin (carbolfuchsin) and heated until steaming (this "melts" the lipid and allows the basic fuchsin to enter). After washing, the stained smear is saturated with 3% hydrochloric acid in ethanol to decolorize nearly all bacteria except the mycobacteria. The smear is washed again and then counterstained with methylene blue to provide a contrasting background. Acid-fast bacilli appear red.

The high lipid content of mycobacteria also helps them to survive both in and out of the body. They are unusually resistant to killing by macrophages, disinfectants and other germicides, dyes (such as Malachite Green, which is put into Lowenstein-Jensen medium to inhibit the growth of other bacteria), many antibiotics, and to drying; however, heating at 60°C for 30 minutes (as is done in the pasteurization of milk) will readily kill them.

Nocardia asteroides is acid-fast and some of the *Actinomyces* are partially or weakly acid-fast. Both groups of organisms are gram-positive rods that often exhibit branching and filamentous forms.

The *Corynebacteria* are gram-positive rods that are related to the *Nocardia*, *Actinomyces*, and mycobacteria. They have a club-shaped morphology and metachromatic granules, which can be easily seen with aniline dyes. True branching is rarely seen in cultures.

Actinobacillus is a small, gram-negative coccobacillus that is frequently present in actinomycosis. It can also cause periodontal disease, abscesses, endocarditis, and osteomyelitis. *Actinobacillus actinomycetemcomitans* is the most common species.

40. The answer is B.   *(Biochemistry)*
A crisis in sickle cell disease occurs when deoxygenated HbS precipitates, deforming (sickling) red blood cells and blocking capillaries. Variables that increase the proportion of HbS in the "deoxy" state tend to increase the probability of a crisis by increasing the extent of sickling. The "deoxy" form of hemoglobin is favored by a decrease in pH (acidosis). An increase in pH (alkalosis), increased oxygen concentration, decreased CO_2 concentration, and decreased 2,3-bisphosphoglycerate concentration would all favor the "oxy" form of hemoglobin.

41. The answer is E.   *(Microbiology)*
Appearance of skin rash, diarrhea, and jaundice are characteristic findings of graft-versus-host disease. The skin, intestinal mucosa, and liver are at high risk because they express large amounts of HLA-DR antigens, the most immunogenic of the class II proteins. If severe, the rash mimics a second-degree burn and becomes desquamative. The diarrhea is caused by malabsorption, gastrointestinal bleeding, and cramps. Liver involvement is caused by inflammation of small bile ducts.

Approximately 30% of bone marrow transplant patients develop acute graft-versus-host disease. This attack, which is primarily by activated $CD8^+$ T lymphocytes of the donor, is against the cells and tissues of the recipient. Biopsy of skin or other affected sites would show intense infiltration of $CD8^+$ cells.

In most other types of transplants, if graft-versus-host disease occurs, it is caused by "passenger" T cells in the graft, which become activated and recruit the recipient's own cells to attack the host.

Cyclosporin A is an effective drug for prevention of graft-versus-host disease. Renal failure and hypertension are the major toxicities associated with its use. These are not mentioned in the case history.

A host-versus-graft rejection is unlikely because patients are greatly immunosuppressed before bone marrow transplants and are able to wage little or no response.

The patient is at greatest risk for infection before engraftment of the bone marrow cells occurs because during that time very few circulating leukocytes are present. Infections with *Staphylococcus* (and other gram-positive cocci), gram-negative bacteria, *Candida*, and *Aspergillus* can progress rapidly and kill the patient.

Recurrence of acute lymphocytic leukemia (ALL) is possible, but unlikely. The recipient's immune system is virtually destroyed by a combination of chemotherapy and whole body radiation treatments. In most bone marrow recipients, all hematopoietic and immune cells are replaced by donor cells.

Whenever possible, an ABO blood group compatible donor bone marrow is selected. If an ABO-compatible donor is not available, the erythrocytes are removed from the marrow in vitro prior to transplantation; however, the recipient will eventually acquire the ABO blood group of the donor in these cases, if engraftment is successful.

42. The answer is B. *(Behavioral science)*
The type of reasoning used by this 5-year-old boy, who believed that something bad he was thinking caused a bad event to occur (i.e., the bicycle accident), is called magical thinking. This type of reasoning is typical of children in Piaget's preoperational stage (age 2–7 years).

43. The answer is C. *(Microbiology)*
Cryptococcus neoformans causes cryptococcus, especially cryptococcal meningitis. *C. neoformans* is an oval, budding yeast surrounded by a large polysaccharide capsule. It occurs widely in nature and grows abundantly in soil containing bird droppings. The organism is most often inhaled and spread hematogenously from the lungs.

Lung infections range from asymptomatic to pneumonia. Cryptococcosis is the most common encapsulated infection in the immunocompromised host. The organism disseminates hematogenously to the central nervous system (meningitis) and other organs. It can be cultured from cerebral spinal fluid (CSF) or diagnosed by serologic tests for either antibody or antigen. Amphotericin B and flucytosine are used to treat cryptococcal meningitis.

44. The answer is B. *(Behavioral science)*
In a triangle, two family members join forces against a third family member, often crossing generational boundary lines. The father and daughter have formed a subsystem although the parents should rightfully form an executive subsystem. In an emotional cutoff, a family member is ignored. In mutual accommodation, family members try to adjust to the needs of other family members. Multigenerational transmission process is the way in which family styles and interactions are passed from one generation to the next.

45. The answer is A. *(Microbiology)*
Tinea (i.e., pityriasis) versicolor is a superficial skin infection of cosmetic importance only. Lesions are usually noticed as hypopigmented or hyperpigmented areas, with possible slight scaling or itching. The lesion contains both the budding yeast cells and hyphae of *Malassezia furfur* (i.e., *Pityrosporon orbiculare*). The diagnosis is usually made by observing this mixture in potassium hydroxide preparations of skin scrapings and noting "spaghetti and meatball" appearance of the hyphae and yeasts. The treatment of choice is topical miconazole.

Histoplasmosis, coccidioidomycosis, blastomycosis, and chromoblastomycosis are all systemic infections with few, if any, skin lesion manifestations. Diagnosis is confirmed by laboratory isolation and identification of these etiologic agents.

46. The answer is D. *(Behavioral science)*
A child with separation anxiety may develop functional abdominal pain on days when he has to go to school. This is because he is fearful of separation from home and mother and knows that illness will keep him at home. Genetic factors, learning disabilities, mental

retardation and developmental immaturity may contribute to separation anxiety but are not the most correct answers.

47-48. The answers are: 47-C, 48-A. *(Microbiology)*

It is likely that the patient has an active disease caused by *Mycobacterium tuberculosis*. His symptoms are typical for tuberculosis. Furthermore, his condition is likely to be the result of reactivation, which almost always begins in the apices of the lungs, where oxygen tension (PO_2) is the highest.

The fact that the patient has had a positive tuberculin skin test for quite some time indicates that he has been infected with *Mycobacterium tuberculosis* and that all viable organisms have not been eradicated. A positive test does not indicate that he is immune to development of the disease.

Mycobacterium tuberculosis is naturally found only in humans. The organisms are readily transmitted by airborne respiratory secretions. People living in urban areas become infected at a younger age than rural dwellers. Homeless individuals, minorities (African-Americans and Hispanics), and the very young and very old are under increased risk. Malnutrition, stress, overcrowding, and declining immunologic status have been associated with reactivation.

Individuals who are seropositive for HIV or who have AIDS are at high risk for developing disease caused by *Mycobacterium tuberculosis* because they have impaired cellular immunity. In addition, the organisms are likely to be disseminated. The lymph nodes, bone marrow, central nervous system, and genitourinary tract may become involved. Tuberculosis in AIDS patients is often fatal; however, in the United States, *Mycobacterium avium-intracellulare* (*M. avium* complex), which is prevalent in the environment (soil, water, food, and birds and other animals), is more common than *Mycobacterium tuberculosis* in patients with AIDS (25% to 50% are infected with this complex).

Mycobacterium scrofulaceum is a saprophyte that is mostly associated with chronic cervical lymphadenitis in children. *Mycobacterium marinum* and *Mycobacterium ulcerans* are found in water and fish. They may produce superficial skin ulcers ("swimming pool granuloma") in humans. *Mycobacterium fortuitum-chelonae* complex is found in soil and water. On rare occasions,

it is isolated from superficial and systemic human disease.

In the great majority of cases, an individual with primary *Mycobacterium tuberculosis* infection acquires a cell-mediated hypersensitivity response against the organisms. This is manifested as a positive reaction in the tuberculin skin test.

A tuberculin test is performed by intradermal injection of a purified protein derivative (PPD) obtained by chemical fractionation from a concentrated broth of the tubercle bacillus ("Old Tuberculin"). The intermediate-strength preparation contains 5 tuberculin units (TU) and is the one which gives the fewest false positives or false negatives.

Once an individual is positive in the tuberculin test, it is generally not given again because the test can provoke an intense and painful reaction in these individuals. Recent converters are usually followed instead with periodic radiographs.

A positive reaction does not always mean that an individual currently has active tuberculosis. It can also indicate that the person has been infected with the organism sometime in the past. In addition, people who have been previously immunized with bacille Calmette-Guerin (BCG—an attenuated strain of *Mycobacterium bovis*) may test positive for a period of 3 to 7 years.

Although antibodies are generated against a variety of components of *Mycobacterium tuberculosis*, they are not responsible for a positive tuberculin skin test. It is not clear what role, if any, the antibodies have in disease progression.

An individual becomes positive in the tuberculin skin test approximately 4 to 6 weeks after a primary infection with *Mycobacterium tuberculosis*. Most people will remain positive for a lifetime; however, some eventually do revert to negative if the organisms are completely eradicated because of host resistance or prompt treatment after conversion.

49. The answer is C. *(Physiology)*

In primary hyperparathyroidism, serum calcium is elevated because parathyroid hormone (PTH) increases bone resorption and intestinal calcium absorption (via increased activation of vitamin D). Although PTH also acts at the renal distal tubule to increase calcium reabsorption, hyperparathyroidism is associated with urinary loss of calcium because the increased filtered load of calcium exceeds the renal capacity for reabsorption. PTH also increases urinary excretion of phosphate by an action primarily at the proximal tubule.

Dietary calcium deficiency and dietary vitamin D deficiency produce hypocalcemia and result in a secondary increase in plasma PTH. The decreased renal filtered load of calcium, together with the action of PTH to increase renal reabsorption of calcium, leads to a decrease in 24-hour urinary excretion of calcium. The action of PTH to increase renal excretion of phosphate could lead to increased 24-hour urinary excretion of this anion.

In primary hypoparathyroidism and pseudohypoparathyroidism (target-cell insensitivity), 24-hour excretion of both calcium and phosphate is decreased.

50. The answer is E. *(Microbiology)*
Sporothrix schenckii is a dimorphic fungus that lives on vegetation. Usually introduced into the skin by thorn puncture, it causes a local pustule or ulcer with nodules along the draining lymphatics. There is little systemic illness, but lesions may become chronic. Diagnosis is made by seeing round or cigar-shaped yeasts.

Mycetoma occurs when soil organisms enter through wounds and cause abscesses, with pus discharged through sinuses. Dermatophytoses (*Trichophyton*) species infect only superficial keratinized structures. *Mucor* infections invade tissues of immunocompromised hosts. They proliferate in the walls of blood vessels and other tissues and result in necrosis.

51. The answer is C. *(Behavioral science)*
Tertiary prevention involves reducing the likelihood of physical and social problems associated with a disorder. Thus, helping a schizophrenic patient learn self-care can improve his social functioning.

52. The answer is B. *(Microbiology)*
Histoplasma capsulatum causes histoplasmosis. A dimorphic fungus, it exists as a mold in soil and as a yeast in tissue. It is endemic to central and eastern United States, especially in the Ohio and Mississippi river valleys. Soils contaminated with pigeon droppings support fungal growth. Inhaled spores (microconidia) are engulfed by macrophages and develop into yeast forms. Most infections are asymptomatic.

For diagnosis, oval yeast cells within macrophages are seen in tissue biopsies or bone marrow aspirates.

Coccidioides is present as a spherule in tissue, and *Blastomyces* is a yeast in tissue with a thick wall and a single, broad-based bud. *Cryptococcus* is normally seen in spinal fluid as a budding yeast with wide capsules. *Mucor* exists as a mold, even in the walls of blood vessels.

53. The answer is C. *(Biochemistry)*
Xeroderma pigmentosum is a rare genetic disorder in which cells cannot repair damaged DNA. In the most common form of the disease, an ultraviolet-specific endonuclease necessary for the process of excision repair is missing. Patients with this disease are not able to remove thymine dimers caused by exposure to the ultraviolet radiation present in sunlight. The mutations, caused by the inability to repair such damage, frequently lead to the development of skin cancer.

54. The answer is C. *(Microbiology)*
Paracoccidioides brasiliensis causes paracoccidioidomycosis. It is a dimorphic fungus that exists as a mold in soil and as a yeast in tissue. The yeast is thick-walled with multiple buds ("ship's wheel" appearance), in contrast to *Blastomyces dermatitides*, which has a yeast with a single bud that has a broad base. *Histoplasma capsulatum* occurs as an oval budding yeast inside macrophages, whereas *Coccidioides* is a spherule in tissue, with many endospores within the spherule. *Sporothrix*, a dimorphic fungus from vegetation, is introduced into the skin and forms a local pustule or ulcer with nodules; round or cigar-shaped budding yeasts are seen in tissue specimens.

55. The answer is A. *(Behavioral science)*
Primary prevention involves decreasing the likelihood that a disorder will develop. Thus, training expectant parents in the principles of child development can reduce the likelihood that a child will have emotional or social disorders. In secondary prevention, early identification of a disorder to reduce its occurrence or duration is the goal. Tertiary prevention is meant to reduce the likelihood of physical and social problems caused by a disorder that is already present.

56. The answer is D. *(Microbiology)*
Virulent strains of *Mycobacterium tuberculosis*, an acid-fast bacteria, have cord factor (trehalose-6,6'-dimycolate), which enables them to stick together and grow in "serpentine cords" (i.e., they align themselves in parallel chains). Cord factor inhibits leukocyte migration, induces chronic granuloma formation, and acts as an immunologic adjuvant. *Mycobacterium tuberculosis* produces a number of lipids, including mycolic acids (long-chain fatty acids, waxes, and phosphatides).

Sulfatides (sulfur-containing glycolipids) are responsible for the neutral red reactivity associated with virulent strains of *Mycobacterium tuberculosis*. They appear to be nontoxic in and of themselves, but can synergistically enhance the activities of cord factor. Sulfatides may also prevent fusion of lysosomes with phagosomes and thus promote survival of the tubercle bacillus within macrophages.

Wax D (actually a family of waxes), or just the muramyldipeptide (MDP) portion of it, can greatly enhance the hypersensitivity response induced by cord factor.

The tubercle bacillus does not have a polysaccharide capsule; however, it does contain a variety of polysaccharides, which can induce an immediate hypersensitivity reaction. Their role in the disease of tuberculosis is unclear.

Injection of proteins of *Mycobacterium tuberculosis*, when bound to a wax fraction, can result in hypersensitivity to tuberculin and induction of specific antibodies. These proteins, however, are not considered to be virulence factors.

Gram-positive and gram-negative microorganisms do not have cord factor.

There are striking differences in the ability of mycobacteria to cause disease in humans, as well as in animals. *Mycobacterium tuberculosis* and *Mycobacterium bovis* are equally pathogenic for humans. The two species are closely related in many respects, including the DNA level.

57. The answer is E. *(Behavioral science)*
The sex-specific mortality rate for tuberculosis (deaths of males/population of males × 1000) cannot be calculated from the data given because no information is provided on how many male and female deaths there were of the total 1000 deaths.

58. The answer is B. *(Microbiology)*
Isoniazid (isonicotinic acid hydrazine, INH) is highly effective against most strains of *Mycobacterium tuberculosis* and is most likely to be included in the treatment. Tubercle bacilli lose their acid-fastness in its presence. Although the drug is relatively nontoxic to the host, sideroblastic anemia caused by pyridoxine (vitamin B_6) deficiency may occur. Patients with this side effect may exhibit peripheral neuritis and seizures. Because resistance to a single drug can easily emerge, subjects with active tuberculosis are routinely given a combination of drugs; a widely used regimen in the United States is pyrazinamide for the first 2 months (until results of drug susceptibility tests become known), followed by INH plus rifampin for an additional 4 months. Arrest of the disease is achieved in 95% or more of cases.

Close contacts (especially children) of patients with active tuberculosis are often given prophylactic therapy with INH for 12 months and are monitored with radiographs and tuberculin skin tests. Patients older than 20 (and especially older than 35) are at increased risk for developing INH-induced hepatitis.

The following table lists drugs approved for use against tuberculosis.

First-line drugs	Second-line drugs
	Streptomycin
	Kanamycin
	Capreomycin
Isoniazid	Ethionamide
Rifampin	Cycloserine
Pyrazinamide	Ofloxacin
Ethambutol	Ciproxacin

59. The answer is C. *(Biochemistry)*
The trivalent form of arsenite (arsenic, AsO_2) has a high affinity for sulfhydryl groups and binds with great avidity to lipoic acid, one of the five cofactors of pyruvate dehydrogenase. The most efficient way to remove this arsenite is by administering a competitive sulfhydryl compound, such as dimercaprol.

Chelating agents such as ethylenediaminetetraacetate (EDTA), penicillamine, or deferoxamine will react with circulating metals and remove them from the body. Yet, they are less effective in competing with sulfhydryl groups than the mercaptans.

60. The answer is E. *(Microbiology)*

There are no serologic tests that are routinely used in the diagnosis of either tuberculosis or leprosy. Clinical presentation, skin testing, and isolation of an acid-fast bacillus (Ziehl-Neelsen staining technique) from sputum or other specimens are the usual methods; however, high levels of immunoglobulin G (IgG) against purified protein derivative (PPD) from *Mycobacterium tuberculosis* can be detected by enzyme-linked immunosorbent assays in patients with active pulmonary disease.

The progression of leprosy is generally very slow. After infection, symptoms may not appear for several years. On the other hand, the speed at which tuberculosis progresses is quite variable and highly dependent upon the innate resistance of the host. Most people who are exposed to *Mycobacterium tuberculosis* are not aware that they have been infected. Approximately 5% to 9% of them eventually develop clinical evidence of disease within 5 years. The pathogenic mycobacteria grow slowly. Their doubling time is often 16 to 24 hours or more, whereas the doubling time for many other bacterial pathogens can be as short as 1 hour.

The incidence of drug-resistant strains of *Mycobacterium tuberculosis* has been increasing in recent years. The organisms are often resistant to many of the approved drugs. The mechanisms leading to resistance are not fully understood. An increased incidence of resistant strains has been noted, even prior to therapy. No drug-resistant *Mycobacterium leprae* have been reported in the United States.

Delayed-type hypersensitivity develops in the great majority of people infected with *Mycobacterium tuberculosis*, including those in which there is no other evidence of disease.

Mycobacterium tuberculosis can be cultured on a variety of artificial media, including Lowenstein-Jensen (whole egg-based medium) and Middlebrook 7H9 and 7H12 (semisynthetic agar media). Colonies will appear on these media in approximately 2 to 8 weeks.

Recently, ^{14}C-palmitic acid has been added to the 7H12 medium (BACTEC culture system for mycobacteria). The organisms utilize the ^{14}C-palmitic acid, thereby releasing $^{14}CO_2$ which can be detected by a machine within approximately 2 weeks. *Mycobacterium leprae* has not yet been cultivated in vitro; however, this species will grow in the mouse footpad and in the nine-banded armadillo.

Methods used to identify the species of a cultured mycobacterium include rate of growth, pigmentation of colonies, colonial morphology, and biochemical profiles. Molecular probes and DNA-amplification techniques are likely to replace these older methods eventually.

61. The answer is D. *(Behavioral science)*

The number of people with multiple sclerosis in the population per 100,000 population per year is the prevalence rate. The number of new cases of multiple sclerosis per 100,000 population per year and number of new cases of cancer of the prostate per 100,000 men per year are examples of incidence rate. The number of 10-year-old children who die of leukemia and the number of men who die per 100,000 population per year are cause-specific and sex-specific mortality rates, respectively.

62. The answer is B. *(Microbiology)*

The disease of leprosy is divided into two basic types: lepromatous and tuberculoid. The lepromatous form is an aggressive disease, whereas the tuberculoid form tends to be self-limiting. Individuals with lepromatous leprosy have an inflammatory skin infiltrate, which consists largely of macrophages that have a characteristic vacuolated or "foamy" appearance (caused by the accumulation of lipids within phagocytes) and intracellular acid-fast bacilli. In the lepromatous form, presence of organisms indicates impaired cellular immunity, unlike the tuberculoid type, which can effectively kill the bacteria.

Differential characteristics of lepromatous and tuberculoid leprosy

	Lepromatous	**Tuberculoid**
Nature of disease	Disseminated	Often self-limiting
Acid-fast bacilli	Abundant	Rare
Bacteremia	Yes	No
Cell-mediated immunity	Low	High
T helpers in skin	No	Yes
T suppressors in skin	Yes	No
Immunoglobulin level	High	Low
Lepromin* reaction	Negative	Positive
Syphilis serology**	Positive (40–60%)	Negative

* Extract of *M. leprae,* used for intradermal skin testing. The test is not useful diagnostically, but assists in determining where the patient is in the immunologic spectrum.

** False positive syphilis serology in screening tests such as VDRL and RPR. Patients have polyclonal hypergammaglobulinemia and antibodies of many different specificities are present.

Mycobacterium leprae grows best in the cooler parts of the body (i.e., skin, nose, fingers, toes). The organisms invade nerves and selectively infect Schwann cells. Cutaneous nerve endings are destroyed, thereby producing anesthesia. Repeated infections of cuts and wounds may result in disfiguration because of bone resorption and scarring.

Humans are the only natural hosts for *Mycobacterium leprae*. Although transmission routes have not been firmly established, the organisms are shed in nasal secretions and are present in ulcer exudates. Leprosy is endemic in Hawaii, Texas, and several other parts of the world.

Leprosy is a good example of a disease in which the outcome of infection is highly dependent upon a T–cell-mediated response against the organisms. In the tuberculoid form, the presence of specific T-cell reactivity against *Mycobacterium leprae* can be readily demonstrated.

Dapsone, rifampin, and clofazimine are used effectively for treatment.

63. The answer is D. *(Biochemistry)*

The addition of a poly A tail to the 3′ end is one of the post-transcriptional modifications that occurs in the processing of eukaryotic messenger RNA (mRNA). A cap consisting of a guanosine derivative is attached to the 5′ end. Intervening sequences (introns) are removed by splicing. All of these processing events occur in the nucleus of eukaryotes. Prokaryotic mRNA undergoes none of these modifications.

64. The answer is A. *(Microbiology)*

Corynebacterium diphtheriae, an aerobic gram-positive rod, is the cause of diphtheria. A hallmark feature of the disease is the development of a grayish "pseudomembrane" over the tonsils, larynx, and pharynx, which can obstruct breathing (hence the cyanosis). The membrane is not a true membrane. It consists of fibrin, red and white blood cells, and the organisms. It is deeply embedded and attempts to remove it may cause extensive bleeding. Intubation or tracheostomy may be required to prevent suffocation. Children with the disease often have dysphonia or difficulty in speaking.

Corynebacterium diphtheriae secretes a potent toxin, which is absorbed into the mucous membranes of the respiratory tract. This toxin causes inflammation, sore throat, and fever. Difficulty in breathing (dyspnea) and prostration follow shortly thereafter. Damage to the heart may occur, leading to cardiac arrhythmia. It may also cause problems with vision, speech, and swallowing. Some individuals may experience difficulty in moving arms or legs. These manifestations generally subside spontaneously.

Children are routinely immunized with diphtheria toxoid that is adsorbed onto aluminum hydroxide or aluminum phosphate as an adjuvant. The toxoid is commonly given together with the pertussis vaccine and tetanus toxoid (i.e., DPT).

In addition to the respiratory tract, *Corynebacterium diphtheriae* can also be recovered from wounds and the skin of healthy individuals, including normal carriers.

Corynebacteria have club-shaped swellings at either one pole or the other and metachromatic granules, which are especially evident after culture on Loeffler's medium and staining with methylene blue. The rods are arranged in acute angles to each other, giving them a characteristic appearance (i.e., like Chinese letters).

Corynebacterium pseudodiphtheriticum, and a number of other species, are known as diphtheroids. They are part of the normal flora of the upper respiratory tract, urinary tract, and conjunctivae. They are rarely associated with disease in humans. In young children, group A *streptococcus* most commonly causes a subacute nasopharyngitis with a thin serous discharge and enlarged lymph nodes. Extension to the middle ear, mastoid, or the meninges is common. If the organisms produce pyrogenic exotoxins A–C and erythrogenic toxin, a scarlet fever rash occurs. *Propionibacterium* species are anaerobic diphtheroids found on the skin. They may participate in the pathogenesis of acne (*P. acnes*). They produce lipases, which split fatty acids from lipids in the skin. The fatty acids, in turn, induce inflammation. *Erysipelothrix rhusiopathiae* is a gram-positive rod that can cause infection of the skin (erysipeloid). It is acquired through contact with contaminated fish ("fish handler's disease"), shellfish, meat, or poultry. It occurs worldwide, especially in swine.

65. The answer is C. *(Behavioral science)*
Approximately 13% of the gross domestic product was spent on health care in 1992. Hospitalization was the most expensive element, accounting for 41% of the total expenditure.

66. The answer is B. *(Microbiology)*
The diphtheria toxin is a heat-labile polypeptide that has a molecular weight of approximately 62,000. It consists of fragment A and fragment B, which are held together by disulfide bonds. Fragment B is not toxic; however, it binds to mammalian cells and facilitates the entry of fragment A, which has the toxic activity.

Fragment A catalyzes a reaction that results in free nicotinamide plus an adenosine diphosphate (ADP)-ribose-elongation factor-2 (EF-2) complex, which is inactive. This leads to immediate inhibition of protein synthesis within the host cell. *Pseudomonas aeruginosa* produces toxin A, which also inhibits protein synthesis by ADP ribosylation of EF-2.

EF-2 is required for translocation of polypeptidyl-transfer RNA (tRNA) from the acceptor to the donor site on ribosomes in the cytoplasmic membrane.

All *Corynebacterium diphtheriae* are not toxigenic. Only those organisms that are infected with a certain bacteriophage can secrete the toxin. The gene for the toxin is carried by the virus.

Effects of the diphtheria toxin are usually restricted to the upper respiratory tract, but lesions may occur in other parts of the body. The most serious complications include effects on the cardiovascular and nervous systems. The toxin causes fatty myocardial degeneration, which may result in cardiac dysfunction and circulatory collapse. Cardiovascular abnormalities account for approximately 20% of deaths caused by the disease. The neurologic effects of the toxin include paralysis of the soft palate and polyneuritis of the lower extremities. Neurologic problems usually disappear with resolution of the disease.

Treatment of diphtheria consists of administration of a specific antitoxin immunoglobulin preparation and erythromycin. The antibodies are produced by hyperimmunization of animals such as horses, rabbits, sheep, and goats. The antitoxin may be given intramuscularly in mild cases or intravenously. The antitoxin should be given as early as possible in order to minimize the chance for severe disease. Antibiotics such as erythromycin and penicillin will inhibit the growth of the microorganisms; however, they have no effect on toxin that is already produced.

Toxin-producing organisms that increase the intracellular level of cyclic adenosine monophosphate (cAMP) include some of the enteric gram-negative rods.

Diphtheria toxin is an exotoxin, not an endotoxin.

67. The answer is B. *(Behavioral science)*
The standardized mortality rate (SMR) is the number of observed deaths divided by the number of expected deaths. Thus, a ratio of 1.0 means that there are equal numbers of observed and expected deaths in a group. Groups with an SMR of less than 1.0, such as office workers in the example given (SMR = 0.95), are less likely to die than those in the general population. An SMR of more than 1.0 indicates that individuals in that group are more likely to die than individuals in the general population.

68. The answer is C. *(Microbiology)*

Listeria monocytogenes, a short gram-positive rod, has an unusual tumbling "end-over-end" motility at 22°C, but not at 37°C. This property is useful in laboratory diagnosis because it rapidly differentiates the organism from all other gram-positive rods. In addition, the organisms produce a small zone of β-hemolysis around and under colonies grown on blood agar.

Listeria monocytogenes can cause perinatal listeriosis (granulomatosis infantiseptica). When symptoms are manifested early, the organisms are thought to have been transmitted in utero. In the early-onset syndrome, the infants are either born dead or die shortly after delivery. The late-onset syndrome is manifested as meningitis within the first 3 weeks after delivery.

Adults, especially those who are immunocompromised, can occasionally develop meningoencephalitis and bacteremia caused by the organisms.

The organisms are believed to be acquired primarily by ingestion of contaminated foods. Recent outbreaks of listeriosis have been linked to raw vegetables, raw and pasteurized milk (the milk was contaminated after pasteurization), and cole slaw. The organisms can invade and multiply within intestinal epithelial cells, as well as in phagocytes.

Listeria monocytogenes is susceptible to ampicillin, penicillin, erythromycin, and trimethoprim-sulfamethoxazole.

Bacteria that are commonly associated with meningitis include:

Bacteria	Age group
Escherichia coli	neonates
β-hemolytic streptococci (*Streptococcus agalactiae*)	neonates (most common)
Haemophilus influenzae	3 months–5 years
Neisseria meningitidis	young adults
Streptococcus pneumoniae	adults

The presence of neutrophils, low glucose, and increased protein in cerebrospinal fluid is suggestive of a bacterial etiology.

69. The answer is C. *(Biochemistry)*

δ-Aminolevulinic acid (ALA) is synthesized in the mitochondrial membrane of all cells, including the red blood cell precursors, by ALA synthase. This enzyme uses succinyl coenzyme A (CoA) and glycine as a substrate and pyridoxal (vitamin B_6) phosphate as a cofactor. Heme synthesis is an anabolic process that requires the energy inherent in the succinyl CoA bond. Succinyl CoA can only be accumulated under high-energy charge conditions, when it is not necessarily used to produce energy. Under these high-energy conditions, isocitrate dehydrogenase, α-ketoglutarate dehydrogenase, and citrate synthetase are inhibited by the high adenosine triphosphate (ATP) and reduced nicotinamide-adenine dinucleotide (NADH) levels. The inhibition of the isocitrate dehydrogenase is reinforced by low levels of adenosine diphosphate (ADP), a required activator. Succinyl CoA amplifies the inhibition of citrate synthase and α-ketoglutarate dehydrogenase. Therefore, under high-energy charge conditions, succinyl CoA is largely formed from succinate, a route made difficult in this case because of the high Michaelis-Menten constant (K_m) for succinate. Consequently, heme synthesis is impaired and a microcytic anemia results.

70. The answer is B. *(Microbiology)*

In the United States, plague is primarily a disease of rodents. There are more than 200 different species of rodents that can harbor the organisms. Among the most common are skunks, field mice, prairie dogs, squirrels, gerbils, and moles. In many other countries rats, which tend to live closer to human populations than most other rodents, are often important hosts.

Rodents are relatively resistant to plague, but can develop disease (septicemia and bacteremia) and die from it.

The plague bacillus is present in wild animal populations in at least 15 different states, most of which are in the western portion of the country.

Plague is caused by *Yersinia pestis*, a gram-negative rod that belongs in the Enterobacteriaceae family; however, because these organisms are not inhabitants of the intestinal tract, they are not considered together with the enteric bacteria.

Fleas are the primary vectors of *Yersinia pestis*. They transmit the organisms from one animal to another, and also to humans, by bite. The classic vector is the rat flea (*Xynopsylla cheopsis*). It is more likely than most other fleas to transmit the organisms to humans. In addition, it can harbor them for more than one season and thus perpetuate plague. The human flea can transmit the organisms from one human to another.

Yersinia pestis multiplies well at the normal body temperature of the flea (28°C) and produces coagulase. Both of these factors result in blockage of the proventriculus ("esophagus") of the flea and regurgitation of the organisms into the wound during a blood meal.

Humans can also become infected by inhalation of aerosols, when in close contact with a plague victim. Direct contact with dead or infected animals or with soil from contaminated burrows are also possible routes of infection.

Control and eradication of plague are difficult because of the many wild animal species that are involved and the variety of transmission routes. Insecticides are helpful. Rodent extermination may be counterproductive, because the fleas will leave in search of another host.

71. The answer is D. *(Behavioral science)*
To assess the strength of association between two variables that are linearly related, the most appropriate test is correlation. The Fisher exact and chi-square tests are nonparametric tests used to evaluate differences between frequencies in two samples. The *t*-test and analysis of variance (ANOVA) are parametric tests designed to assess significant differences between the means of two samples (*t*-test) or more than two samples (ANOVA).

72. The answer is B. *(Biochemistry)*
Both lactase and the peptidases are mucosal cell (brush border) enzymes, which are lost in inflammation, particularly after rotavirus infections. Loss of these enzymes results in maldigestion of lactose to glucose plus galactose and small peptides to free amino acids. The only other conversion listed that is catalyzed by a mucosal enzyme is the breakdown of maltose to glucose. However, there is no problem with converting milk albumin into polypeptides by trypsin and chymotrypsin, enzymes that are synthesized and released from the pancreas rather than the brush border. The conversion of starch to limit dextrin is done mostly by α-amylase, another pancreatic enzyme.

73. The answer is B. *(Behavioral science)*
The average life expectancy for all Americans at birth is approximately 75.5 years. The average life expectancy for American men is 72.1 years and for American women, 79.0 years.

74. The answer is B. *(Biochemistry)*
The vast majority of people in Africa and Asia lose their lactase activity during early childhood. In yogurt and cheese, the lactose is prefermented by a lactobacillus to form lactic acid. Unlike cheese, the yogurt spoils in a tropical country without refrigeration. Therefore, cheese is used throughout the world as a staple product. Milk and cream, dried or not, create bloating and other digestive problems in a lactase-deficient population and are not acceptable as a nutritional source. Butter lacks lactose and most of the other nutrients such as calcium and protein, which give milk its nutrient value.

75. The answer is C. *(Physiology)*
Ketoacidosis is associated with severe insulin deficiency. A patient with untreated type I diabetes mellitus has low plasma levels of insulin and C peptide caused by β cell destruction. Type I diabetes is also associated with increased protein breakdown (negative nitrogen balance), increased lipolysis and ketogenesis, and decreased blood volume caused by the glucose-induced osmotic diuresis.

Type II diabetes is rarely associated with ketoacidosis because the insulin resistance is not severe enough, and there is enough insulin effect to prevent ketogenesis but not hyperglycemia.

76. The answer is C. *(Behavioral science)*
When compared with men, women are more likely to seek medical attention. Men are more likely than women to show aggressive behavior and be involved in accidents that result in spinal cord injury. Men and women show equivalent levels of hypochondriasis. The incidence of homosexuality in men is 3% to 10%, whereas the incidence of homosexuality in women is 1% to 3%.

77. The answer is D. *(Behavioral science)*
Medicaid is financed by both federal and state governments and pays for health care for low-income people.

The percentage of costs that the federal government pays ranges from 40% to 79%, depending on the per capita income in each state.

78. The answer is C. *(Biochemistry)*
DNA replication in bacteria is a complicated process involving many different enzymes. All newly synthesized strands are made in the 5′ → 3′ direction and are complementary, not identical, to the template. This allows the "leading strand" to be made in one long piece, whereas the "lagging strand" is made as a series of small pieces called "Okazaki fragments." Synthesis of each Okazaki fragment begins with an RNA primer. Proofreading is provided by the 3′ → 5′ exonuclease activity of the DNA polymerase. DNA topoisomerase provides a swivel. DNA ligase seals nicks in the backbone of DNA and joins together the Okazaki fragments, following replacement of the RNA primers with DNA.

79. The answer is D. *(Behavioral science)*
A 55-year-old white woman is more likely to attempt suicide than a 55-year-old African-American woman. The African-American woman is more likely to be obese and to have diabetes, heart disease, and hypertension. There is no racial difference in the occurrence of schizophrenia.

80. The answer is A. *(Pharmacology)*
The fluoroquinolones are known to damage growing cartilage in animals, causing juvenile arthropathy. There is little evidence that this occurs in humans; however, until further studies are conducted, it seems prudent to avoid this drug in children unless alternative drugs are unavailable.

Tetracyclines should be avoided in children up to age 8 because they deposit in growing teeth and may cause permanent staining. Macrocytic anemia is an adverse effect of trimethoprim and is most likely to occur in pregnant women who have inadequate folate in their diet. Ototoxicity may be caused by vancomycin or the aminoglycosides, particularly in combination with furosemide. Hyperpyrexia is a dangerous adverse effect of atropine overdose in children.

81. The answer is A. *(Behavioral science)*
Because primary prevention involves decreasing the likelihood that a disorder will develop, improving the

nutrition of a pregnant woman can improve her chance of having a healthy child.

82. The answer is B. *(Pharmacology)*
The most serious side effect of zidovudine is bone marrow suppression. Ganciclovir (Cytovene) may also cause these adverse effects, but acyclovir (Zovirax) usually does not. Didanosine and zalcitabine (other dideoxynucleosides used for HIV) are less likely to cause bone marrow suppression than zidovudine and are more frequently associated with pancreatitis and sensorimotor neuropathy.

83. The answer is A. *(Behavioral science)*
The probability that both patients will develop side effects is the chance of one of the patients developing side effects (10%) multiplied by the chance of the other patient developing side effects (10%) = 1%.

84. The answer is D. *(Pathology)*
Fibronectin is a glycoprotein secreted by fibroblasts and some epithelial cells. Fibronectin binds to collagen and glycosaminoglycans and, thus, has important roles in cell adhesion and migration. Fibronectin is linked to the surface of cells by a transmembrane protein. In cancer, this connection is severed, and fibronectin is lost from the cell surface, leading to loss of adhesive properties.

Laminin is a glycoprotein of the basal lamina and can bind collagen, proteoglycan, and glycosaminoglycan. Integrin is a transmembrane receptor protein that links fibronectin to the cell allowing for internal (cellular) control of fibronectin arrangement. The glycocalyx is the carbohydrate coating of the cell membrane, which is found on microvilli. Hyaluronic acid is a nonsulfated glycosaminoglycan that is found in the extracellular matrix. It binds to collagen via linking proteins, serving to stabilize the extracellular matrix and hydrate it for buoyancy.

85. The answer is B. *(Microbiology)*
Hepatitis B virus (HBV) presents as an acute or a chronic type of infection. Approximately 10% of the total infections may progress to chronic status. Chronic carriers may have symptoms ranging from subclinical to active disease. The definition for chronic infection is the presence of HBV surface antigen

(HBsAg) for more than 6 months. Antibodies to HBsAg may be present, but apparently are not sufficient to neutralize all HBV particles present.

Demonstration of hepatitis Be antigen (HbeAg), which is not usually measured, indicates active virus growth, which is quite contagious. The presence of HBsAg antibody only indicates protection acquired by either vaccination or recovery from natural infection. The presence of HbsAg alone in a patient indicates a "healthy carrier" because the patient is not infectious.

86. The answer is D. *(Biochemistry)*
Phosphatidylinositol derivatives play several distinct roles in the cell membrane, one of which is that they anchor several cell surface proteins. Cell surface proteins bound to phosphatidylinositol are also found in several parasitic protozoa. By altering these proteins, these protozoa can change their antigenic properties and avoid immunosurveillance. Being attached via a relatively long chain to the membrane via phosphatidylinositol, rather than being a part of the membrane itself, allows these proteins lateral movement on the cell surface. The proteins can be cleaved from the membrane by the action of phospholipase C. The other compounds listed are also phospholipids, but they do not anchor proteins in the membrane.

87. The answer is C. *(Behavioral science)*
To estimate the adult height of a 2-year-old, the height is doubled; therefore, a 2-year-old girl who is 33 inches tall can be expected to be 66 inches tall in adulthood.

88. The answer is B. *(Behavioral science)*
The risk attributable to smoking to bladder cancer in men is equal to the incidence rate in men exposed to smoking (48.0/100,000) minus the incidence rate in men not exposed to smoking (25.4/100,000). Thus, the attributable risk of smoking to bladder cancer in men is 22.6 per 100,000 men per year.

89. The answer is B. *(Behavioral science)*
This man is suffering from depression. Symptoms of depression include overwhelming guilt, hopelessness, severe weight loss, and absence of attempts to return to a normal life style. The most effective treatment for depression is antidepressant medication. In a normal grief reaction, although the patient may feel sad and have an initial loss of appetite, he shows attempts to return to a normal life style. While encouraging the patient to see friends and family and increasing doctor–patient contact can be helpful in a normal grief reaction, these interventions will have little effect on the symptoms of depression.

90-91. The answers are: 90-C, 91-D. *(Microbiology)*
Brucellosis is also known as undulant fever, thus the daily periodicity of fever and chills is an important clue. Undulation of the fever is seen primarily with *Brucella melitensis*, which is found in goats and sheep. In addition, the slow insidious onset of symptoms and granulomatous lesions in the liver are classic manifestations. Farmers, veterinarians, and abatoir (slaughterhouse) workers are at greatest risk.

The other two major species involved in human infections are *Brucella abortis* (cattle) and *Brucella suis* (swine). *Brucella canis* is responsible for outbreaks of disease in kennels, especially among beagle dogs. A few rare cases of human brucellosis caused by this species have been documented.

Brucella is transmitted primarily by direct contact with tissues of infected animals or by ingestion of raw, unpasteurized milk (and cheeses that are made from the milk). Aerosol transmission has been documented in meat-packing plants. The organisms can remain viable in dry soil for 40 to 60 days. Person-to-person transmission is rare.

Brucellae are short, pleomorphic, nonmotile gramnegative coccobacilli that occasionally exhibit bipolar staining and need air for growth. A small capsule, which is present in primary isolates, is lost upon subculture (smooth to rough colonial variation is observed). They are intracellular parasites.

In animals, *Brucella* can cause contagious abortion. The organisms may be carried for years and shed in the milk of apparently healthy hosts. They localize in the mammary glands and in the pregnant uterus. Other animals who eat, or even lick, aborted fetuses can become infected. Brucellae are highly invasive.

Francisella tularensis, *Salmonella typhi*, and *Mycobacterium bovis* are unlikely to be correct because the case history does not fit the diseases caused by these organisms.

The macrophage is considered to be the most important cell in determining the outcome of brucellosis, as shown in the following flow chart.

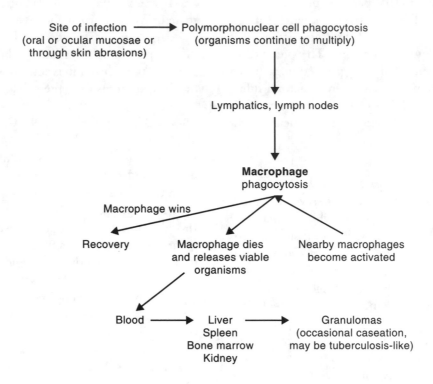

Most infections with brucellae remain asymptomatic; however, after an incubation period of 1 to 6 weeks, the disease may be acute, subacute, or chronic. There are species differences regarding clinical manifestations.

- *B. melitensis*—acute, severe
- *B. abortus*—mild, noncaseating
- *B. canis*—mild, noncaseating
- *B. suis*—chronic

Results of the dye sensitivity test (ability to grow in the presence of thionine and basic fuchsin) and evidence of the production of H$_2$S help differentiate species.

Signs and symptoms that may be present, in addition to those mentioned in the case history, are: splenomegaly, hepatomegaly, gastrointestinal disturbances, weakness, and depression.

92. The answer is B. *(Behavioral science)*
In countertransference, doctors have special feelings toward patients with whom they are personally associated, such as friends and relatives. As such, physicians may minimize the severity of an illness in that patient.

In transference, the patient views the doctor as a parent or other close person. Rationalization, displacement, and projection are defense mechanisms. In rationalization, an irrational feeling is made to appear normal. Displacement involves transfer of emotions from an unacceptable to an acceptable idea, while projection refers to attribution of unacceptable ideas to others.

93. The answer is E. *(Biochemistry)*
N-linked glycosylation of a protein begins in the endoplasmic reticulum, where a core oligosaccharide is transferred from the lipid dolichol to the side chain of an asparagine residue on the protein. The oligosaccharide is trimmed and then modified by the addition of other sugar residues as the protein moves through

the endoplasmic reticulum and the Golgi apparatus. The lysosome is the final destination of some glycosylated proteins. Cytoplasmic and nuclear proteins are usually not glycosylated.

94. The answer is D. *(Microbiology)*
The Epstein-Barr virus (EBV) causes infectious mononucleosis in young adults of college age, especially when they are stressed. The clinical findings described in the short case history are typical of the disease. Laboratory diagnosis is often based on the heterophile agglutination test, which detects antibodies against sheep or horse erythrocytes. Identification of EBV antigens on immortalized B lymphocytes, which may be recovered from patient specimens, such as lymphoid tissues and peripheral blood, is done by nucleic acid hybridization. EBV markers are present on approximately 1% of circulating lymphocytes during the acute phase of the disease.

EBV has also been linked to "chronic fatigue syndrome," which is characterized by extreme fatigue that may persist for months, low-grade fever, sore throat, swollen lymph nodes, myasthenia, and mild memory loss.

B lymphocytes are infected after the EBV binds to the CD21 surface molecule. CD21 protein is also found on follicular dendritic cells and epithelial cells of the pharynx.

After infection with EBV, atypical CD8$^+$ T lymphocytes appear in the blood circulation. They are activated cells that are unusual in two respects: most of them are not specific for antigens of the EBV, and they are not major histocompatibility complex (MHC)-restricted. The T lymphocytes become activated when they bind to EBV-infected B cells, which express the lymphocyte-determined membrane antigen (LYDMA); however, there are some virus-specific, MHC-restricted cytotoxic CD8$^+$ T cells that are also present.

HIV-1 and HTLV-I both infect CD4$^+$ T lymphocytes.

The human herpes virus type 6 (HHV-6) infects immature T lymphocytes, B cells, monocyte-macrophages, and several other cell types. Infection with this virus usually occurs in early infancy and is characterized by high fever and skin rash (exanthem subitum, roseola infantum, or "sixth disease"). It is considered to be a mild disease of childhood. In adults, the virus has been associated with persistent lymphadenopathy and possibly hepatitis.

Cytomegalovirus (CMV) infection produces a generalized depression of cell-mediated immunity. The mechanisms are unclear, but recognition of infected cells by virus-specific T-cytotoxic lymphocytes may be impaired, presumably because of selective interference with MHC class I presentation.

95. The answer is B. *(Pathology)*
Malignant cells with focal areas of gland formation and mucin production revealed through sections of the tumor indicate the grade of the cancer, which in this case would be well-differentiated (low-grade) adenocarcinoma. The grade of a tumor is based primarily on the degree of differentiation of the tumor (how much it resembles its parent tissue) and on the amount of mitotic activity, which indirectly indicates its growth rate. Grading terms include low grade (or well-differentiated), intermediate grade, or high grade (poorly differentiated, or anaplastic).

Tumor stage is based on the size of the primary tumor and the presence or absence of lymph nodal or hematogenous dissemination. The prognosis is closely related to the grade and stage of the cancer. The stage of a cancer is the most important factor determining the prognosis, not only in breast cancer but other cancers as well. Lymph node status is the single most important factor that determines the prognosis in women with breast cancer.

The size of the tumor, condition of margins, and number of lymph nodes involved are all factors that influence staging. The presence of malignant cells in a liver biopsy also refers to staging, because it indicates tumor in sites other than lymph nodes.

96. The answer is C. *(Behavioral science)*
Smoking is the single most important risk factor contributing to increased mortality in the United States. It is also the single most important cause of premature death in the United States, accounting for one of every six deaths. The risk factors that follow smoking are diet, alcohol, and accidents.

97. The answer is B. *(Pathology)*
The most common primary cancer in the lung is an adenocarcinoma. Malignant tumors arising from

epithelial origin are called carcinomas. The epithelium can be derived from ectoderm (squamous carcinoma, transitional cell carcinoma), endoderm (colon adenocarcinoma), or mesoderm (e.g., renal adenocarcinoma).

Cervical cancers are most commonly squamous cancer. Most are related to human papillomavirus type 16, 18, 31. Smoking and immunosuppression are other predisposing causes.

Esophageal cancers are most commonly squamous. Predisposing causes include achalasia, lye strictures, diverticular diseases, the Plummer-Vinson syndrome (esophageal webs, iron deficiency, achlorhydria), smoking, alcohol, and nitrosamines.

True vocal cord cancers are most commonly squamous. Predisposing causes include smoking and alcohol.

Bladder cancers are most commonly transitional carcinoma. Predisposing causes include smoking, aniline dyes, benzidine, and cyclophosphamide.

98. The answer is A.   (Pathology)
Neuroblastoma is associated with a deletion on chromosome 1 and inactivation of a suppressor gene.

Wilm's tumors of the kidney have an abnormality on chromosome 11, with loss of a suppressor gene.

Osteogenic sarcoma has an abnormality on chromosome 17, particularly a point mutation with inactivation of a p53 suppressor gene.

Retinoblastoma (Rb) has an abnormality on chromosome 13, with inactivation of a Rb-suppressor gene that normally inhibits the growth of retinal cells.

Neurofibromas have an abnormality on chromosome 17, in which there is a neurofibromatosis-1 gene that down regulates the function of the ras oncogene in producing second messengers.

99. The answer is D.   (Pathology)
The grade of a tumor is based primarily on the degree of differentiation of the tumor and on the amount of mitotic activity, which indirectly indicates its growth rate. Grading terms include

- low grade, or well differentiated, in which the pathologist can tell that the tumor is squamous (e.g., keratin present), transitional, or an adenocarcinoma (e.g., glands with mucin)
- intermediate grade

- high grade, poorly differentiated, or anaplastic, in which the pathologist cannot tell whether the tumor is squamous, glandular, or sarcomatous

Tumor stage is based on the size of the primary tumor and the presence or absence of lymph nodal or hematogenous dissemination. The prognosis is closely related to the grade and stage of the cancer (stage is the most important factor). The TNM system is frequently used for staging. T stands for characteristics of the primary tumor (e.g., size, skin involvement), N refers to the lymph node status and the localization of those involved (e.g., mediastinal, axillary), and M refers to distant metastasis. There are other staging systems used including the modified Dukes' classification for colon cancer or the Columbia system for breast cancer.

In the pathologist's description. only information relating to the grade of the tumor is given. Because the tumor is forming glands, it is a low-grade, or well-differentiated endometrial carcinoma. It is also associated with benign squamous epithelium; therefore, the correct diagnosis is a low-grade endometrial carcinoma, with focal areas of benign squamous epithelium. Not enough squamous epithelium is present to warrant the diagnosis of adenoacanthoma.

Atypical endometrial hyperplasia with focal areas of squamous metaplasia is incorrect, because the tumor is malignant by virtue of the fact that there are atypical mitotic spindles and glandular crowding. High-grade cancer of the endometrial glands with focal invasion into the cervix is incorrect, because glands are forming (low grade) and the squamous epithelium is part of the tumor, rather than an invasion into the cervix. Well-differentiated squamous cancer infiltrating into the endometrial cavity is incorrect only in that no information is given about the depth of invasion into the myometrium, because none was present in the specimen. Anaplastic endometrial cancer with squamous cell carcinoma (adenosquamous carcinoma) is incorrect, because the tumor is low grade and the squamous component is benign, not malignant.

100. The answer is D.   (Biochemistry)
A high insulin–glucagon ratio is characteristic of the fed state, in which insulin is the key hormone. Insulin

enhances the storage of glycogen in the liver and triac-ylglycerol in the adipose. Insulin enhances glycolysis, so that intermediates, such as glucose-6-phosphate (starting point for the pentose phosphate shunt and glycogenesis), dihydroxyacetone phosphate (forms glycerol 3-phosphate, the carbohydrate backbone of triglyceride), and acetyl CoA (for fatty-acid synthesis) are formed. The main rate-controlling enzyme in gly-colysis is phosphofructokinase-1 (PFK-1), which con-verts fructose 6-phosphate into fructose 1,6-bisphos-phate. Insulin release is stimulated by gastric inhibitory peptide and hyperglycemia in the fed state. Hypergly-cemia inhibits glucagon release, which normally stimu-lates adenylate cyclase to generate cyclic adenosine monophosphate (cAMP). Therefore, the cAMP con-centration is low in the fed state, deactivating protein kinase A and permitting dephosphorylated PFK-2. Accumulation of the non-phosphorylated form of

PFK-2 favors the production of fructose 2,6 bisphos-phate, the most potent stimulator of PFK-1 in the glycolytic cycle. Fructose 2,6-bisphosphate also inhib-its the gluconeogenic enzyme, fructose bisphosphatase, thus preventing gluconeogenesis.

During gluconeogenesis the insulin–glucagon ratio is low and glucagon is the key hormone. This increases cAMP levels. The cAMP activates protein kinase A, which phosphorylates PFK-2. Phospho-PFK-2 no longer phosphorylates fructose 6-phosphate; instead, it hydrolyzes fructose 2,6-bisphosphate. The resulting decrease in fructose 2,6-bisphosphate permits PFK-1 to be inhibited by adenosine triphosphate and citrate and, therefore, inhibits glycolysis. The decrease in fruc-tose 2,6-bisphosphate levels also de-inhibits fructose 1,6-bisphosphatase and stimulates gluconeogenesis. The following chart is a comparison of these two processes:

	Fed State (High insulin–glucagon ratio)	Fasting State (Low insulin–glucagon ratio)
Adenylate cyclase synthesis of cAMP	Low	High
Protein kinase A activity	Decreased	Increased
Phosphofructokinase-2 activity	Increased	Decreased
Fructose 2,6-bisphosphatase activity	Decreased	Increased
Formation of fructose 2,6-bisphosphate	Increased	Decreased
Phosphofructokinase-1 activity	Increased	Decreased
Fructose 1,6-bisphosphatase activity	Decreased	Increased
Glycolysis	Increased	Decreased
Gluconeogenesis	Decreased	Increased

101. The answer is D. *(Microbiology)*
The following diagram represents the growth stages of a typical, resting bacterium introduced into a new environment contain nutrients and subsequent growth of the bacterial culture.

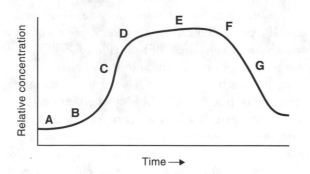

The stages are:

(A) Lag: resting bacteria; minimum metabolism
(B) Acceleration: induction of new enzymes needed to metabolize the nutrients
(C) Exponential (or logarithmic) stage: cell growth is occurring at the fastest rate; numbers increase exponentially, not additively

(D) Deceleration I: metabolism slowing; nutrients being consumed and wastes building up
(E) Stationary: During this time, there is slow loss of cells through death, which is balanced by the formation of new cells through growth and division (binary fusion). When this occurs, the total cell count slowly increases, although the viable count stays constant.
(F) Deceleration II: more bacteria die than are produced by binary fusion
(G) Death: Most bacteria die because of nutrient exhaustion and/or waste buildup. Cell numbers return to a low level, with minimal metabolism occurring (lag phase).

102. The answer is D. *(Behavioral science)*
A low-income 45-year-old man is least likely to make an office visit to a private physician. Patients who visit physicians in their private offices are more likely to be affluent; low-income patients are more likely to seek help in emergency departments of hospitals. Women are more likely than men to visit physicians.

103. The answer is A. *(Biochemistry)*
Acetyl CoA is not a fuel for gluconeogenesis because the reaction that converts pyruvate into acetyl CoA via pyruvate dehydrogenase is irreversible, as shown in the following figure.

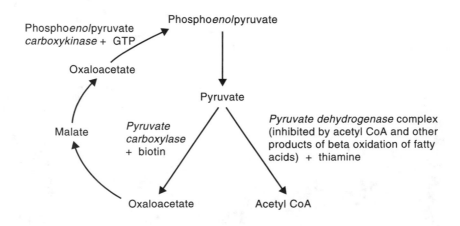

Acetyl CoA, however, does participate in the inactivation of pyruvate dehydrogenase, so that pyruvate preferentially forms oxaloacetate via pyruvate carboxylase. Oxaloacetate is then converted into malate, which is transported from the mitochondria into the cytoplasm where it is converted back into oxaloacetate. The oxaloacetate is then converted into phosphoenolpyruvate using phosphoenlopyruvate carboxykinase and GTP, thus completing the first step in the gluconeogenic process.

Glycerol is only metabolized by the liver, which has glycerol kinase. Glycerol kinase converts glycerol into glycerol 3-phosphate, which is converted into dihydroxyacetone phosphate, a three-carbon intermediate for gluconeogenesis.

Lactate is converted back into pyruvate, the key substrate for gluconeogenesis, by lactate dehydrogenase.

The oxidation of odd-chained fatty acids produces propionyl CoA, which is eventually converted into succinyl CoA in the tricarboxylic acid cycle. Succinyl CoA is eventually converted into succinate→ malate→ oxaloacetate→ glucose.

104. The answer is E. *(Pathology)*
In general, malignant cells have a longer cell cycle than their normal counterpart. Acute leukemias and small cell carcinomas of the lung are exceptions to this rule and commonly have shorter cell cycles than their parent tissue. Malignancy is a problem with greater accumulation rather than removal of malignant cells (more cells are produced than die). Not all of the malignant cells are in the proliferative pool. The majority (97%) of the proliferating cells die. It takes at least 30 doubling times for a malignant tumor to become clinically detectable (1 cm:1 cm^3 = 10^8 - 10^9 cells). Malignant lymphomas, leukemias, and small cell carcinomas of the lung have very high proliferation rates.

Inactivation of suppressor genes and failure to check the growth-promoting oncogenes are common mechanisms in oncogenesis. Inactivation of a suppressor gene for retinal growth (Rb gene) on chromosome 13 is operative in retinoblastoma.

Activation of growth-promoting oncogenes involved in the synthesis of growth-promoting factors (e.g., sis oncogene—platelet derived growth factor), growth factor receptors (e.g., erb oncogenes—epidermal growth factor receptors), generation of signal transducing proteins (second messengers; ras oncogene—GTP binding), or nuclear regulatory proteins (myc oncogenes—translocation and amplification functions) are operative in oncogenesis. Activation occurs by point mutations, chromosome translocations, and gene amplification. Activation of the ras oncogene is the most common oncogene associated with human cancer.

105. The answer is C.   *(Biochemistry)*
Pyruvate, an α-ketoacid, is transaminated into alanine (not aspartate) by alanine aminotransferase.

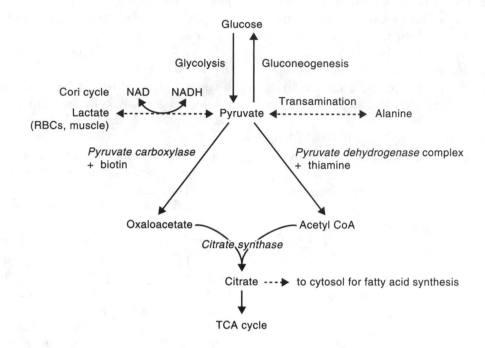

Pyridoxal phosphate is a cofactor in that reaction. Oxaloacetate is transaminated into aspartate using aspartate aminotransferase. Pyruvate is operative in the Cori cycle, wherein lactate derived from red blood cells and muscle is converted into pyruvate by lactate dehydrogenase. Pyruvate is used to generate glucose, which can be used by muscle and red blood cells for fuel. Pyruvate is at the gateway to the tricarboxylic acid cycle. Pyruvate is converted into acetyl CoA via the pyruvate dehydrogenase reaction, using thiamine as a cofactor. It is also converted into oxaloacetate by pyruvate carboxylase, using biotin as a cofactor. Acetyl CoA and oxaloacetate condense to form citrate via citrate synthase. Citrate either remains in the tricarboxylic acid cycle or diffuses into the cytoplasm. In the cytoplasm of the liver, it is converted back into acetyl CoA and oxaloacetate, and the acetyl CoA is used for fatty-acid synthesis.

106. The answer is E.   *(Microbiology)*
Fungi (yeasts and molds) are eukaryotic organisms and differ significantly in structure from prokaryotes.

Bacteria (prokaryotes) have peptidoglycan cell walls, whereas fungi do not.

The fungal cell wall consists primarily of chitin, which is insensitive to penicillins, cephalosporins, and vancomycin. The fungal cell membrane contains ergosterol and zymosterol, in contrast to the human cell membrane, which contains cholesterol. The mechanism of action of amphotericin B is based on this difference. As eukaryotes, the ribosomes are 80S in size, in contrast to the 70S bacterial ribosome.

107. The answer is C.   *(Biochemistry)*
The genetic code is a triplet code. Sixty-one of the sixty-four possible codons represent amino acids, whereas the remaining three codons represent chain termination. The genetic code is degenerate, because a given amino acid can have more than one possible codon. However, the genetic code is not ambiguous, because a given codon always represents only a single amino acid. The codons on a messenger RNA molecule are commaless, or nonoverlapping. The genetic code is said to be universal, because it is the same in

almost all organisms. Mitochondria and a few simple organisms use a slightly modified genetic code.

108. The answer is E. *(Pathology)*
Smoking is the greatest risk factor for lung cancer. Age is the most important risk factor for breast cancer, coronary artery disease, prostate cancer, and colon cancer.

The top three contributors to increased mortality in the United States, in decreasing order of importance, are smoking, diet/exercise, and alcohol.

109. The answer is D. *(Behavioral science)*
Although some 3-year-old children can draw sticklike figures, it is not until approximately the age of 4 that a child can draw a detailed figure of a person. A 3-year-old child can put on shoes without tying the laces, follow a three-step command, and ride a tricycle. Gender identity, the sense of being male or female, develops between 2 and 3 years of age.

110. The answer is D. *(Microbiology)*
Although there are some conflicting data, the consensus is that presentation of antigen by cells of the monocyte-macrophage lineage is impaired in AIDS patients. Antigen presentation is an important accessory function performed by these cells and elicits specific immune responses from lymphocytes.

HIV-1 infects macrophages and persists intracellularly. It either does not multiply or multiplies at a reduced rate compared with CD4$^+$ T lymphocytes.

Migration of HIV-1 infected macrophages in response to chemotactic signals is diminished. Normally, macrophages are highly motile cells and will move to the site of highest concentration of a chemotactic agent.

HIV-1 infected macrophages secrete an inhibitor of interleukin-1, which is called contra-interleukin-1. In healthy individuals, interleukin-1 is secreted by macrophages and other antigen-presenting cells when they come into contact with the antigen and the MHC class II molecule on the T-helper cell surface. Interleukin-1 is a costimulatory signal for T-lymphocyte activation.

The macrophages are thought to be the main reservoir cells for the virus in vivo. Nonactivated, resting CD4$^+$ T lymphocytes can also serve as a reservoir.

Macrophage phagocytosis and killing of bacteria and other ingested materials are also deficient in AIDS patients.

111. The answer is D. *(Behavioral science)*
The factor least likely to be affected by this drug discovery is the incidence rate because discovery of the new drug will not affect the number of new cases of this type of cancer appearing per year (incidence rate). The drug discovery will, however, affect the number of people who die of this cancer per year and, thus, will affect the crude mortality rate (all deaths during a calender year/population at midyear × 1000) and the cause-specific mortality rate (deaths caused by this form of cancer/population × 1000). The point and period prevalence rate (number of people with this form of cancer in the population at a specific point in time or during a specific period of time/ total population) will also be affected when a cure is discovered.

112. The answer is E. *(Microbiology)*
Antibodies specific for p24, the major core protein of the virus, are low at the terminal stage of AIDS and are indicative of a poor prognosis. Their decline is caused by increasing immune complex formation as p24 rises.

Proliferation of T lymphocytes in response to mitogens, such as phytohemagglutinin (PHA), concanavalin A (Con A), and pokeweed is low in HIV-1 infected individuals. In patients with AIDS, the response is especially depressed. Stimulation of the T cells with antigens shows a similar pattern of declining ability to proliferate; response to hepatitis B, influenza, and pneumococcal vaccines decreases as the disease progresses. Proliferation of B lymphocytes incubated with T-independent antigens (such as certain strains of formalinized *Staphylococcus aureus*) also becomes low.

After infection, anti-HIV-1 antibodies are generally not detectable for approximately 2 to 8 weeks. Thus, there can be a relatively long period of time when an individual is infected, but tests negatively for antibodies. The immunoglobulin M (IgM) class appears first and is followed by immunoglobulin G (IgG). These early antibodies are directed against p24 and gp41 (the transmembrane glycoprotein of the virus).

The titer of p24 antigen in the blood (HIV antigenemia) is high early after infection and precedes seroconversion to positive for anti-HIV-1 antibodies.

The level of p24 antigen is high again at the terminal stages of AIDS. The rise of p24 after a period of low levels is a sign of poor prognosis.

113. The answer is E. *(Behavioral science)*
The specialty least likely to have a surplus of physicians by the end of the century is emergency medicine. Shortages are expected in psychiatry, preventive medicine, and hematology/oncology. Physician surpluses are projected in obstetrics and gynecology, internal medicine, ophthalmology, surgery, and neurosurgery.

114-116. The answers are: 114-A, 115-C, 116-E. *(Microbiology)*
The patient is most likely undergoing a type I (anaphylactic) immediate hypersensitivity reaction. The venom of Hymenoptera insects (e.g., wasps, honeybees, hornets, fire ants) is a common allergen. The sting of a single insect may be sufficient to induce a life-threatening reaction.

Other common allergens include pollens (e.g., ragweed), grasses, mold spores, animal danders, dust (actually the airborne feces of the house dust mite), foods (e.g., egg whites, milk, seafood, nuts), and drugs and their metabolic products (e.g., penicillin).

The patient's history, combined with the rapid onset and type of symptoms, strongly suggests that this is a type I reaction; however, a variety of symptoms and various degrees of severity can be seen. The clinical manifestations may include rhinitis and conjunctivitis ("hay fever"), asthma, urticaria (hives), eczema, and gastrointestinal disturbances (vomiting, diarrhea, pain). The symptoms may be localized or systemic.

In type II (cytotoxic) hypersensitivity, antibody binds directly to cells and results in tissue damage because of complement activation or through effector cells with Fc or C3b receptors.

Type III (immune complex) hypersensitivity involves the lodging of immune complexes in the walls of blood vessels, activation of complement, and infiltration of polymorphonuclear cells.

Type IV (delayed-type) hypersensitivity is a T–cell-mediated response against an antigen, which is often persistent and cannot be easily removed or destroyed.

Complement is important in type II and III hypersensitivity reactions, but not in type I or IV.

During the sensitization phase, individuals with type I hypersensitivity produce a high level of immunoglobulin E (IgE) in response to an allergen. This may be caused by an imbalance between IgE helper and suppressor T cells. The response may be partly under the control of major histocompatibility complex (MHC) genes, because type I has a tendency to occur in families. Through its Fc portion, the IgE binds to high-affinity receptors (FcεRI), present in large numbers on mast cells and basophils. Mast cells are significantly more important than basophils in type I hypersensitivity. They are present in high numbers in the skin, mucous membranes, and around blood vessels in connective tissue. The binding of IgE is strong and may persist for weeks.

The activation phase begins upon re-exposure to the allergen. The allergen crosslinks the Fab of two adjacent IgE molecules and causes receptor aggregation. The cells degranulate and release preformed pharmacologically active mediators including histamine, eosinophil chemotactic factor of anaphylaxis (ECF-A), and serotonin. Mediators formed during the late phase reaction via the lipoxygenase pathway of arachidonic acid metabolism include the leukotrienes (LTB_4, LTC_4, LTD_4, and LTE_4; the latter three mediators are sometimes collectively referred to as SRS-A or slow-reacting substance of anaphylaxis). Prostaglandins and thromboxanes are formed via the cyclooxygenase pathway of arachidonic acid metabolism.

The effector phase is mediated by the factors; their effects are summarized below.

Mediator	Effects
Histamine (binds to H1 and H2 receptors)[a]	Smooth muscle contraction Vasodilation Increased vascular permeability
ECF-A	Attracts eosinophils, which release histaminase (degrades histamine) and arylsulfase (degrades SRS-A)
Serotonin (minor importance in humans)	Capillary dilatation Increased vascular permeability Smooth muscle contraction
Leukotrienes (SRS-A)	Increased vascular permeability Smooth muscle contraction
Prostaglandins	Increased vascular permeability Smooth muscle contraction
Thromboxanes	Platelet aggregation

(NOTE: leukotrienes are major mediators of asthma)

[a] Antihistamines compete with histamine for H1 and H2 receptors.

Epinephrine (adrenalin) is the drug of choice in life-threatening systemic anaphylaxis. It relaxes smooth muscle and decreases vascular permeability. It is fast acting.

Topical corticosteroids may work well in patients with small areas of eczema. Large areas of skin involvement may require a course of systemic corticosteroids. Topical corticosteroids will not reverse systemic anaphylaxis.

Cyclosporin A inhibits synthesis and secretion of interleukin-2 by T-helper cells. It is used extensively for immunosuppression of organ transplant patients, but is not very effective in treating type I hypersensitivity.

Methotrexate, an early anticancer drug, inhibits DNA synthesis by blocking dehydrofolate reductase. It is used in patients with autoimmune diseases and for immunosuppression of transplant patients.

Cromolyn sodium is a mast-cell stabilizer. It binds to the membranes of the cells and inhibits the release of pharmacologically active mediators. The drug is used prophylactically by asthmatics and is often present in inhalers. It does not reverse an acute anaphylactic reaction.

Comparison of type I-IV hypersensitivity reactions

Reaction	Mechanism	Result	Treatment
Type I (immediate, anaphylactic)	IgE, mast cells, basophils, histamine, leukotrienes, PGD2, other mediators	Bronchoconstriction, increased vascular permeability, shock, urticaria, eczema, etc.	Antihistamines, epinephrine, cromolyn sodium, hyposensitization, corticosteroids
Type II (cytotoxic)	IgG/IgM, Ag on cells/tissues complement	Cell lysis, tissue damage, transfusion reaction, anemia, erythroblastosis fetalis	Corticosteroids
Type III (immune complex)	Intermediate-size immune complexes, IgG/IgM, complement, PMNs	Arthus, serum sickness, vasculitis, tissue damage, autoimmunity	Aspirin, antihistamines, plasmapheresis, corticosteroids
Type IV (delayed)	T cells, lymphokines, macrophages (later)	Granulomas, contact dermatitis	Corticosteroids

117. The answer is A.   *(Physiology)*
Target-tissue insensitivity to parathyroid hormone (PTH) produces symptoms related to hypoparathyroidism (i.e., decreased serum calcium, increased serum phosphate, decreased activity of 1α-hydroxylase). Furthermore, bone resorption is decreased. However, because of the hypocalcemia, PTH secretion is increased leading to elevated serum levels of the hormone. Target-tissue insensitivity to PTH (pseudohypoparathyroidism) can result from diminished G_s and, therefore, diminished cyclic adenosine monophosphate (cAMP) production.

118. The answer is C.   *(Behavioral science)*
The average income of Native Americans is lower than that of white Americans. Native Americans have higher rates of alcoholism, suicide, emotional problems, and infant mortality than white Americans.

119. The answer is C.   *(Biochemistry)*
DNA replication or DNA synthesis occurs during the S phase of the cell cycle. G_1, S, and G_2 make up interphase. Mitosis completes the cell cycle and is composed of prophase, metaphase, anaphase, and telophase. Cytokinesis is the division of the cell cytoplasm that occurs in telophase and is orchestrated by the microfilaments. Chromatids separate and move toward the poles of the cell in anaphase. The nuclear membrane and nucleolus disappear during metaphase.

120. The answer is B.   *(Behavioral science)*
In aging, there is increased fat relative to muscle. Other physiologic changes associated with aging include impaired immune responses, decreased brain weight, enlarged brain ventricles, and decreased blood flow to the gastrointestinal system.

121. The answer is D.   *(Microbiology)*
Epidermophyton floccosum is the only organism listed that is a dermatophyte [i.e., it infects only superficial, keratinized structures (skin, hair and nails)].

The other fungi listed represent organisms involved in systemic mycoses. *Coccidioides, Blastomyces,* and *Histoplasma* are often dimorphic (i.e., have yeast and fungal forms), with saprophytic mold forms in the soil. Within the lungs, the spores differentiate into yeasts or other specialized forms. Lung infections are most common with these organisms. *Aspergillus* exists only as molds, which can grow in old pulmonary cavities (e.g., posttuberculin) and produce a "fungus ball," which can be seen on a radiograph. It is seen as a complication primarily in immunocompromised individuals.

122. The answer is B.   *(Behavioral science)*
The patient least likely to experience erectile dysfunction is a 65-year-old male Parkinson patient who is taking L-dopa. In contrast to L-dopa, which has a stimulatory effect on sexuality, disulfiram and guanethidine have negative effects on sexual performance. Patients who have had myocardial infarctions often have fears about having another heart attack when they engage in sexual activity and are, thus, likely to experience erectile dysfunction. Patients who have diabetes have circulatory and neurologic problems, which can result in erectile dysfunction.

123. The answer is E.   *(Biochemistry)*
Trehalase breaks down the disaccharide trehalose, which is found only in young mushrooms and insects.

α-Amylase chews disaccharide moieties off the ends of starch until it approaches an α-1,6-glucosidic linkage, producing maltose and limiting dextrans. Isomaltase breaks the 1,6 bonds allowing the α-amylase to continue its work. Maltase hydrolyzes the disaccharide maltose into two glucose moieties. Glucoamylase is an exoglucosidase that chews off terminal glucose molecules. The net result of the action of these four enzymes is that starch is converted to free glucose.

124. The answer is E.   *(Behavioral science)*
By 2 weeks of age, infants show stepping, palmar grasp, the rooting reflex, and the copying of facial expressions. The Babinski reflex is normally positive until a child is approximately 12 months of age.

125. The answer is A. *(Biochemistry)*

Glucose 1-phosphate has no known regulatory function in the glycolytic pathway.

Fructose 6-phosphate is a regulator of glucokinase activity in liver cells. This metabolite inhibits glucokinase activity by promoting the binding of an inhibitory protein to the enzyme. The inhibitory effect is countered by fructose 1-phosphate. These effects are limited to the liver, one of the few organs expressing glucokinase. Most other organs phosphorylate glucose through hexokinase, which is inhibited by glucose 6-phosphate.

Citrate and adenosine triphosphate (ATP) are allosteric inhibitors, and fructose 2,6-bisphosphate is an allosteric activator of phosphofructokinase-1. In the liver, fructose 2,6-bisphosphate overrides the negative effects of ATP and citrate in the hepatocyte, under fed conditions. This permits glycolysis in the liver under high-energy charge conditions when the concentrations of ATP and citrate are high.

This figure illustrates the synthesis of fatty acids from glucose.

phosphofructokinase 1

Glucose → → fructose 6 phosphate ⎯⎯⎯⎯⎯⎯⎯⎯⎯⎯⎯⎯→ fructose 1,6-bisphosphate → → → pyruvate →
acetyl CoA → → citrate → acetyl CoA → malonyl CoA → → → fatty acid

If phosphofructokinase 1 is inhibited, glucose cannot be converted into fatty acids.

126. The answer is D. *(Behavioral science)*

Intelligence is not a characteristic of an individual's temperament. Rather, characteristics of temperament include the level of motor activity, emotional intensity, adaptability to change, and biological predictability.

127. The answer is E.   *(Microbiology)*

Mycobacterium tuberculosis can multiply in virtually all organs of the body; however, the lungs are the primary site of involvement in immunocompetent individuals. In the United States., pulmonary tuberculosis accounts for 85% of active cases, but the majority of infected persons have no evidence of disease except for a positive tuberculin (PPD) skin test. An intense inflammatory response in some patients results in the formation of granulomatous lesions, which eventually are surrounded by a calcified capsule (tubercles). A very small percentage of individuals exhibits little or no resistance to the organisms and the disease progresses rapidly to death.

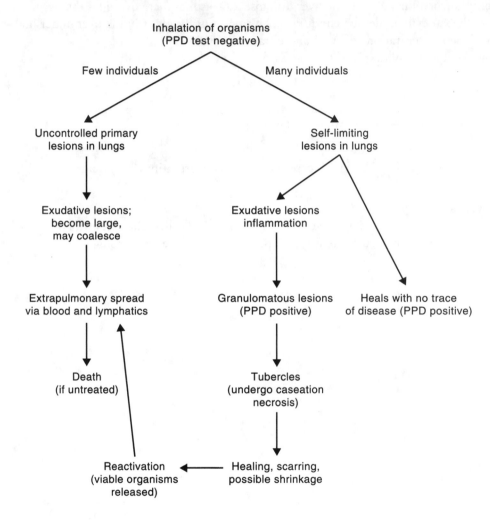

Major determinants in the outcome of infection are the number of inhaled tubercle bacilli, and the resistance and hypersensitivity of the host.

128. The answer is A. *(Behavioral science)*
Adolescents (11–20 years) rather than latency age (6–11 years) children tend to engage in risky behavior. Nine-year-olds typically show interest in artistic projects, are industrious and hard working, and enjoy telling riddles and jokes. Nine-year-olds also understand the concept of conservation, the idea that the quantity of a substance remains the same no matter what size container it is in.

129. The answer is B. *(Biochemistry)*
DNA is found in the eukaryotic cell nucleus; therefore, DNA replication and transcription must occur there. RNA processing events, including the capping of messenger RNA (mRNA) and the removal of introns, also occur in the nucleus. Mature mRNA only moves from the nucleus to the cytoplasm after processing is completed. Translation of the mRNA molecule into the amino acid sequence of a protein occurs in the cytoplasm.

130. The answer is D. *(Microbiology)*
Each molecule of immunoglobulin G (IgG) contains two identical heavy chains and two identical light chains. The two identical antigen-binding sites are each formed by the folding together of the variable portion of one heavy chain and one light chain. These variable portions are located in the amino terminal portion of each polypeptide chain. Although there are many different antibody-producing cells in the body, each individual cell produces just one type of antibody.

131. The answer is C. *(Pathology)*
Lichen sclerosis et atrophicus is a type of vulvar dystrophy characterized by atrophy of the squamous epithelium, unlike the hypertrophic variant, which has hyperplasia (often atypical). The latter type is a risk for vulvar squamous carcinoma.

Koilocytic atypia (vacuolated squamous cells with condensed nuclei) with human papilloma virus types 16, 18, 31 is a precursory lesion for squamous cell carcinoma in the cervix or any other location it is noted in (e.g., anus).

Barrett's esophagus is a precursor lesion for adenocarcinoma of the distal esophagus.

Vaginal adenosis is a precursor lesion for clear cell carcinoma of the vagina. It has a relationship with diethylstilbestrol exposure in the mother.

Intestinal metaplasia in chronic atrophic gastritis is a precursory lesion for adenocarcinoma of the stomach.

132. The answer is A. *(Pathology)*
Xeroderma pigmentosum is an autosomal recessive disease with an abnormality in DNA-repair enzymes and the excision repair of thymidine dimers formed by ultraviolet light damage of DNA. This renders the patients susceptible to basal cell carcinoma, squamous cell carcinoma, and malignant melanomas of the skin.

Ataxia telangiectasia is an autosomal recessive disease with defects in DNA repair to damage induced by ionizing radiation resulting in an increased risk for lymphoid malignancies, cerebellar ataxia, and telangiectasias in the eye. Fanconi syndrome is an autosomal recessive disease involving a defect in DNA-repair enzymes necessary for the removal of crosslinks that form after exposure to certain agents. These syndromes predispose an individual to acute leukemia, aplastic anemia, and carcinomas of the mouth and anus. In addition, they are associated with hypoplasia of the thumbs and radii. A third disease, Bloom syndrome, is also autosomal recessive and has a DNA-repair enzyme defect for damage induced by both ultraviolet light and irradiation. This syndrome predisposes patients to acute leukemia, colon cancer, and growth retardation. These three diseases are part of the chromosome instability syndrome.

Patients with Bruton agammaglobulinemia, a sex-linked recessive disease with a pure B–cell-immunodeficiency state, have a high incidence of autoimmune and immunoproliferative disease (B- and T-cell lymphomas). In general, all patients with immunodeficiency conditions or autoimmune diseases have an increased incidence of malignant lymphomas.

133. The answer is A. *(Pathology)*
Anal carcinoma in homosexuals is related to the human papilloma virus types 16, 18, and 31.

Viruses are potential carcinogens. Acute transforming retroviruses (RNA viruses) already have activated oncogenes (v-oncs) in their genome. These represent captured proto-oncogenes from a host cell that have been activated, so that their reintroduction into a host cell's genome results in a transformed cell. Both RNA and DNA viruses have been implicated in cancer.

Viruses	Cancer relationship
RNA	
Human T-lymphocyte virus-1 (HTLV-1)	HTLV-1 adult T-cell leukemia/lymphoma
HTLV-II	? Hairy cell leukemia
HIV	Kaposi sarcoma
Hepatitis C	Hepatocellular carcinoma
DNA	
Hepatitis B (HBV)	Hepatocellular carcinoma
Epstein-Barr virus (EBV)	Burkitt lymphoma, nasopharyngeal carcinoma, polyclonal malignant lymphoma
Human papilloma virus (HPV)	Squamous carcinoma of the cervix, vagina, and vulva; anus in homosexuals

Retroviruses are RNA viruses that have reverse transcriptase (an RNA-dependent DNA polymerase). Reverse transcriptase converts RNA of the virus into DNA, which is then inserted into the host cell's genome. Acute transforming retroviruses already have activated oncogenes (v-oncs) that directly transform a host cell when it is infected. Slow-transforming viruses do not have v-oncs. Some of them activate proto-oncogenes (normally functioning oncogenes) in the host cell by inserting their genome above or below a proto-oncogene, causing them to overexpress their gene product (gene amplification). Other viruses inactivate suppressor genes. HTLV-1 retroviruses are associated with T-cell leukemia/ lymphomas. Once integrated into the T-cell genome, they code for a gene product that stimulates the formation of interleukin 2 and granulocyte/macrophage colony-stimulating factors. This results in T-cell proliferation and increases the chances of mutation, leading to full-blown T-cell leukemia/lymphoma. HPV apparently inactivates suppressor genes, leading to squamous cell carcinoma.

DNA viruses differ from retroviruses in that they do not require reverse transcriptase. They cannot both integrate and replicate themselves at the same time without killing the cell. DNA viruses are oncogenic by either inactivating a suppressor gene or activating a proto-oncogene.

Unlike chemically induced tumors that have different tumor antigens for every tumor, virally induced tumors have tumor antigens that are the same in all the tumors.

134. The answer is D. *(Biochemistry)*
Sphingomyelin is formed by adding phosphorylcholine to ceramide. Ceramide is formed by adding a fatty acid to sphingosine. Sphingosine is formed by condensing palmitic acid with a decarboxylated serine and then reducing the product. Glycerol never is involved in the structure of sphingomyelin.

Phosphotidylethanolamine, cardiolipin, phosphotidylcholine, and phosphotidylinositol are synthesized using phosphatidic acid as the basic building block. Phosphatic acid is diacylglycerol with a phosphate ester on carbon three; therefore, glycerol is the backbone of all of these compounds.

135-138. The answers are: 135-C, 136-B, 137-A, 138-D. *(Pathology)*
Bromocriptine is a dopamine agonist. Because dopamine is a prolactin-inhibiting hormone, treatment with bromocriptine should diminish prolactin secretion by pituitary adenomas.

Menopause results from exhaustion of ovarian follicles and hence decreased secretion of estrogen. The low estrogen level removes feedback inhibition of the secretion of follicle-stimulating hormone (FSH) and luteinizing hormone (LH). Therefore, the blood level of both gonadotropins increases. The increase in FSH is greater than the increase in LH.

In pregnancy, estrogen and progesterone levels rise throughout the 40 weeks. Progesterone is made in the placenta from maternal cholesterol. Estrogen (primarily estriol) is made in the placenta from fetal 16-OH dehydroepiandrosterone sulphate (DHEAS). Feedback inhibition by estrogen and progesterone keeps serum levels of LH and FSH low.

Sheehan syndrome results from anterior pituitary infarction associated with hemorrhage during parturition.

139-143. The answers are: 139-B, 140-A, 141-E, 142-H, 143-C. *(Pharmacology)*

Isoproterenol activates cardiac beta$_1$ receptors to increase heart rate, and propranolol is an antagonist at these receptors. Both drugs also bind to beta$_2$ receptors.

Skeletal muscle relaxation is produced by pancuronium, which is a competitive antagonist of acetylcholine at the skeletal neuromuscular junction.

Phenylephrine produces vasoconstriction by activating adrenergic alpha$_1$ receptors—an effect that is blocked by the receptor antagonist prazosin.

Histamine acts to increase the permeability of vascular endothelial cells—an effect that can be blocked by diphenhydramine.

Pupillary constriction (miosis) is produced by acetylcholine, and is blocked by the muscarinic receptor antagonist atropine.

144-149. The answers are: 144-E, 145-E, 146-H, 147-D, 148-G, 149-D. *(Biochemistry)*

Phosphatidylinositol 1,4,5-trisphosphate is cleaved at the phosphate ester bond of glycerol by membrane-bound phospholipase C, producing inositol-1,4,5, trisphosphate and diacylglycerol. Both products are second messengers (intracellular molecules, relaying information carried by hormones that interact with cell surface receptors to enzymes, which act to alter metabolic function). Inositol 1,4,5,-trisphosphate serves to increase intracellular free calcium levels, while diacylglycerol, in the presence of calcium ion, serves as an allosteric activator of protein kinase C.

The fatty acid on the second carbon of phosphatidylinositol and its phosphorylated derivatives is usually arachidonic acid, which is liberated by the action of phospholipase A$_2$. This reaction is inhibited by corticosteroids.

The plasmalogens are phospholipids in which the fatty acid on carbon 1 is linked to the glycerol moiety by an ether, rather than an ester bond. This difference is noted in their names by the use of an "al," rather than "yl." (Note the difference in spelling between choices C and H.) The plasmalogens and their derivatives are important biologic compounds. Myelin contains considerable ethanolamine plasmalogen and heart contains much choline plasmalogen. The platelet-activating factor (PAF) is a plasmalogen derivative, which serves as a major mediator of hypersensitivity, acute inflammatory reactions, and anaphylactic shock.

Dipalmitoylphosphotidylcholine serves as the major lung surfactant. It decreases the surface tension of the extracellular fluid surrounding the alveoli, preventing their collapse. Respiratory distress syndrome is associated with a deficiency of this compound. Glucocorticoids and thyroxine enhance its synthesis by type II pneumocytes. Insulin inhibits its synthesis.

Cardiolipin is an important phospholipid found in the inner mitochondrial membrane. It is also the only human phospholipid that is antigenic. Anticardiolipin antibodies are associated with vascular thrombosis, frequently responsible for fetal wastage.

The three methyl groups of phosphatidylcholine (lecithin) must be derived from S-adenosylmethionine (SAM). Because methionine is an essential amino acid often present in limited amounts in the diet, the presence of preformed choline in the diet can be of clinical significance.

150-154. The answers are: 150-B, 151-D, 152-C, 153-A, 154-E. *(Pharmacology)*

Both acylovir and ganciclovir are activated by a viral kinase, making them selective for virus-infected cells. Acylovir is less active against cytomegalovirus, whereas ganciclovir is more active against this virus (and more toxic to host cells). Zidovudine (AZT, Retrovir) is one of several inhibitors of reverse transcriptase and is active against retroviruses including HIV. Ribavirin is a guanosine analog that blocks guanosine phosphate formation and is active against a wide range of viruses, particularly respiratory syncytial virus that causes pneumonia in neonates.

155-160. The answers are: 155-G, 156-A, 157-E, 158-D, 159-B, 160-F. *(Biochemistry)*

When blood glucose levels are low, glucagon levels increase and insulin levels decrease. Glucagon binds to a membrane receptor. This changes the conformation of a G$_s$ protein in the membrane, which in turn activates adenylate cyclase (A) to produce cyclic adenosine monophosphate (cAMP). The cAMP activates protein kinase A (B), which phosphorylates many proteins, including glycogen synthetase A (E) and phosphorylase kinase (G). Phosphorylated glycogen synthetase is inactive; phosphorylated phosphorylase kinase is active. Because this latter enzyme phosphorylates inactive phosphorylase, activating it, this mechanism serves to inhibit glycogen synthesis and activate glycogenolysis in a synchronous fashion, producing from glucose 1-phosphate and inhibiting its utilization to form more glycogen. In the liver, this glucose 6-phosphate formed from glucose 1-phosphate is hydrolyzed to free glucose, which is released into the blood. The enzyme catalyzing this reaction is glucose-6-phosphatase.

Once blood glucose levels are restored, the glucagon levels decrease and insulin levels increase. The decrease in glucagon inhibits the cascade, whereas the increase in insulin activates phosphatases, which reverse the phosphorylations. In this way, protein phosphatase 1 is activated (D), converting the inactivated glycogen synthetase back to active nonphosphorylated synthetase and the active phosphorylase kinase back to the inactive nonphosphorylated phosphorylase kinase. The decrease in the glucagon:insulin ratio also activates cAMP diesterase (F), converting it to AMP. The latter reaction is inhibited by methylxanthines, such as caffeine and theophylline.

161-165. The answers are: 161-C, 162-B, 163-A, 164-C, 165-D. (Pharmacology)

Aminoglycosides such as streptomycin bind to the 30S ribosomal subunit and block the formation of the initiation complex. They also cause misreading of messenger RNA (mRNA) and the insertion of incorrect amino acids into the growing peptide. Tetracyclines and chloramphenicol prevent the binding of transfer RNA (tRNA) to the 30S subunit, a reaction that is reversible and consistent with their bacteriostatic effects. Chloramphenicol and erythromycin inhibit peptidyl transferase and the addition of a new amino acid to the peptide chain, whereas erythromycin and clindamycin block the translocation step whereby the peptide chain is transferred to the peptidyl site from the aminoacyl site in preparation for the addition of the next amino acid. Both chloramphenicol and erythromycin bind to the 50S subunit to exert their effects.

166-168. The answers are: 166-C, 167-E, 168-A. (Physiology)

An adrenocorticotropic hormone (ACTH)-secreting tumor produces elevated plasma levels of ACTH, which act at the zona fasciculata and zona reticularis of the adrenal cortex to increase steroidogenesis. Cortisol secretion increases, but aldosterone secretion is usually normal.

Secondary adrenal insufficiency results from decreased secretion of ACTH from the anterior pituitary. Therefore, plasma ACTH and cortisol levels are decreased. Because ACTH is not the long-term regulator of aldosterone secretion from the zona glomerulosa of the adrenal cortex, secondary adrenal insufficiency is not usually associated with decreased aldosterone or symptoms of mineralocorticoid deficiency.

In Addison disease, adrenal dysfunction usually includes all zones of the adrenal cortex. Therefore, plasma levels of both cortisol and aldosterone are decreased. Plasma ACTH is increased because of loss of feedback inhibition by cortisol.

169-172. The answers are: 169-D, 170-C, 171-A, 172-E. (Biochemistry)

Apolipoprotein-E is transferred from high-density lipoprotein (HDL) to the nascent chylomicron and to nascent very low-density lipoprotein (VLDL) particles. Apolipoprotein E serves as a recognition site for receptors in the liver that induce endocytosis of spent chylomicrons (remnants). In the absence of apolipoprotein E, these remnant chylomicrons accumulate in the blood.

Intermediate-density lipoproteins (IDL) also accumulate. Ordinarily, apolipoprotein E is passed from IDL to HDL when IDL is converted to low-density lipoprotein (LDL). The absence of apolipoprotein E inhibits the conversion of IDL to HDL and results in an accumulation of the former.

Individuals with this disorder develop palmar xanthomas and often have coronary or vascular disease by middle age because of increased levels of triglycerides and cholesterol from the accumulated chylomicron and IDL remnants.

Apolipoprotein C-II is transferred from HDL to the nascent chylomicrons and VLDL particles, along with apolipoprotein E. Apolipoprotein C-II activates capillary lipoprotein lipase, an extracellular enzyme, which degrades triacylglycerol and cholesterol esters, permitting cholesterol and fatty acids to be taken up by surrounding tissues.

This disorder results in a massive accumulation of triacylglycerol-rich lipoproteins (chylomicrons) in the plasma. A more common mechanism for a syndrome having a very similar phenotype is lipoprotein lipase deficiency.

Most cells have a receptor that recognizes apolipoprotein B-100 on the surface of circulating LDL particles. These receptors reside in a clathrin-coated pit on the surface of a cell. When they bind to an LDL particle, the coated pit with the LDL moiety is engulfed and internalized as an endosome. The receptor is then removed and returned to the surface. The endosome is converted into a lysosome, in which the proteins are broken down into amino acids and the esters into free fatty acid and cholesterol.

Phosphatidylcholine:cholesterol acyltransferase (PCAT) (also called lecithin:choline transferase [LCAT]) is a plasma enzyme, synthesized in the liver. It transfers the fatty acid from carbon 2 of lecithin to cholesterol. This traps the resulting cholesterol ester in the HDL, thus preventing its possible transfer to a membrane, where it may contribute to plaque formation. Levels of PCAT are increased by modest intake of ethanol.

173-177. The answers are: 173-C, 174-B, 175-G, 176-D, 177-E. *(Pharmacology)*
α_2-Adrenergic receptors are primarily presynaptic autoreceptors that mediate feedback inhibition of neurotransmitter release by inhibiting adenylyl cyclase and decreasing cyclic adenosine monophosphate (cAMP) formation.

α_1-Adrenergic receptors mediate vasoconstriction through the formation of inositol triphosphate (IP_3) and the subsequent release of calcium from the sacroplasmic reticulum.

Bronchoconstriction is mediated by muscarinic receptors via formation of IP_3 and the subsequent release of calcium.

β_1- and β_2-Adrenergic receptors activate adenylyl cyclase and increase cAMP levels in smooth muscle and cardiac muscle, leading to smooth muscle relaxation (vasodilation) and cardiac stimulation, respectively.

178-180. The answers are: 178-E, 179-D, 180-C. *(Biochemistry)*
Homeotic proteins contain a homeodomain and regulate development in all eukaryotes. The homeodomain binds to specific DNA sequences and regulates gene expression. Because these proteins function by binding to DNA, they are specifically found in the cell nucleus.

Carbamoylphosphate synthetase I synthesizes carbamoylphosphate from CO_2, NH_4^+, and adenosine triphosphate (ATP) in the mitochondrion. The enzyme requires N-acetylglutamate for activity, and it provides carbamoylphosphate for the urea cycle. The formation of carbamoylphosphate and its reaction with ornithine to form citrulline occur in the mitochondrion. The remainder of the urea cycle occurs in the cytosol. A related enzyme, carbamoylphosphate synthetase II, is located in the cytosol and provides carbamoylphosphate for the synthesis of pyrimidines.

Glycosylation of secretory proteins is a posttranslational modification that begins in the endoplasmic reticulum. Further modification of the oligosaccharide structures occurs as the protein moves from the endoplasmic reticulum to the Golgi apparatus. Terminal glycosylation, or addition of the sugar residues at the end of each oligosaccharide branch, occurs in the Golgi apparatus before the protein is secreted from the cell.

Test 2

QUESTIONS

DIRECTIONS:

Each of the numbered items or incomplete statements in this section is followed by answers or by completions of the statement. Select the ONE lettered answer or completion that is BEST in each case.

1.   A psychiatrist hypothesizes that the extent of physical disability following a stroke is related to personality type. To test this hypothesis, a study is designed in which 500 patients are classified according to their physical deficit as mildly or severely affected and assigned to one of two personality groups. The statistical test that is most appropriate for analyzing these data is the

(A)   independent t-test
(B)   chi-square test
(C)   correlation
(D)   analysis of variance
(E)   paired t-test

2.   Which one of the following statements is true regarding generalized transducing phages (e.g., phage P1)?

(A)   Bacterial DNA is carried in every phage particle
(B)   The entire bacterial chromosome is carried within a single phage particle
(C)   Only particular host genes are carried in the phage particle
(D)   The phage particle integrates into the host chromosome at one specific site
(E)   The phage will only affect genes that are near each other in the host chromosome

Questions 3-4

The diagram below represents a mature messenger RNA (mRNA) molecule coding for the heavy chain of an immunoglobulin.

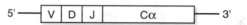

3.   Which type of immunoglobulin would contain the product from this message?

(A)   Immunoglubulin A (IgA)
(B)   Immunoglobulin D (IgD)
(C)   Immunoglobulin E (IgE)
(D)   Immunoglobulin G (IgG)
(E)   Immunoglobulin M (IgM)

4.   Which one of the following statements is true regarding this message?

(A)   The 5′ end contains poly A
(B)   The message contains introns
(C)   The C (α) portion codes for part of the antigen binding site
(D)   The VDJ portion will be translated before the C (α) portion
(E)   Translation of this message will be initiated in the lumen of the endoplasmic reticulum

5.   Which one of the following statements concerning plasmids is true?

(A)   All plasmids possess the information for their own transfer by conjugation
(B)   Much of the information coded in the plasmid is essential to the survival of the bacteria cell
(C)   R plasmids carry genes for antibiotic resistance
(D)   R plasmids cannot be transferred to other bacterial cells
(E)   Plasmids lack an origin of replication

6.   In which of the following sites is a tumor more likely to occur in adults than in children?

(A) Soft tissue
(B) Lungs
(C) Central nervous system
(D) Bone
(E) Kidney

7.   How do tetracyclines inhibit bacterial growth?

(A) They prevent protein synthesis at the 30S ribosomal subunit
(B) They prevent protein synthesis at the 50S ribosomal subunit
(C) They inhibit bacterial RNA polymerase
(D) They prevent peptide bond formation
(E) They interfere with folic acid metabolism

8.   In the Ames test, a chemical compound to be studied is incubated with a rat liver extract and then used to treat histidine-deficient mutants of *Salmonella typhimurium*. The purpose of the rat liver extract is to

(A) provide histidine for bacterial growth
(B) metabolically convert the tested compound to a mutagenic derivative
(C) make the bacteria competent for transformation
(D) help the tested compound penetrate the bacterial cell wall
(E) provide growth factors necessary for *Salmonella* cell division

9.   Which of the following types of cancers is most common in organ transplant recipients?

(A) Skin cancer
(B) Breast cancer
(C) Lung cancer
(D) Prostate cancer
(E) Pancreatic cancer

10.   Tumor size is most often associated with malignancy potential in

(A) renal adenocarcinoma
(B) breast adenocarcinoma
(C) prostate adenocarcinoma
(D) colon adenocarcinoma
(E) squamous cell carcinoma of the lung

11.   The following serologic test results for hepatitis were reported: hepatitis A virus immunoglobulin M (HAV IgM), negative; hepatitis B surface antigen (HBsAg), positive; antibody to HBsAg, positive. What is the patient's status?

(A) Susceptible to hepatitis B virus infection
(B) Immune to hepatitis B virus infection
(C) Immune to hepatitis C virus infection
(D) Chronic carrier of hepatitis B virus
(E) Requires a hepatitis B virus vaccination booster

12.   Which of the following statements about collagen is correct?

(A) Collagen has a compact, globular structure
(B) Collagen has a double-helical structure
(C) The ribosome incorporates hydroxyproline and hydroxylysine into the polypeptide chain as the messenger RNA is translated
(D) The N- and C-terminal propeptides are cleaved before the molecule enters the endoplasmic reticulum
(E) Collagen normally functions outside the cell

13.   Which one of the following Gram-negative rods produces no reaction on triple-sugar iron agar, is oxidase positive, and produces blue-green pigments?

(A) *Neisseria gonorrhoeae*
(B) *Branhamella catarrhalis*
(C) *Escherichia coli*
(D) *Salmonella typhi*
(E) *Pseudomonas aeruginosa*

14. Compared with a healthy 30-year-old man, laboratory test results in a healthy 80-year-old man have

(A) similar creatinine clearance
(B) slightly increased hemoglobin concentration
(C) similar partial pressure of arterial oxygen (PaO$_2$)
(D) increased serum alkaline phosphatase
(E) similar forced expiratory volume 1 second

15. Fraction I antigen is associated with both virulence and immunity in

(A) *Francisella tularensis*
(B) *Brucella melitensis*
(C) *Yersinia enterocolitica*
(D) *Yersinia pseudotuberculosis*
(E) *Yersinia pestis*

16. Which of the following laboratory test results would a healthy 30-year-old woman have when compared with those of a healthy 30-year-old man?

	Hemoglobin concentration	Serum high-density lipoproteins (HDL)	Serum ferritin
(A)	Equal	Equal	Equal
(B)	Equal	Increased	Decreased
(C)	Decreased	Increased	Equal
(D)	Decreased	Decreased	Decreased
(E)	Decreased	Increased	Decreased

17. In the Ziehl-Neelsen acid-fast staining procedure, the carbolfuschin dye stains mycobacteria which color?

(A) Blue
(B) Red
(C) Green
(D) Yellow-orange
(E) No color

18. Which of the following statements concerning the Recommended Dietary Allowance (RDA) is correct?

(A) There is one RDA recommendation that is designed to meet the caloric requirements of 95% of the men in the United States population
(B) There is one RDA recommendation that usually fits the needs of 95% of both men and women in the United States population
(C) The RDA recommendations are designed to meet the minimal daily requirement for most individuals, after making allowances for gender and age
(D) The RDA recommendations are designed to meet the optimal requirement for 95% of the United States population, after making allowances for gender and age
(E) The RDA recommendations are designed to prevent well-recognized deficiency syndromes in 95% of the United States population, after making allowances for gender and age

19. Which of the following laboratory test results would a healthy 5-year-old child have when compared with those of a healthy adult?

	Hemoglobin concentration	Serum alkaline phosphatase	Serum phosphorus
(A)	Equal	Equal	Equal
(B)	Increased	Increased	Increased
(C)	Decreased	Increased	Increased
(D)	Decreased	Increased	Equal
(E)	Equal	Increased	Increased

20. Following a major traffic accident, Jane Doe (blood group B) and John Doe (blood group A) are rushed to the emergency room. Donor blood for Jane is erroneously transfused into John. Within minutes, John develops a fever, chills, dyspnea, and a dramatic decrease in blood pressure. This reaction is most likely because of

(A) immunoglobulin M (IgM) production by the recipient in response to the B antigen
(B) anti-B isohemagglutinin of the IgM class preformed in the recipient
(C) a cell-mediated response against the A antigen of the recipient
(D) immunoglobulin G (IgG) production by the recipient in response to the infused red blood cells
(E) anti-A isohemagglutinin of the IgM class present in the recipient

21. When blood is collected in a clot tube (red top) and spun down the centrifuge, the liquid above the clot contains

(A) fibrinogen
(B) factor V
(C) factor VIII
(D) platelets
(E) factors VII, IX, and X

22. A 25-year-old male stockbroker prefers to wear women's sexy underclothing beneath his pinstriped suit. Which one of the following statements is most likely to be true about this man?

(A) He has a male gender identity
(B) He has sexual interest in other men
(C) He would like to have a sex-change operation
(D) He is very distressed about this preference
(E) He has a female gender role

23. Which of the following statements about preanalytic variables affecting laboratory test results is correct?

(A) In patients who are having a lipid profile, fasting is required to obtain an accurate serum cholesterol and high-density lipoprotein concentration
(B) Diurnal analytes, such as serum iron and cortisol, are typicallly collected in the afternoon when they are at peak concentration
(C) The serum lactate dehydrogenase and serum potassium levels are falsely elevated in hemolyzed samples
(D) A sample of blood that is visibly turbid has an increase primarily in the low-density lipoprotein fraction
(E) Collecting venous blood from above an intravenous line containing 5% dextrose and water has no significant effect on the patient's serum glucose or electrolyte results

Questions 24-25

A 28-year-old woman in labor is rushed to the hospital by her husband. It is quickly determined she has blood group type A and is Rh negative. She has a 3-year-old child who is Rh positive, and the father is Rh positive.

24. The infant is most likely at risk for developing

(A) drug-induced hemolytic anemia

(B) neutropenia

(C) an autoimmune disease

(D) Rh hemolytic disease of the newborn

(E) ABO incompatibility

25. Which of the following agents will most likely protect the baby from developing the disease?

(A) Rh-positive erythrocytes

(B) Plasma from randomly selected donors

(C) Albumin from Rh-positive donors

(D) A transfusion of platelets

(E) Anti-Rh antibody (Rh immunoglobulin)

26. The mechanism of cellular swelling in tissue hypoxia is most closely associated with

(A) free radical injury of the cell

(B) a dysfunctional adenosine triphosphate (ATP)–dependent sodium–potassium pump

(C) calcium entering the mitochondria

(D) irreversible injury to the cell membrane

(E) the detachment of ribosomes from the rough endoplasmic reticulum

27. A patient presents with the classic symptoms of mild but chronic beriberi. He takes a multivitamin and mineral supplement daily, which contain minimum Recommended Daily Allowance (RDA) levels for all known micronutrients. A blood sample is sent for enzymatic studies. The most logical finding consistent with his symptoms is

(A) a white blood cell pyruvate dehydrogenase with a high K_m value for thiamine pyrophosphate

(B) a red blood cell transketolase with a high K_m value for thiamine pyrophosphate

(C) a red blood cell glucose-6-phosphate dehydrogenase with a high K_m value for oxidized nicotinamide adenine dinucleotide phosphate ($NADP^+$)

(D) a white blood cell cytoplasmic isocitrate dehydrogenase with a high K_m value for $NADP^+$

(E) a red blood cell α-ketoglutarate dehydrogenase with a high K_m value for thiamine pyrophosphate

28. Which of the following cell organelles and their associated biochemical processes is most affected during the early phase of tissue hypoxia?

(A) Mitochondria—β-oxidation of fatty acids

(B) Rough endoplasmic reticulum—protein synthesis

(C) Mitochondria—oxidative phosphorylation

(D) Smooth endoplasmic reticulum—cytochrome system

(E) Nucleus—DNA synthesis

29. *Streptococcus pyogenes* and *Staphylococcus aureus* produce "beta" and "clear zone" hemolysis, which is caused by

(A) hemolysins completely destroying the red blood cells

(B) hemolysins incompletely destroying the red blood cells

(C) released hemoglobin from red blood cells, causing a green discoloration

(D) the bacteria attaching to red blood cells, causing hemagglutination

(E) hemolysins with no effect on red blood cells, causing no lysis

30. Fibrinoid necrosis is most likely found in which of the following biopsy specimens?

(A) Damaged cardiac tissue secondary to an acute myocardial infarction
(B) Punch biopsy from the skin of a patient with palpable purpura
(C) Renal biopsy tissue from a patient with diabetic nephropathy
(D) Section of terminal ileum from a patient with Crohn disease
(E) Lung biopsy of a solitary coin lesion in the right upper lobe

31. An overweight patient has a daily caloric expenditure of 2000 cal. He is placed on a diet of 1000 cal per day. Assume that 1kg = 2 lbs. If the patient adheres to this diet, how long will it take him to lose 2 lbs of fat?

(A) 1 day
(B) 3 days
(C) 5 days
(D) 7 days
(E) 9 days

32. Which of the following growth alterations is an example of hyperplasia rather than metaplasia?

(A) Increased goblet cells in the mainstem bronchus of a smoker
(B) Squamous epithelium in the bladder of a patient with *Schistosoma haematobium*
(C) Distal esophagus with glandular epithelium intermixed with squamous epithelium
(D) Goblet and Paneth cells in the glands of the gastric mucosa
(E) Squamous epithelium in the mainstem bronchus of a smoker

33. The major problem of a person with an antisocial personality disorder is most likely to be in the part of the mind that Freud called the

(A) id
(B) ego
(C) superego
(D) preconscious
(E) unconscious

34. Which of the following growth alterations is an example of hypertrophy rather than hyperplasia?

(A) Thickened bladder wall in a patient with urethral obstruction
(B) Increased reticulocyte count in a patient with a hemolytic anemia
(C) Breast tissue in a woman with a prolactinoma
(D) Biopsy of the endometrium taken a few days before ovulation
(E) Prostate enlargement in an elderly man with difficulty initiating his urinary stream

35. Energy consumption is used to support basal metabolism, the thermic effect of food (i.e., specific dynamic action), and activity. Which of the following statements most accurately describes one or more of these functions?

(A) The basal metabolic rate (BMR) is invariant in a given individual at a given time; it cannot be influenced by diet or exercise
(B) The thermic effect of food accounts for 30% to 50% of the caloric expenditure of most individuals
(C) Physical activity accounts for 50% or more of the caloric expenditure in most sedentary individuals
(D) The greatest variability in caloric expenditure is through physical activity
(E) Mental activity, such as studying, increases the caloric expenditure by the brain to a significant extent

36. In which of the following combinations are both abnormalities reversible?

(A) Enzymatic fat necrosis in the pancreas—fat necrosis in the previously traumatized breast tissue of a woman
(B) Cellular swelling in ischemic myocardial tissue—myocardial tissue exhibiting eosinophilia, absent cross striations, and karyolysis
(C) Fatty change in the liver of an individual with alcoholism—mild cervical dysplasia
(D) Squamous metaplasia in the vocal cords of a smoker—carcinoma in situ of the cervix
(E) Small airway disease in bronchial asthma—centrilobular emphysema in a smoker

37. A man driving from San Diego, California, to Bar Harbor, Maine, using the southern route across the United States, presents to a physician in Maine with fever, nonproductive cough, and flu-like symptoms. The physician would strongly suspect that the patient has which one of the following infections?

(A) Histoplasmosis
(B) Aspergillosis
(C) Sporotrichosis
(D) Coccidioidomycosis
(E) Mycetoma

38. In which of the following combinations do both diseases involve either a different type of pigment or of accumulation?

(A) Vitiligo and albinism
(B) Stasis dermatitis and hemochromatosis
(C) Pompe and McArdle diseases
(D) Gaucher and von Gierke diseases
(E) Xanthelasma and Achilles tendon xanthoma

39. Which of the followings statements concerning fat in the diet is the most accurate?

(A) Coconut and palm oils have a higher percentage of saturated fatty acids than lard or butter
(B) If an individual consumes sufficient unsaturated fatty acid from only linoleic, he will receive all the essential fatty acids required for optimal health
(C) Margarine is an important source of essential fatty acids, because it is derived from oils that are rich in polyunsaturated fatty acids
(D) Potatoes fried in oils that are rich in unsaturated fatty acids have greater nutritional value than those cooked in monounsaturated or saturated oils
(E) According to the dietary goals for the American public set by various agencies, the fat content of an individual's diet should be about 30% of his total diet by weight

40. In which of the following pathologic processes does apoptosis play a dominant role?

(A) Acute myocardial infarction
(B) Acute appendicitis
(C) Ischemic atrophy in the brain
(D) Type III hypersensitivity reactions
(E) Formation of a venous thrombus

41. The stage of the sexual response cycle likely to differentiate most between men and women is

(A) excitement
(B) plateau
(C) orgasm
(D) resolution
(E) anticipation

42. An alcoholic with chronic obstructive lung disease takes theophylline as prescribed to improve his breathing. If a blood sample is drawn immediately before his next dose of theophylline, a low serum theophylline would most likely be caused by

(A) decreased uptake in the gastrointestinal tract
(B) increased uptake in the body fat
(C) decreased excretion in the urine
(D) alcohol blocking the reabsorption of the drug
(E) increased metabolism of the drug in the liver

43. A 35-year-old man who enjoys hunting jackrabbits has a sudden onset of headache, fever, chills, and swollen lymph nodes. He also experiences nausea, vomiting, and abdominal discomfort. A painful papule on his left hand heals over a period of about 6 weeks, and his lymphadenopathy subsides approximately 4 months later. No microorganisms are seen in lymph node aspirates, and routine blood cultures are negative. Which of the following organisms is the most likely causative agent?

(A) *Yersinia pestis*
(B) *Yersinia enterocolitica*
(C) *Francisella tularensis*
(D) *Pasteurella multocida*
(E) *Brucella melitensis*

44. A 45-year-old man is taking theophylline for chronic obstructive lung disease and cimetidine for duodenal ulcer disease. He is taking the medications as prescribed. If a blood sample is drawn before his next doses, a toxic level of theophylline would most likely be caused by

(A) decreased metabolism in the liver
(B) decreased uptake in the body fat
(C) decreased excretion in the urine
(D) decreased uptake in the liver
(E) increased reabsorption in the gastrointestinal tract

45. Renal impairment necessitates reducing the dose or increasing the dosage interval of which of the following antibiotics?

(A) Azithromycin
(B) Gentamicin
(C) Doxycycline
(D) Ceftriaxone
(E) Nafcillin

46. Which one of the following organisms is the most common cause of neonatal meningitis?

(A) *Streptococcus pyogenes*
(B) *Listeria monocytogenes*
(C) *Staphylococcus aureus*
(D) *Streptococcus pneumoniae*
(E) *Streptococcus agalactiae*

47. Of the following male sexual dysfunctions, the most common dysfunction is

(A) premature ejaculation
(B) male orgasmic disorder
(C) sexual desire disorder
(D) primary erectile disorder
(E) dyspareunia

48. Which one of the following diseases is most likely to be diagnosed by performing a blood culture?

(A) *Staphylococcus* food poisoning
(B) Toxic shock syndrome
(C) Rheumatic fever
(D) Infant botulism
(E) Meningococcemia

49. Which one of the following enzymes can seal "nicks" in DNA?

(A) DNA polymerase I
(B) DNA ligase
(C) Helicase
(D) DNA polymerase III
(E) Endonuclease

50. A 49-year-old woman is bitten by her cat on the dorsal aspect of her right index finger at 8:00 am. By 4:30 pm, she has a temperature of 38°C, and the finger and the dorsum of her right hand are red, swollen, and painful. An oxidase- and catalase- positive, gram-negative rod with bipolar staining is recovered from an aspirate of the abscess on her finger. The organism most likely responsible is

(A) *Brucella canis*
(B) *Pasteurella multocida*
(C) *Haemophilus influenzae*
(D) *Francisella tularensis*
(E) *Yersinia pseudotuberculosis*

51. Which one of the following reflexes describes the tendency for an infant to turn its head in the direction of the cheek that is stroked?

(A) Babinski reflex
(B) Rooting reflex
(C) Grasp reflex
(D) Moro reflex
(E) Knee reflex

52. In which of the following diseases can the causative agent be identified in a peripheral blood smear?

(A) Relapsing fever
(B) Syphilis
(C) Pinta
(D) Leptospirosis
(E) Yaws

53. Which one of the following antibiotics is believed to pose the least risk to the fetus when used to treat an infection in a pregnant patient?

(A) Tetracycline
(B) Cephalexin
(C) Amikacin
(D) Griseofulvin
(E) Streptomycin

54. Which of the following statements about syphilis is correct?

(A) A single injection of penicillin cures the disease in early stages
(B) A hypersensitivity reaction to penicillin is called Jarisch-Herxheimer reaction
(C) The incidence of the disease is declining in the United States
(D) Treponemes are easily eradicated from the central nervous system
(E) Drug-resistant strains of *Treponema pallidum* have been isolated

55. Gender identity is normally established by which of the following age ranges?

(A) 0 to 1 years
(B) 1 to 2 years
(C) 2 to 3 years
(D) 3 to 4 years
(E) 4 to 5 years

56. Which of the following statements about *Mycoplasma* is correct?

(A) They are the smallest organisms capable of multiplying in cell-free media
(B) They are wall-defective organisms that can revert back to their parental forms
(C) Humans are the only natural hosts
(D) They are primarily associated with disease in the elderly
(E) They are genetically related to L-forms

57. Myelosuppression caused by large doses of methotrexate can be prevented by which one of the following actions of leucovorin?

(A) It acts as a methotrexate receptor antagonist
(B) It accelerates maturation of granulocyte precursors
(C) It decreases formation of polyglutamate derivatives
(D) It is an active form of folic acid
(E) It inhibits the activation of methotrexate

58. Which of the following is a gram-negative, oxidase-positive rod associated with outbreaks of pneumonia that are traced to air conditioners?

(A) *Acinetobacter*
(B) *Calymmatobacterium granulomatis*
(C) *Legionella pneumophila*
(D) *Afipia felis*
(E) *Streptobacillus moniliformis*

59. In a cohort study, the ratio of the incidence rate of miscarriage among women who previously took oral contraceptives to the incidence rate of miscarriage among women who did not previously take oral contraceptives is described as

(A) attributable risk
(B) odds-risk ratio
(C) incidence rate
(D) prevalence rate
(E) relative risk

60. A gram-negative rod is isolated from the sputum of a 22-year-old woman who is hospitalized with cystic fibrosis. Laboratory tests show that the bacterium is an aerobic "nonfermenter" that is highly resistant to numerous antibiotics. The organism is most likely

(A) *Escherichia coli*
(B) *Klebsiella pneumoniae*
(C) *Mycoplasma pneumoniae*
(D) *Pseudomonas aeruginosa*
(E) *Mycobacterium*

61. Which one of the following symptoms is most likely to occur in menopausal women in all countries and cultures?

(A) Dysphoria
(B) Memory problems
(C) Hot flashes
(D) Anxiety
(E) Depression

62. The most common opportunist isolated from patients with AIDS in the United States is

(A) *Mycobacterium kansasii*
(B) *Mycobacterium avium-intracellulare* complex
(C) *Mycobacterium bovis*
(D) *Mycobacterium fortuitum-chelonae* complex
(E) *Mycobacterium scrofulaceum*

63. The strength of an association between a factor and a disease is best measured by which one of the following methods?

(A) Prevalence of the disease in the total population
(B) Incidence of the disease in the total population
(C) Attributable risk
(D) Relative risk
(E) Reliability

64. Which of the following characteristics applies to the toxin produced by *Corynebacterium diphtheriae*?

(A) It has only local effects
(B) It consists of lipid
(C) It is a poor antigen
(D) It is an exotoxin
(E) It is encoded by a chromosomal gene

65. Compared with males aged 20 to 30 years, males aged 70 to 80 years are less likely to

(A) use prescription drugs
(B) have no health insurance
(C) visit physicians
(D) suffer from depression
(E) suffer from dementia

66. Which of the following organisms is most likely to cause watery diarrhea?

(A) *Campylobacter jejuni*
(B) *Yersinia pseudotuberculosis*
(C) *Salmonella typhi*
(D) *Shigella sonnei*
(E) *Vibrio cholerae*

67. When infants do not have a primary attachment figure, they commonly display

(A) infantile autism
(B) Asperger syndrome
(C) childhood schizophrenia
(D) anaclitic depression
(E) bipolar illness

68. A 19-year-old phenotypically female patient shows no secondary sex characteristics, has not menstruated, and has short stature and a thick neck. The best way to obtain diagnostic information about this patient is by using which one of the following diagnostic methods?

(A) A gonadal hormone profile
(B) A buccal smear
(C) A determination of her gender identity
(D) A determination of her sexual preference
(E) A determination of her gender role

69. An enzyme increases the rate of a chemical reaction through which one of the following effects?

(A) Decreasing the free energy of the substrate
(B) Increasing the free energy of the product
(C) Decreasing the free energy of the transition state
(D) Shifting the equilibrium of the reaction toward the product
(E) Altering the free energy change of the reaction

70. The DNA component cytosine is best described as a

(A) purine base
(B) pyrimidine base
(C) purine nucleoside
(D) pyrimidine nucleoside
(E) nucleic acid

71. During the process of protein synthesis, which one of the following actions occurs?

(A) The initiator transfer RNA (tRNA) enters the "A site" on the ribosome
(B) Both prokaryotic and eukaryotic polypeptide chains are initiated with formylmethionine (fmet)
(C) UAG serves as the chain initiation codon
(D) The peptidyl transferase activity is located in both the elongation and termination steps
(E) The 28S ribosomal RNA (rRNA) is translated to form the proteins of the large ribosomal subunit

72. The *uvr*ABC endonuclease is involved in which one of the following processes?

(A) DNA replication
(B) RNA splicing
(C) DNA repair
(D) DNA recombination
(E) DNA ligation

73. Both histamine and serotonin act to cause which one of the following effects?

(A) Vasoconstriction, except in skeletal muscle and heart
(B) Intense itching by stimulating sensory nerve endings
(C) Relaxation of vascular smooth muscle
(D) Bronchodilation
(E) Gastric acid secretion

74. Saralasin and losartan share which one of the following properties?

(A) They both inhibit renin release
(B) They both inhibit angiotensin-converting enzyme
(C) They both inhibit bradykinin degradation
(D) They both block angiotensin II receptors
(E) They both are orally effective

75. Early intervention programs for children with emotional disorders is an example of

(A) primary prevention
(B) secondary prevention
(C) tertiary prevention
(D) active prevention
(E) retroactive prevention

76. Mesothelium and endothelium contain which one of the following intermediate filament types?

(A) Desmin
(B) Keratin
(C) Actinin
(D) Vimentin
(E) Desmoplakin

77. In the United States, children at day care centers have been observed to have a higher rate of infection by which one of the following sets of organisms when compared to those who do not attend day care centers?

(A) *Giardia lamblia* and *Isospora belli*
(B) *Enterobius vermicularis* and *Entamoeba histolytica*
(C) *Giardia lamblia* and *Enterobius vermicularis*
(D) *Dientamoeba fragilis* and *Necatur americanus*
(E) *Taenia saginata* and *Balantidium coli*

78. Which one of the following statements concerning choline is true?

(A) It is an essential nutrient
(B) It is negatively charged
(C) It is a constituent of lung surfactant
(D) It is a constituent of ceramide
(E) It is a constituent of cardiolipin

79. The enzymes in the three irreversible reactions of glycolysis that are bypassed in gluconeogenesis are:

(A) hexokinase, phosphofructokinase-2, and pyruvate kinase
(B) hexokinase, phosphofructokinase-1, and pyruvate kinase
(C) hexokinase, phosphoglycerate kinase, and pyruvate kinase.
(D) hexokinase, glyceraldehyde-3-phosphate dehydrogenase, and pyruvate kinase
(E) hexokinase, glyceraldehyde dehydrogenase, and phosphoglycerate kinase

80. When comparing glycosphingolipids and phosphosphingolipids, the only difference is that glycosphingolipids, but not phosphosphingolipids, have which one of the following characteristics?

(A) They are found in membranes of nervous tissues
(B) They contain ceramide
(C) They contain sugar moieties
(D) They contain fatty acid
(E) They cause mental retardation and other symptoms when they accumulate

81. The number of health care workers who have been infected with HIV during the past 14 years is approximately

(A) 1
(B) 14
(C) 40
(D) 230
(E) 950

82. In most female adolescents, the time from the appearance of breast buds to the first menstruation is approximately

(A) 2 months
(B) 6 months
(C) 12 months
(D) 24 months
(E) 36 months

83. An adolescent has a large peer group that appears to totally dictate his dress and behavior. His teacher informs his physician that he is disruptive in school and does not listen to her. The age of this adolescent is most likely to be

(A) 12 years
(B) 15 years
(C) 17 years
(D) 18 years
(E) 19 years

84. DNA replication occurs in which phase of the eukaryotic cell cycle?

(A) M phase
(B) S phase
(C) G_0 phase
(D) G_1 phase
(E) G_2 phase

85. The following serum values were obtained from a patient before and after drug therapy. Which one of the following drugs was most likely administered?

	Before	After
Serum aldosterone	High	Low
Serum potassium	3.5 mEq/L	4.5 mEq/L
Plasma renin activity	Normal	High
Angiotensin II	High	Low

(A) Hydrochlorothiazide
(B) Propranolol
(C) Captopril
(D) Spironolactone
(E) Hydralazine

86. Which one of the following sequences is the correct sequence of junctions at 1, 2, and 3 in the figure below?

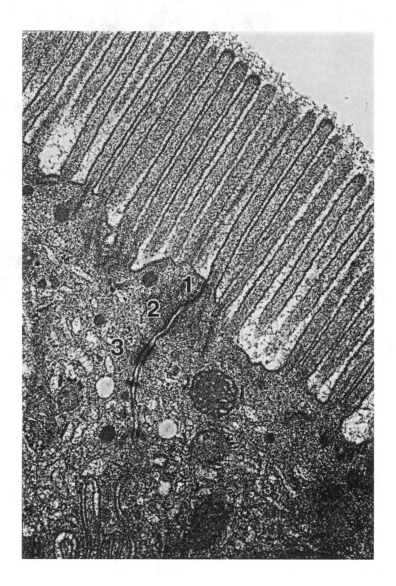

(A) Tight junction, zonula adherens, macula adherens
(B) Tight junction, macula adherens, gap junction
(C) Zonula adherens, macula adherens, gap junction
(D) Zonula adherens, tight junction, macula adherens
(E) Zonula adherens, macula adherens, hemidesmosome

87. Which of the following virus families has double-stranded DNA in four different isomers?

(A) Poxviruses
(B) Herpesviruses
(C) Rabiesviruses
(D) Orthomyxoviruses
(E) Retroviruses

88. Which of the following groups is most likely to be involved in the formation of a peptide bond in a protein molecule?

(A) The hydroxyl group on the side chain of serine
(B) The sulfhydryl group on the side chain of cysteine
(C) The amino group on the side chain of lysine
(D) The amide group on the side chain of glutamine
(E) The α-amino group of alanine

89. Cyclosporin A is used in transplant patients to reduce the risk for graft rejection. Which of the following statements best describes its mechanism of action?

(A) It inhibits cytotoxic lymphocyte activity
(B) It inhibits DNA synthesis in all proliferating cells
(C) It inhibits the maturation of T-cell precursors
(D) It inhibits DNA synthesis in antigen-presenting cells
(E) It inhibits the synthesis of interleukin-2 (IL-2) and its receptor

90. In newborns, tumors derived from all three germ cell layers are most commonly located in the

(A) central nervous system
(B) ovaries
(C) testicles
(D) mediastinum
(E) sacrococcygeal area

Questions 91-93

The following shows the biosynthetic pathway in the metabolism of two amino acids. The *letters* and *numbers* represent substrates and key enzymes.

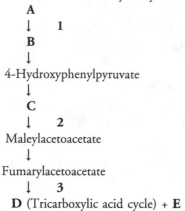

A
↓   1
B
↓
4-Hydroxyphenylpyruvate
↓
C
↓   2
Maleylacetoacetate
↓
Fumarylacetoacetate
↓   3
D (Tricarboxylic acid cycle) + **E**

91. Which of the following intermediates shown in the biosynthetic pathway turns black in urine when exposed to light and deposits in cartilage to produce a crippling degenerative joint disease?

(A) A
(B) B
(C) C
(D) D
(E) E

92. Which of the following enzymes, when deficient, causes the buildup of a substrate leading to mental retardation and the formation of intermediate compounds that give the individual's sweat a mousy odor?

(A) 1
(B) 2
(C) 3
(D) 1 and 2
(E) 1 and 3

93. Which of the following is an amino acid that can be used to synthesize hormones derived from the adrenal medulla?

(A) A
(B) B
(C) C
(D) D
(E) E

94. What occurs when a temperate bacteriophage enters a state called "lysogeny"?

(A) Most viral genes are expressed
(B) The bacterial cell is lysed
(C) Many new viruses are produced
(D) Most normal bacterial functions are turned off
(E) The virus may become integrated into the host genome

DIRECTIONS:

Each of the numbered items or incomplete statements in this section is negatively phrased, as indicated by a capitalized word such as NOT, LEAST, or EXCEPT. Select the ONE lettered answer or completion that is BEST in each case.

95. All of the following are functions of the ego EXCEPT

(A) regulation of instinctual drives
(B) adaptation to reality
(C) reality testing
(D) representing moral values
(E) sustaining interpersonal relationships

96. All of the following are viruses containing positive-sense, single-stranded linear RNA genomes EXCEPT

(A) polioviruses
(B) rhinoviruses
(C) flaviviruses
(D) retroviruses
(E) rhabdoviruses

97. Glycosaminoglycans are important in all of the following EXCEPT

(A) lysosomal storage diseases
(B) negative charge of the glomerular basement membrane
(C) joint lubrication
(D) matrix of bone, skin, tendons, and cartilage
(E) production of blood group antigens

98. All of the following cell types have the potential for both hyperplasia and hypertrophy EXCEPT

(A) smooth muscle cells
(B) renal tubular cells
(C) skeletal muscle cells
(D) hepatocytes
(E) thyroid follicle cells

99. Acetyl coenzyme A (acetyl CoA) is LEAST directly used in which of the following processes

(A) ketone body synthesis
(B) fatty acid synthesis
(C) cholesterol synthesis
(D) pyruvate formation
(E) citrate formation

100. All of the following characteristics describe infections caused by *Entamoeba histolytica* EXCEPT

(A) flask-shaped ulcers in the cecum
(B) erythrophagocytosis by trophozoites
(C) liver abscess
(D) contraction by ingesting contaminated water or food
(E) treatment with trimethoprim and sulfa drugs

101. The following schematic depicts a series of biochemical reactions that occur in different tissues throughout the body. The letters refer to compounds and the numbers refer to key enzymes.

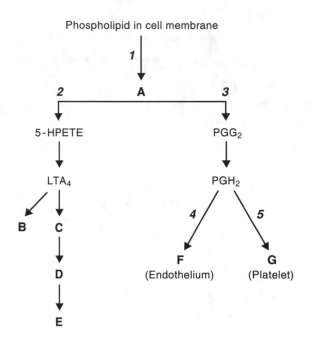

Which one of the following statements is INCORRECT?

(A) Compound A is synthesized from linoleic acid; its liberation may be blocked by corticosteroids

(B) Compound B is a potent chemotactic agent and increases adhesion molecule synthesis in leukocytes

(C) Compounds C, D, and E play a key role in bronchial asthma and asthma associated with aspirin sensitivity

(D) Compounds F and G inhibit and enhance platelet aggregation and vasodilate and vasoconstrict vessels, respectively

(E) Enzyme 1 is blocked by corticosteroids and enhanced by calcium, whereas enzyme 5 is blocked by both aspirin and nonsteroidal agents

102. Which of the following factors is LEAST likely to influence whether an infarct will occur in tissue?

(A) Size of the vessel obstructed

(B) Extent of collateral circulation

(C) Presence or absence of a dual blood supply

(D) Presence or absence of preexisting disease in that tissue

(E) Hemoglobin concentration

103. The following schematic depicts ethanol metabolism. The letters represent key compounds and the numbers represent enzymes.

$$\text{Alcohol} \xrightarrow{\textcircled{1}} \textbf{A} + \text{NADH} \xrightarrow{\textcircled{2}} \text{Acetate} + \textbf{B} \longrightarrow \textbf{C}$$

Which one of the following statements is INCORRECT?

(A) Enzyme 1 can also catalyze reactions involving methyl alcohol and ethylene glycol, which would reduce the maximum velocity (Vmax) of the enzyme without affecting the substrate concentration at one-half the Vmax (Km)

(B) Enzyme 2 is relatively inactive in Asians, causing the effects of drinking alcohol to be more pronounced in Asians

(C) Enzyme 2 is blocked by disulfiram

(D) Compound B aids in the conversion of pyruvate to lactate and acetoacetate to β-hydroxybutyrate

(E) Compound C can be used in ketone body formation

104. Which one of the following is LEAST characteristic of sexuality in a 75-year-old male patient?

(A) Decreased sexual interest
(B) Decreased ejaculation intensity
(C) Increased refractory period
(D) Decreased opportunity
(E) Delayed ejaculation

105. All of the following are mechanisms for the neutralization of free radicals EXCEPT

(A) superoxide dismutase
(B) catalase
(C) glutathione peroxidase
(D) vitamins C and E
(E) cytochrome oxidase system

106. All of the following statements about exotoxins produced by enteric, gram-negative bacteria are correct EXCEPT

(A) they consist primarily of lipids
(B) they often consist of multiple subunits
(C) they are secreted by the bacteria
(D) they are encoded most often by extrachromosomal genes
(E) they mediate their effects by binding to specific receptors

107. Which of the following sets of laboratory tests are NOT considered stat tests in the emergency room?

(A) Serum glucose and electrolytes
(B) Complete blood cell count and serum amylase
(C) Gram stain and urinalysis
(D) Erythrocyte sedimentation rate and serum transaminases
(E) Arterial blood gases and urine drug screen

108. All of the following peptides produce vasodilation in most vascular beds EXCEPT

(A) endothelin
(B) bradykinin
(C) vasoactive intestinal peptide
(D) calcitonin gene-related peptide
(E) substance P

109. All of the following statements regarding hydatid disease are true EXCEPT

(A) man is an accidental intermediate host
(B) entrapped larvae grow slowly into a large unilocular cyst
(C) filariform larvae from dog feces penetrate the skin and migrate to the liver
(D) daughter cysts develop within the hydatid cyst and these produce brood capsules
(E) hydatid sand is a term applied to the individual scolices in hydatid cyst fluid

110. Which one of the following methods is the LEAST effective treatment for enuresis in a 6-year-old child?

(A) Restriction of fluids before bedtime
(B) Punishment
(C) Bed-wetting alarms
(D) Midsleep awakening for voiding
(E) Antidepressant medication

111. With appropriate laboratory technique, microorganisms that may be cultured from the nose and throat of a healthy individual may include all of the following organisms EXCEPT

(A) *Corynebacterium pseudodiphtheriticum*
(B) *Neisseria sicca*
(C) *Streptococcus mitis*
(D) *Treponema macrodentium*
(E) *Staphylococcus epidermidis*

112. A 24-year-old patient has been diagnosed with androgen-insensitivity (testicular feminization) syndrome. The patient is likely to have all of the following signs EXCEPT

(A) an XY chromosome complement
(B) menstruation
(C) female external genitalia
(D) heterosexuality
(E) breast development

113. Regarding both *Bacteroides fragilis* and *Bacteroides melaninogenicus*, which of the following statements is LEAST accurate?

(A) Both are gram-negative rods that do not form spores
(B) Both organisms produce an exotoxin that increases cyclic adenosine monophosphate (AMP), which plays an important role in pathogenesis
(C) *B. fragilis* causes disease primarily below the diaphragm, whereas *B. melaninogenicus* causes disease primarily about the diaphragm
(D) Although *B. fragilis* typically causes disease in a mixed infection with facultative gram-negative rods, it can cause disease by itself, as well
(E) Both species do not respond equally well to penicillin therapy

114. All of the following substances are products of arachidonic acid metabolism EXCEPT

(A) leukotrienes
(B) thromboxane
(C) endothelin
(D) prostacyclin
(E) lipoxins

115. All of the following statements concerning streptococci are correct EXCEPT

(A) M proteins are responsible for the virulence and antiphagocytic properties in group A streptococci

(B) susceptibility to optochin separates *Streptococcus pneumoniae* from viridans streptococci

(C) the CAMP test is useful in identifying *Streptococcus agalactiae*

(D) the quellung reaction (capsular swelling) is a diagnostic feature of group A streptococci

(E) group A streptococci are beta hemolytic on sheep blood agar

116. Prostaglandins E_1 or E_2 produce all of the following EXCEPT

(A) renal vasodilation

(B) gastric cytoprotection

(C) platelet aggregation

(D) bronchodilation

(E) induction of labor

117. All of the following statements about immigrants to the United States are true EXCEPT

(A) they are at increased risk for psychiatric problems

(B) they are at greater risk for psychiatric problems if they are women than if they are men

(C) they show a higher incidence of paranoid symptoms than the general population

(D) they have a relatively good prognosis when they show paranoid symptoms

(E) they have fewer emotional problems if they can associate with people of their own culture

118. During the endogenous phase (schizogony) of *Plasmodium malariae*, which one of the following life cycle aspects is NOT related or observed?

(A) Obligate intracellular stage

(B) Intracellular stage in liver parenchymal cells

(C) Ring stage trophozoites in mature blood cells (RBCs)

(D) Merozoites released by mature schizonts

(E) Sporozoites in stained, thin smears of human RBCs

119. Which one of the following characteristics is LEAST normal in a 5-year-old girl?

(A) Hopping on one foot

(B) Preference for using the right hand

(C) The use of the future tense in speech

(D) Following a three-step command

(E) Parallel play

120. Which one of the following classes of drugs is LEAST likely to cause sexual dysfunction?

(A) Antiparkinson drugs (e.g., L-dopa)

(B) Selective serotonin reuptake inhibitors (SSRIs)

(C) Antipsychotics

(D) MAO inhibitors

(E) Tricyclic antidepressants

121. Which one of the following substances is NOT a component of the gram-positive bacterial cell wall?

(A) Peptidoglycan

(B) Lipid A

(C) Lipoteichoic acid

(D) *N*-acetyl muramic acid

(E) *N*-acetyl glucosamine

122. All of the following associations for growth-promoting proto-oncogenes are correct EXCEPT

(A) *Sis* —synthesis of growth factor

(B) *Ras*—suppressor gene–inhibiting DNA synthesis

(C) *Abl*—non-receptor associated tyrosine kinase activity for generating second messengers

(D) *Myc*—synthesis of nuclear regulatory proteins

(E) *Erb* —growth factor receptor synthesis

123. In the biosynthetic pathway below, *A, B,* and *C* represent key substrates, and *1* represents a key enzyme.

$$\text{Methionine} \rightarrow \mathbf{A} \rightarrow S\text{-adenosylhomocysteine} \xrightarrow{\;1\;} \mathbf{B} \rightarrow \text{Cystathionine} \rightarrow \mathbf{C}$$

All of the following statements are correct EXCEPT

(A) substrate A is a high-energy compound
(B) substrate A can be used for 1-carbon transfers
(C) substrate B accepts methyl groups from vitamin B_{12} and can transfer them to methionine
(D) substrate B, when it accumulates from a deficiency of enzyme 1, produces the autosomal recessive disease alkaptonuria
(E) substrate C is a major component of α-keratin

124. Which one of the following does NOT occur during the eclipse period of a viral life cycle?

(A) Adsorption (virus–cell interaction)
(B) Penetration (entry of the virus into the cytoplasm)
(C) Uncoating (release of the genome from the cytoplasm)
(D) Decreased infectivity
(E) Increased infectivity

DIRECTIONS:

Each set of matching questions in this section consists of a list of four to twenty-six lettered options (some of which may be in figures) followed by several numbered items. For each numbered item, select the ONE lettered option that is most closely associated with it. To avoid spending too much time on matching sets with large numbers of options, it is generally advisable to begin each set by reading the list of options. Then for each item in the set, try to generate the correct answer and locate it in the option list, rather than evaluating each option individually. Each lettered option may be selected once, more than once, or not at all.

Questions 125-128

Match each of the following descriptive phrases with the most appropriate term regarding classical conditioning.

(A) Unconditioned stimulus
(B) Conditioned stimulus
(C) Unconditioned response
(D) Conditioned response
(E) Extinction

125. The smell of pizza baking in the cafeteria oven at lunchtime

126. Salivating in response to the smell of pizza baking

127. Salivating in response to hearing the lunch bell at 12 P.M.

128. Two weeks after your lunch time was changed to 2 P.M., you stop salivating in response to the 12 P.M. lunch bell.

Questions 129-134

For each of the following antibiotics, select the drug's pharmacologic classification.

(A) Carbapenem
(B) Third-generation cephalosporin
(C) Second-generation cephalosporin
(D) First-generation cephalosporin
(E) Monobactam

129. Ceftazidime

130. Imipenem

131. Aztreonam

132. Cefaclor

133. Cefazolin

134. Ceftriaxone

Questions 135-137

Match each of the following descriptions with the appropriate steroid.

(A) Cholesterol
(B) Androstenedione
(C) Estradiol
(D) Pregnenolone
(E) Testosterone
(F) Corticosterone
(G) Progesterone
(H) 11-Deoxycorticosterone
(I) Aldosterone
(J) 17-α-Hydroxyprogesterone
(K) 11-Deoxycortisol
(L) Cortisol

135. It is the C21 precursor of many active steroids and the major final product in the corpus luteum

136. It is the hormone that increases gluconeogenesis

137. It is a C18 compound derived from testosterone

Questions 138-140

Match each of the following clinical uses with the proper prostaglandin.

(A) Misoprostol
(B) Thromboxane A$_2$
(C) Alprostadil
(D) Dinoprostone or carboprost (Prostin 15M)

138. Maintenance of patent ductus arteriosus before surgery

139. Prevention of gastric ulcers caused by nonsteroidal antiinflammatory drugs

140. Induction of labor or abortion

Questions 141-142

The following graph shows the changes in energy when a reactant is converted to a product. Match each of the following descriptions with its representative letter on the graph.

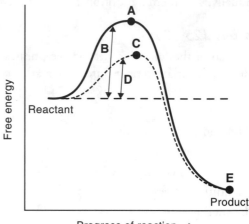

141. The energy level of the transition state for the uncatalyzed reaction

142. The free energy of activation of the catalyzed reaction

Questions 143-147

Match each of the following developmental milestones with the age at which it commonly first appears.

(A) 0 to 3 months
(B) 4 to 6 months
(C) 6 to 8 months
(D) 12 to 14 months
(E) 16 to 24 months

143. Sitting unassisted

144. Stranger anxiety

145. Rapproachment

146. Social smile

147. Walking unassisted

Questions 148-150

For each patient described, select the parasite most likely to have caused the conditions noted.

(A) *Ascaris lumbricoides*
(B) *Diphyllobothrium latum*
(C) *Dracunculus medinensis*
(D) *Necatur americanus*
(E) *Onchocerca volvulus*
(F) *Strongyloides stercoralis*
(G) *Taenia solium*
(H) *Entamoeba histolytica*

148. Microscopic examination of fresh, warm feces from a diarrheic stool reveals trophozoites containing ingested red blood cells

149. A 26-year-old male from Central America is being treated with diethylcarbamazine and suramin for ocular lesions and skin nodules on his head

150. A 17-year-old female is transported to the local clinic from her village in Tanzania (Africa). She has a fever, cough and pneumonia. Laboratory results show eosinophilia. Thiabendazole is prescribed.

Questions 151-155

Match each of the following statements with the appropriate acids.

(A) Linoleic acid
(B) Palmitic acid
(C) *Cis*-oleic acid
(D) α-Linolenic acid
(E) Arachidic acid
(F) Butyric acid
(G) Arachidonic acid
(H) Trans-oleic acid
(I) Eicosapentaenoic acid

151. An essential dietary factor that functions as a precursor of prostaglandins of the 1 and 2 series

152. A product of partial hydrogenation

153. A common constituent of phosphatidylinositol and phosphatidylcholine that is released from the cell membrane by the action of phospholipase A_2

154. A product found in fish oils.

155. A saturated fatty acid that increases serum cholesterol levels

Questions 156-157

Match each of the following descriptions with the appropriate organism.

(A) *Fusobacterium* species
(B) *Treponema pallidum*
(C) *Spirillum minus*
(D) *Borrelia recurrentis*
(E) *Borrelia burgdorferi*

156. This organism readily evades the immune system because of antigenic variation

157. This organism causes an infection that is characterized by a "bulls-eye" skin lesion

Questions 158-162

Match each of the following research examples with the appropriate statistical test.

(A) Independent *t*-test
(B) Paired *t*-test
(C) Chi-squared test
(D) Correlation
(E) Analysis of variance

158. Used to evaluate the relationship between the scores of medical students on USMLE Step 1 and their parents' income

159. Used to evaluate differences among scores on USMLE Step 1 of medical students in three age groups

160. Used to evaluate the difference in the percentage of medical students who pass USMLE Step 1 versus those who pass USMLE Step 2 on their first attempt

161. Used to evaluate differences between a group of medical students' scores on USMLE Step 1 and the same students' scores on USMLE Step 2

162. Used to evaluate differences between USMLE Step 1 scores of medical students in two different medical schools

Questions 163-166

Match each of the following descriptions with the appropriate compounds.

(A) Alanine
(B) Asparagine
(C) Aspartate
(D) Cysteine
(E) Cytosine
(F) Glutamine
(G) Glycine
(H) Guanine
(I) Histidine
(J) Ornithine
(K) Proline
(L) Serine
(M) Thymine
(N) Urea
(O) Glutamate
(P) Tryptophan
(Q) Phenylalanine

163. Negatively charged at physiologic pH

164. Essential amino acids

165. Its degradation product is uric acid

166. It is involved in disulfide bond formation

Questions 167-171

For each of the following pharmacologic effects, select the appropriate synergistic pair of drugs.

(A) Probenecid—penicillin G
(B) Imipenem—cilastatin
(C) Sulbactam—ampicillin
(D) Rifampin—isoniazid
(E) Trimethoprim—sulfamethoxazole

167. Inhibits renal metabolism

168. Inhibits tandem steps in a synthetic pathway

169. Inhibits renal tubular secretion

170. Inhibits bacterial inactivation

171. Prevents emergence of bacterial resistance

Questions 172-173

Match the following clinical scenarios with the laboratory test results that best represent how the test is interpreted.

(A) True positive
(B) True negative
(C) False positive
(D) False negative

172. When tested for syphilis, a patient has a positive rapid plasma reagin (RPR) test and a negative fluorescent treponemal antibody absorption (FTA-ABS) test

173. When tested for human immunodeficiency antibody, a patient has a positive enzyme-linked immunosorbent assay (ELISA) and a positive Western blot

Questions 174-175

The diagram below illustrates a transfer RNA (tRNA) molecule. Match each description with the appropriate point on the diagram.

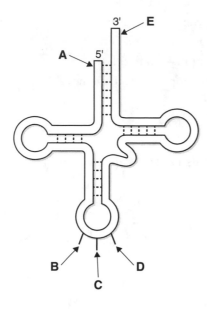

174. The point at which an amino acid becomes covalently bound

175. The wobble position

Questions 176-180

For each description, select the appropriate virus.

(A) Hepatitis B virus
(B) Influenza A virus
(C) Mumps virus
(D) Adenovirus
(E) Coxsackievirus
(F) Papillomavirus
(G) Rotavirus

176. Circular, double-stranded DNA with a virion DNA polymerase

177. Single-stranded RNA virus with no envelope, replicates in cytoplasm

178. Linear, double-stranded DNA with no envelope

179. Unsegmented single-stranded RNA with a virion RNA polymerase

180. Segmented single-stranded RNA, replicates in the host cell nucleus and cytoplasm

ANSWER KEY

1. B	31. E	61. C	91. C	121. B	151. A
2. E	32. A	62. B	92. A	122. B	152. H
3. A	33. C	63. D	93. B	123. D	153. G
4. D	34. A	64. D	94. E	124. E	154. I
5. C	35. D	65. B	95. D	125. A	155. B
6. B	36. C	66. E	96. E	126. C	156. D
7. A	37. D	67. D	97. E	127. D	157. E
8. B	38. D	68. B	98. C	128. E	158. D
9. A	39. A	69. C	99. D	129. B	159. E
10. A	40. C	70. B	100. E	130. A	160. C
11. D	41. D	71. D	101. E	131. E	161. B
12. E	42. E	72. C	102. E	132. C	162. A
13. E	43. C	73. B	103. A	133. D	163. C, O
14. D	44. A	74. D	104. A	134. B	164. I, P, Q
15. E	45. B	75. B	105. E	135. G	165. H
16. E	46. E	76. D	106. A	136. L	166. D
17. B	47. A	77. C	107. D	137. C	167. B
18. E	48. E	78. C	108. A	138. C	168. E
19. C	49. B	79. B	109. C	139. A	169. A
20. B	50. B	80. C	110. B	140. D	170. C
21. E	51. B	81. C	111. D	141. A	171. D
22. A	52. A	82. D	112. B	142. D	172. C
23. C	53. B	83. B	113. B	143. C	173. A
24. D	54. A	84. B	114. C	144. C	174. E
25. E	55. C	85. C	115. D	145. E	175. B
26. B	56. A	86. A	116. C	146. A	176. A
27. A	57. D	87. B	117. B	147. D	177. E
28. C	58. C	88. E	118. E	148. H	178. D
29. A	59. E	89. E	119. E	149. E	179. C
30. B	60. D	90. E	120. A	150. F	180. B

ANSWERS AND EXPLANATIONS

1. The answer is B. *(Behavioral science)*
The most appropriate statistical test to analyze 500 patients in one of two physical groups and assigned to one of two personality groups is the chi-square test. The chi-square test evaluates differences between percentages of patients in each category (i.e., mildly affected or severely affected by stroke in each of the two personality categories). An independent (nonpaired) t-test evaluates the difference between the means of two samples that are unrelated. A dependent (paired) t-test evaluates the difference between the means of two samples that are related. Analysis of variance examines differences between the means of more than two samples, and correlation focuses on the relationship between two different variables.

2. The answer is E. *(Microbiology)*
During a standard lytic infection, the phage DNA is packaged into the capsid before being released from the cell. Sometimes, the host cell DNA becomes degraded and a small fragment of the bacterial DNA is packaged into a phage particle, forming a "transducing particle." Only a small fraction of the progeny phages carry host DNA. Due to their small size, each transducing particle can carry only a tiny fragment of the bacterial chromosome. The host DNA is fragmented randomly, so that any host gene can be loaded into a transducing particle. A generalized transducing phage does not become integrated into the host chromosome, whereas a specialized transducing phage becomes integrated at one specific site. Because only one small fragment of DNA can be carried in each particle, only genes that are located very close to each other can be cotransduced.

3-4. The answers are: 3-A, 4-D. *(Biochemistry)*
Antibody molecules contain two identical heavy chains and two identical light chains. Antibody class is determined by the constant region of the immunoglobulin's heavy chains. The variable portion of the heavy chain is encoded by the VDJ region of the messenger RNA (mRNA) molecule, while the constant portion is encoded by the C region. This message encodes an α heavy chain, which defines the immunoglobulin as immunoglobulin A (IgA). Immunoglobulin D (IgD) contains a δ heavy chain, immunoglobulin E (IgE) contains an ε heavy chain, immunoglobulin G (IgG) contains a γ heavy chain, and immunoglobulin M (IgM) contains μ heavy chains.

Because this is a mature eukaryotic message, it has already been fully processed. It contains a "cap" at the 5′ end and a poly A tail at the 3′ end. Introns have been removed by splicing. The VDJ portion codes for the variable region of the heavy chain, which, together with the variable region of the light chain, makes up the antigen binding site. Translation of messages occurs in the cytosol. Translation of messages occurs in the 5′ to 3′ direction, so that the VDJ portion would be translated before the C α portion.

5. The answer is C. *(Microbiology)*
Plasmids are small, circular, supercoiled DNA molecules found in some bacteria. They usually do not carry essential genes, but some plasmids, such as R (resistance) plasmids, carry genes coding for antibiotic resistance. All plasmids have their own origin of replication, so that they are replicated along with the host chromosome and passed along to progeny cells. Only some plasmids possess genes that allow for their transmittal to other bacteria by the process of conjugation.

6. The answer is B. *(Pathology)*
The lungs are a more common primary site for a tumor in adults than in children. Other tumor sites that are more common in adults than in children are the skin (e.g., basal cell carcinoma, malignant melanoma), the breast (e.g., infiltrating ductal carcinoma), the prostate, and the colon. The most important risk factor for breast, prostate, and colon cancer is age. Skin exposure to ultraviolet light increases the risk of skin cancer.

7. The answer is A. *(Microbiology)*
Tetracyclines are readily absorbed from the intestinal tract and are distributed widely in the tissues. They do not penetrate the cerebrospinal fluid well. Tetracyclines are concentrated by susceptible bacteria and inhibit protein synthesis by inhibiting the binding of aminoacyl-transfer RNA (tRNA) to the 30S subunit

of bacterial ribosomes. Resistant bacteria fail to concentrate the drug; this resistance is under the control of transmissible plasmids. Erythromycin and chloramphenicol inhibit protein synthesis at the 50S ribosomal subunit and prevent peptide bond formation. Rifampin directly inhibits bacterial RNA polymerase activity. Sulfa drugs are metabolic antagonists of para-aminobenzoic acid (PABA), a necessary component of tetrahydrofolate. Use of sulfonamides and trimethoprim together results in the inhibition of sequential metabolic steps (i.e., they have a synergistic antibacterial effect).

8. The answer is B. *(Biochemistry)*
The Ames test is used to identify potential carcinogens by assessing their ability to cause mutations. The test measures the ability of such mutagens to revert auxotrophic histidine-deficient mutants of *Salmonella* back to prototrophic histidine-synthesizing organisms. Some potentially dangerous compounds are not mutagenic themselves, but are metabolically converted to mutagenic byproducts by the liver. The rat liver extract used in the Ames test contains liver enzymes and is designed to allow the *in vitro* conversion of the tested compound to its metabolic derivatives.

9. The answer is A. *(Pathology)*
Carcinomas of the skin are the most common cancers in organ transplant recipients. There is a 4- to 21-fold higher incidence than that of the general population. The skin cancers differ from the carcinomas in the general population because they have increased aggressiveness, are of a squamous cell origin, and occur more frequently in relatively young patients.

Other common cancers in transplant recipients are anogenital cancer (e.g., carcinoma of the cervix, vulva, perineum, penis, and anus, possibly associated with the human papilloma viruses); non-Hodgkin lymphoma, particulary large cell and immunoblastic (most non-Hodgkin lymphomas are of B cell origin and are commonly associated with central nervous system involvement); and Kaposi sarcoma, which has a 400 to 500 times higher incidence than that of the general population. Kaposi sarcoma has an endothelial cell origin and is highly aggressive.

10. The answer is A. *(Pathology)*
The distinction between a benign renal adenoma and renal adenocarcinoma is commonly made on the basis of size; tumors less than 2 cm are rarely malignant and those greater than 3 cm behave in a malignant fashion. This distinction is also made for carcinoid tumors, which most commonly occur in the appendix. These tumors rarely metastasize because they are less than 2 cm. Carcinoids in the small intestine, however, commonly metastasize because they are greater than 2 cm. Although size is an important criterion in staging breast, prostate, colon, and lung cancers, the relationship of tumor size with malignancy potential is more dramatic for renal adenocarcinoma and carcinoid tumors.

11. The answer is D. *(Microbiology)*
This patient is most likely a chronic carrier of the hepatitis B virus. The classic definition for chronic carrier status is the demonstration of hepatitis B surface antigen (HBsAg) on serologic studies for longer than 6 months. In acute hepatitis B virus infection, HBsAg disappears approximately 3 months after infection and then antibody to HBsAg appears 1–2 months later. The simultaneous appearance of HBsAg and antibody to that antigen is typical of chronic viral infection. Small numbers of hepatitis B virus continue to be produced in infected hepatocytes. Although antibody is also produced at the same time, the viruses are not eliminated. The patient would be susceptible to hepatitis A virus infection if he or she encountered the virus, because it would appear that no antibodies to the virus can be found in the patient's serum. No information is given regarding the patient's immune status to hepatitis C virus, so no assessment of immunity or susceptibility to the hepatitis C virus can be made. Finally, because the patient already has antibodies to hepatitis B virus (as a result of infection), a booster vaccination for hepatitis B virus would be of no value.

12. The answer is E. *(Biochemistry)*
Collagen is a fibrous protein that has structural functions in the body outside the cell. Each collagen molecule consists of three polypeptides that are wrapped around each other to form a triple helix. Only the typical 20 amino acids are incorporated when collagen

is synthesized by the ribosome; however, some of the prolines and lysines become hydroxylated during post-translational modification of the molecule. Amino-terminal and carboxy-terminal propeptides are cleaved from procollagen by a protease to form collagen after the molecule has been secreted from the cell.

13. The answer is E.   *(Microbiology)*
Pseudomonas aeruginosa is an obligate aerobe that grows readily on many kinds of media. It produces two pigments, pyocyanin and pyoverdin, which impart a blue-green color to the medium on which it grows. It is oxidase positive and does not ferment carbohydrates, which explains the negative reaction on triple-sugar iron agar (1% lactose and sucrose, 0.1% glucose). *P. aeruginosa* is usually identified on the basis of the oxidase reaction and pigment production. A sweet or fruit-like odor is produced as well. *Neisseria gonorrhoeae* is a Gram-negative diplococcus that is oxidase positive and ferments several carbohydrates, producing acid and no gas. It is lactose negative, but glucose positive. No pigments are produced. *Branhamella catarrhalis* is also oxidase positive, but glucose, lactose, and sucrose negative. The Gram stain reaction would be a significant test to determine organism shape. *Escherichia coli* is lactose positive and oxidase negative. *Salmonella typhi* is lactose negative, oxidase negative, and most often produces hydrogen sulfide (H_2S), which turns triple-sugar iron medium black. *S. typhi* is able to ferment glucose as well.

14. The answer is D.   *(Pathology)*
 In geriatric patients, mild glucose intolerance occurs because of increased adipose tissue, which downregulates the number of insulin receptors available for insulin. Alkaline phosphatase is increased, secondary to an increase in osteoarthritis, which wears down the articular cartilage and increases reactive bone formation at the margins of the joints, causing osteophytes, or spurs. Bone formation increases the alkaline phosphatase, which is concentrated primarily in osteoblasts.

Low testosterone levels in geriatric males reduce erythropoietin stimulation, thus decreasing the plasma hemoglobin concentration to that of a normal adult female.

Pulmonary function studies in the elderly are similar to those of individuals with obstructive lung disease.

Vital capacity, forced expiratory volume 1 second, elasticity, diffusing capacity, and partial pressure of arterial oxygen (PaO_2) decrease with age, whereas compliance (i.e., the ability of the lung to stretch on inspiration), residual volume ("senile emphysema"), and functional residual capacity increase with age.

The glomerular filtration rate and the creatinine clearance decrease with age.

15. The answer is E.   *(Microbiology)*
Fraction I is the major envelope protein of *Yersinia pestis*. It is antiphagocytic, and it also activates complement. Individuals who recover from plague tend to be resistant to a second attack or develop a milder form of the disease. Antibodies against fraction I as well as against endotoxin and exotoxin appear to be important in resistance.

Other *Yersinia* species, *Francisella tularensis*, and *Brucella melitensis* do not produce Fraction I.

16. The answer is E.   *(Pathology)*
Women have slightly lower hemoglobin and hematocrit concentration than men because of menses and child bearing; without iron supplements, there is a net loss of 500 mg per pregnancy. Also, women have less testosterone, which is a potent stimulator of erythropoiesis.

The normal iron stores in a man are approximately 1000 mg, whereas in a woman iron stores are only 400 mg. Because the iron stores are typically represented by a small, circulating fraction of ferritin, the normal serum ferritin reference intervals are lower in women than they are in men.

The serum high-density lipoproteins (HDL) are higher in women than in men because of the presence of estrogen. HDL has a protective effect against the formation of atheromatous plaques by aiding in the elimination of low-density lipoprotein (LDL) in the liver (reverse cholesterol transport). In addition to preventing osteoporosis, estrogen replacement in the menopausal woman helps prevent coronary artery disease.

17. The answer is B.   *(Microbiology)*
Mycobacteria are aerobic, rod-shaped organisms that do not stain well in the Gram stain procedure because of the high lipid content in the mycobacterial cell

wall. The organism will take up carbolfuschin dye quite well by either the Ziehl-Neelsen procedure (heating) or the Kinyoun technique (detergent added; no heating). Once stained, the mycobacteria resist destaining with acid-alcohol. Any other bacteria present will destain and take up the blue color of the methylene blue counterstain. Therefore, mycobacteria appear as thin, red bacteria. If mycobacteria in sputum or tissue samples are stained by auramine or rhodamine and observed using fluorescence microscopy, they appear yellow-orange. The mycobacteria would never appear as green or colorless when stained by procedures using carbolfuschin dye.

18. The answer is E. (Biochemistry)

The Recommended Daily Allowance (RDA) is an estimate of the amount of nutrient required to meet the needs of 95% of the United States population. The RDA is not set at the minimal requirement for individuals. However, although it is intentionally set to provide a safety margin for most individuals, the RDA does not attempt to meet the optimal requirement of an individual. There is considerable controversy concerning the optimal quantity of many nutrients. For example, the minimal daily requirement of vitamin C is 10 mg, which is the amount required to prevent symptoms of scurvy. The RDA of vitamin C is 60 mg per day, which is a six-fold excess; however, there is a popular school of thought that the optimal amount is 1000 mg or more per day.

To allow for their greater muscle mass, the dietary allowances for men are set about 20% higher than they are for women. However, the dietary allowance for iron is an exception; women need to replace iron that is lost during menstruation.

There is no RDA single standard for caloric intake. If caloric intake is set at a level that meets the requirements of 95% of the population, 94% would be obese and 4% would be thin.

19. The answer is C. (Pathology)

Children are in the continuous process of laying down bone. Osteoblasts contain alkaline phosphatase; therefore, excessive osteoblastic activity is accompanied by an increase in alkaline phosphatase that is 2 to 5 times greater than adult values.

Phosphorus is the primary force for driving calcium into unmineralized osteoid to form bone. To facilitate the rapid bone growth in children, the serum phosphorus concentration is typically increased in children. Another benefit of increased phosphate concentration is an increased concentration of 2,3-bisphosphoglycerate in red blood cells, which decreases the affinity of hemoglobin for oxygen, thus increasing the delivery of oxygen to tissue. More oxygen is delivered to tissue in children than in adults; therefore, there is less stimulus for the release of erythropoietin to increase red blood cell production and hemoglobin concentration, resulting in a slightly decreased hemoglobin concentration in children.

20. The answer is B. (Microbiology)

Jane Doe, who is in blood group A, has preformed immunoglobulin M (IgM) against the B antigen on the transfused erythrocytes. The IgM binds to the cells, activates complement, and lysis occurs (type II hypersensitivity). The antibody–antigen complexes on the erythrocyte surface also activate Hageman factor, which leads to production of kinins (i.e., vasoactive peptides that cause hypotension and shock by increasing capillary permeability). If the infusion of ABO-incompatible blood is not stopped promptly, kidney failure caused by renal vasoconstriction and intravascular thrombi may occur.

IgM isohemagglutinins begin to appear shortly following birth, presumptively because of colonization of the gastrointestinal and respiratory tracts by normal flora, which have oligosaccharide antigenic determinants that are similar to those on the A and B antigens. However, an individual will produce antibodies only against those antigens that are different from self.

Group	Antigen	Antibody
A	A	anti-B
B	B	anti-A
O	. . .	anti-A + anti-B
AB	AB	. . .

The term *isohemagglutinin* refers to antibodies in one species that are directed against major antigens on erythrocytes of other individuals of the same species.

21. The answer is E. (Pathology)

Plasma contains all coagulation factors and platelets; therefore, an anticoagulant is added to a collection tube to prevent clotting. Anticoagulants include chelating agents and heparin. Because calcium is important in binding activated clotting factors, adding chelating agents such as ethylenediaminetetraacetic acid (EDTA), citrate, and oxalate prevents clot formation. Heparin prevents clotting by enhancing antithrombin III activity, which neutralizes many of the clotting factors that are serine proteases. When blood is spun down anticoagulated tubes, plasma is harvested. If anticoagulant is not added to a tube, the blood clots and serum is the end product following centrifugation. Serum is deficient in factor V, factor VIII, factor II (prothrombin), and platelets, all of which are consumed in the clot. The vitamin K–dependent factors are factors II, VII, IX, and X, as well as proteins C and S. Except for factor II, these factors are not consumed in a clot and, therefore, are present in serum.

22. The answer is A. *(Behavioral science)*

This stockbroker, who prefers to wear women's sexy underclothing under his pinstriped suit, is an individual who is showing transvestic fetishism, which is a sexual paraphilia characterized by sexual pleasure derived from wearing women's clothing (particularly underclothing). Individuals with transvestic fetishism commonly have a male gender identity, are of heterosexual orientation, are not interested in having a sex-change operation, are content with their sexual orientation, and have a male gender role in society.

23. The answer is C. *(Pathology)*

Variables that influence laboratory testing are designated as preanalytic, analytic, and postanalytic. Preanalytic variables include the patient's age, gender, and habits (e.g., smoking, alcohol intake) as well as factors affecting the collection of the sample (e.g., venipuncture, 24-hour urine collection). Analytic variables refer to laboratory instrumentation and the effect of sample abnormalities (e.g., serum turbidity) that may interfere with the proper performance of the test. Postanalytic variables refer primarily to accurate laboratory data reporting to the clinician (e.g., potential for transcription errors).

A hemolyzed blood sample falsely elevates the serum potassium (the major intracellular cation) and lactate

dehydrogenase, both of which have a high concentration in red blood cells.

A fasting specimen is required for accurate glucose and triglyceride levels, because they are normally elevated after eating.

Turbidity of blood is caused by the presence of triglycerides, not cholesterol. Because triglyceride is carried primarily in the chylomicron and very-low-density lipoprotein (VLDL) fractions, if either or both of these fractions are increased, the plasma is frequently turbid. Chylomicrons have less protein and more triglyceride, so they float on the serum to form a supranate; whereas VLDL has slightly more protein and less triglyceride than chylomicrons, thus producing a turbid infranate. Turbidity markedly interferes with certain types of laboratory tests, particularly those involving the measurement of enzyme activity.

Some analytes, such as serum iron and cortisol, have a significant diurnal variation in that they have higher concentration in the blood from 7 A.M. to 8 A.M. than they have from 3 P.M. to 4 P.M.

Collecting venous blood from above an intravenous line containing 5% dextrose and water falsely increases a patient's serum glucose and falsely decreases electrolytes. Venous blood flows back to the heart, so blood collected above an intravenous line is composed of a mixture of the intravenous fluid and the patient's blood.

24-25. The answers are: 24-D, 25-E. *(Pathology)*

The infant is at risk for developing hemolytic disease of the newborn. The mechanism involves passage of Rh-positive erythrocytes from the fetus into the blood circulation of an Rh-negative mother, which usually occurs near the time of delivery. The mother becomes sensitized and may begin producing anti-Rh antibodies. The firstborn child is generally not at great risk, because it is born before an appreciable level of immunoglobulin G (IgG) antibody is formed. However, in a subsequent pregnancy with an Rh-positive fetus, the mother can have a strong secondary immune response. Maternal anti-Rh antibody of the IgG isotype crosses the placenta and binds to the fetal red blood cells, which are removed by macrophages (type II hypersensitivity). IgG antibodies against the Rh antigen are the major cause of hemolytic disease of the newborn.

The intramuscular administration of high-titer anti-Rh antibodies, also known as anti-Rh immunoglobulin, into an Rh-negative mother within 72 hours following delivery is effective in preventing development of hemolytic disease of the newborn. The mechanism of action of this prophylaxis is not entirely understood, but it is believed that the anti-Rh antibodies attach to the fetal Rh-positive cells in the mother's circulation and thus prevent sensitization.

This type of prophylaxis also is used for Rh-negative women following abortion and amniocentesis. Large doses of the antibody can suppress sensitization following accidental transfusion of Rh-positive blood into an Rh-negative recipient, if administered within 72 hours.

Infusion of Rh-positive red blood cells could further increase the risk for the mother producing anti-Rh antibodies.

Plasma from randomly selected donors is useful in immunodeficiency diseases. Some preparations could conceivably contain anti-Rh antibodies, but this is not the best choice.

Albumin from Rh-positive donors or platelet transfusion would not protect the infant against anti-Rh antibodies.

26. The answer is B. (Pathology)

Hypoxia refers to inadequate oxygenation of tissue, which ultimately results in decreased synthesis of adenosine triphosphate (ATP) by oxidative phosphorylation in the mitochondria, which requires oxygen in the last reaction of the electron transport chain. Because oxidative phosphorylation is inoperative in the anaerobic state, ATP is available only through anaerobic glycolysis, which provides only 2 ATP per glucose molecule. The 2 NADH + 2 H$^+$ that are also generated are used to convert 2 pyruvates into 2 lactates plus 2 NAD$^+$. The 2 NAD$^+$ are used to replenish the 2 NAD$^+$ that are consumed in the conversion of 2 glyceraldehyde 3-phosphates into two 1,3 bisphosphoglycerates. Replenishing NAD$^+$ in this fashion allows generation of two more ATPs. Unfortunately, the buildup of lactate in the cell lowers intracellular pH, which eventually denatures both structural and enzymic proteins. This is primarily responsible for the findings in coagulation necrosis, which refers to cell death characterized by the preservation of the cellular outline in dead tissue. Elevation of plasma lactate is indirect evidence of tissue hypoxia. Depletion of ATP results in the loss of the ATPase–dependent sodium–potassium pump, resulting in the ingress of sodium and water into the cell and cellular swelling (hydropic swelling).

27. The answer is A. (Biochemistry)

A functional deficiency of thiamine pyrophosphate causes beriberi-like symptoms, including congestive cardiomyopathy and neurologic abnormalities. Four enzymes use thiamine pyrophosphate as a cofactor: the pyruvate dehydrogenase complex, the α-ketoglutarate dehydrogenase complex, the branched chain α-keto acid complex, and transketolase. The first three of these enzymes are analogous oxidative decarboxylation reactions, in which a keto acid is decarboxylated. In the transketolase reactions of the pentose phosphate shunt, two carbon ketomoieties are transferred from one sugar to another. The classic symptoms of beriberi are believed to reflect the effect of these malfunctioning enzymes on adenosine triphosphate (ATP) production, primarily due to inhibition of the pyruvate dehydrogenase and α-ketoglutarate dehydrogenase, both located in the mitochondria.

An aberrant transketolase is less likely to produce the symptoms of thiamine deficiency than is an aberrant pyruvate dehydrogenase.

Because the red blood cell lacks mitochondria, α-ketoglutarate dehydrogenase is not present and cannot be measured.

Glucose-6-phosphate dehydrogenase and isocitrate dehydrogenase do not use thiamine pyrophosphate as a cofactor.

Despite taking the Recommended Daily Allowance (RDA) of thiamine, this individual's symptoms indicate that he is among the 5% of the population who need greater than the RDA. In this case, his need is based on his high K_m value for pyruvate dehydrogenase—i.e., because the enzyme's affinity for the cofactor is reduced, a higher concentration of cofactor and its precursor vitamin is required.

28. The answer is C. (Pathology)

The mitochondria house the oxidative phosphorylation process, which is responsible for the generation of adenosine triphosphate (ATP). Mitochondria are the most important cellular organelles affected in early tissue hypoxia.

β-Oxidation of fatty acids, protein synthesis, the cytochrome system, and DNA synthesis are also affected by tissue hypoxia; however, these processes have no value if ATP is unavailable to the cell.

29. The answer is A. *(Microbiology)*
Many microorganisms grow on nutritional agar enriched with 5% red blood cells. Many bacteria produce enzymes (hemolysins) that may produce complete or partial destruction of the red blood cells (RBCs). Such reactions become important in the diagnosis and identification of microorganisms isolated from clinically significant situations.

Beta (clear-zone) hemolysis refers to complete destruction of the RBCs. The microorganisms produce an enzyme or several enzymes that are capable of completely destroying the membrane of the RBC and, in effect, solubilizing the contents. Such an action provides a readily available "food" source for the growing organisms. Such complete hemolysis results in a zone around the bacterial colony that becomes clear and all of the red color disappears as the hemoglobin breaks down. The clear zone is easy to see through, when compared with the opaque, red medium with intact RBCs.

Alpha (incomplete) hemolysis is produced by many streptococci. Enzymes partially destroy the RBC, but hemoglobin is released into the medium. This results in a green or brown zone around the bacterial colony. Again, such destruction provides nutrients for growing organisms. "Gamma" hemolysis describes the lack of hemolytic destruction of RBCs. No change in color or texture occurs in the agar around the colonies.

30. The answer is B. *(Pathology)*
Fibrinoid necrosis is an alteration in injured blood vessels or tissue (e.g., heart valves, synovium) that is characterized by an increase in eosinophilic staining, which is caused by the influx of plasma proteins into the vessel wall or tissue. This necrosis is often associated with immune complexes consisting of immunoglobulins, complement, or both and occurs in disorders such as systemic lupus erythematosus, rheumatic fever, and rheumatoid arthritis. Fibrinoid necrosis involving postcapillary venules produces hypersensitivity vasculitis syndromes (e.g., Henoch-Schönlein purpura), which are clinically recognized by the presence of

palpable purpura caused by the vessel inflammation. Other examples of fibrinoid necrosis are the vegetations on the mitral valve in rheumatic fever and the histologic changes in a rheumatoid nodule.

Damaged cardiac tissue secondary to an acute myocardial infarction is an example of coagulation necrosis. A renal biopsy with diabetic nephropathy exhibits hyaline arteriolosclerosis of the afferent and efferent arterioles, which has an eosinophilic appearance but is not associated with immune complexes. A section of terminal ileum in Crohn disease is likely to reveal noncaseating granulomas, which is a type IV hypersensitivity reaction. A lung biopsy of a solitary coin lesion in the right upper lobe is most commonly caused by granulomatous disease, which is also a type IV hypersensitivity reaction.

31. The answer is E. *(Biochemistry)*
The combustion of 1 g of fat produces 9 cal. Two pounds of fat is equivalent to 1,000 g, or 9,000 cal. Because his daily caloric intake is decreasing by 1,000 cal, it will take 9 days to burn 1,000 g, or 2 lbs of fat.

32. The answer is A. *(Pathology)*
Hyperplasia is an increase in cell number, whereas metaplasia is the replacement of one adult cell type by another adult cell type. Hyperplasia occurs when there is increased trophic stimulation (e.g., hormones, growth factors), increased functional demand, or persistent cell injury. Only labile and stable cells undergo hyperplasia; labile cells have stem cells that frequently divide, and stable cells have resting cells that are stimulated to enter the cell cycle. The presence of increased goblet cells in the mainstem bronchus of a smoker is an example of hyperplasia, because goblet cells are normally present in this area. However, their presence in the terminal bronchiole or gastric mucosa, where they are not normally found, is an example of metaplasia.

Squamous epithelium in the bladder of a patient with *Schistosoma haematobium* is an example of metaplasia, because the epithelium of a normal bladder is transitional. Irritation from the eggs of the schistosomes induces squamous metaplasia and the potential for dysplasia and squamous carcinoma.

A distal esophagus with glandular epithelium intermixed with squamous epithelium is an example of

Barrett esophagus. Chronic acid injury to the distal esophagus from gastroesophageal reflux stimulates the formation of mucous-secreting glandular epithelium, which is a type of glandular metaplasia and predisposes the patient to adenocarcinoma.

Goblet and Paneth cells in the glands of the gastric mucosa is called intestinal metaplasia and is commonly seen in chronic atrophic gastritis of the body and fundus (type A) or pylorus and antrum (type B). It is a precursor lesion of adenocarcinoma of the stomach.

Squamous epithelium in the mainstem bronchus of a smoker is squamous metaplasia, because normal epithelium is pseudostratified, ciliated, and columnar. The squamous epithelium is a reaction to injury induced by cigarette smoke. It predisposes the patient to squamous dysplasia and carcinoma.

33. The answer is C.   *(Behavioral science)*
Individuals with antisocial personality disorders know the difference between right and wrong but do not care. The internal sense of right and wrong characterizes the superego. The ego maintains a relationship to the outside world, whereas the id represents instinctive sexual and aggressive drives. The id, ego, and superego are constructs of Freud's structural theory of the mind. The unconscious mind contains repressed thoughts and feelings that are unavailable to the consciousness, whereas the preconscious mind contains memories that can be easily brought to consciousness. The unconscious, preconscious, and conscious minds are constructs of Freud's topographic theory of the mind.

34. The answer is A.   *(Pathology)*
Hypertrophy is a reversible increase in cell size, whereas hyperplasia is a reversible increase in cell number. Hypertrophy is caused by an increased functional demand, increased trophic signals (e.g., hormones, growth factors), or both. A thickened bladder wall in a patient with urethral obstruction is an example of hypertrophy that is caused by an increase in functional demand imposed by the increased afterload.

Increased reticulocyte count in a patient with a hemolytic anemia, breast tissue in a woman with a prolactinoma, biopsy of the endometrium taken a few days before ovulation, and prostate enlargement in an elderly man with difficulty initiating his urinary stream are all examples of hyperplasia.

35. The answer is D.   *(Biochemistry)*
In the average sedentary individual, about 60% of the caloric expenditure is due to basal metabolic rate (BMR), 10% is due to the thermic effect of food, and the remaining 30% is spent in physical activity. An individual engaged in strenuous physical activity may increase the daily caloric muscular expenditure to greater than twice the BMR. Routine physical activity will also increase the BMR to a small but significant degree. This increase in the BMR is most likely caused by increased circulation and other nonspecific effects. Diet and the timing of physical activity influence contribution of the thermic effect of foods. For example, energy converts carbohydrate to fat. Therefore, fewer calories are required to store fat when the calories are derived from fat than are required to store an equivalent quantity of fat when the calories are derived from carbohydrate or protein.

Although the brain consumes about 25% of the calories used in the resting individual, the amount consumed does not increase during mental activity.

36. The answer is C.   *(Pathology)*
Repair of injured tissue is dependent on the type of tissue involved (e.g., labile, stable, or permanent), whether the scaffolding of the tissue is still intact (e.g., the basement membrane), the presence of preexisting disease in the tissue (e.g., cirrhosis), deficiencies in growth-promoting factors (e.g., hormone deficiencies), and the availability of substrate (e.g., protein, iron, vitamin B_{12}).

Both fatty change in the liver and mild cervical dysplasia are reversible. The most common cause of fatty change is alcoholism. It is related to a buildup of triglyceride in the hepatocytes, which is caused by an increase in glycerol 3-phosphate, the carbohydrate backbone of triglyceride, or an increase in fatty acids. Both of these are normally increased in the metabolism of alcohol. Fatty change is reversible if the individual stops drinking. Persistent intake of alcohol can lead to alcoholic hepatitis, cirrhosis, or hepatocellular carcinoma, the latter two conditions representing irreversible changes.

Mild cervical dysplasia is reversible if the irritant (e.g., human papilloma virus) is removed.

37. The answer is D. *(Microbiology)*
Coccidioides immitis is a dimorphic fungus that exists as a mold in soil and as a spherule in tissue. It is endemic in arid regions of the Southwestern United States. In soil, it forms hyphae with alternating arthrospores and empty cells. The arthrospores are inhaled, and they establish areas of infection in the lungs. Endospores form spherules that can spread virtually to any organ. Some infected persons have an influenza-like fever and cough. The history of travel through the southwest and symptom complex are typical for "valley fever." In fewer than 1% of infected persons, the disease disseminates. The lesions are typical granulomas with a predilection for the lower lobes. Erythema nodosum, which is a localized inflammation of subcutaneous fat, commonly occurs on the lower extremities.

38. The answer is D. *(Pathology)*
Gaucher disease is an autosomal recessive disease characterized by a deficiency of the lysosomal enzyme, glucocerebrosidase, leading to an accumulation of glucocerebroside. It is a sphingolipidosis characterized by lipids containing sphingosine, which is converted into ceramide. When ceramide combines with glucose, it forms glucocerebroside. Von Gierke disease is an autosomal recessive glycogenosis characterized by deficiency of the gluconeogenic enzyme, glucose-6-phosphatase. This enzyme converts glucose 6-phosphate into glucose. Because gluconeogenesis is impaired, patients have a fasting hypoglycemia. There is a build-up of glucose 6-phosphate, which activates glycogen synthetase and glycogen synthesis. Because the gluconeogenic enzymes are located only in the liver and kidneys, the excess formation of normal glycogen is primarily in the liver and kidneys.

Vitiligo refers to the autoimmune destruction of melanocytes and their melanosomes, resulting in depigmentation of the skin. Albinism is an autosomal recessive disease characterized by an absence of tyrosinase, resulting in the inability to convert tyrosine into dopamine and the latter into melanin.

Stasis dermatitis is a deep saphenous vein thrombosis that leads to a back flow of venous blood into the penetrating branches around the ankles with subsequent rupture of the vessels. This rupture of vessels causes ulceration and a bronzed discoloration of the skin because of the excess of hemosiderin released by the red blood cells. Hemochromatosis is an autosomal recessive disease characterized by an excessive absorption of iron from the small intestine with subsequent parenchymal deposition of iron and malfunction of that tissue (e.g., liver, heart, pancreas). The Prussian-blue stain demonstrates the presence of hemosiderin in tissue.

Pompe and McArdle diseases are two autosomal recessive glycogenoses. Pompe disease is the only lysosomal storage disease in the glycogenoses group. It is characterized by a deficiency of the lysosomal enzyme, acid maltase. This deficiency results primarily in glycogen deposition in the heart and a restrictive cardiomyopathy, causing premature death. McArdle disease is caused by a deficiency of muscle phosphorylase, which is needed to break down glycogen for energy purposes. Patients have muscle fatigue and are unable to generate lactic acid in muscle after exercise, because they are unable to retrieve glucose from the glycogen that is needed for glycolysis.

Xanthelasmas and Achille tendon xanthomas are both characterized by an increased deposition of cholesterol in the tissue. They are usually signs of type II hyperlipidemia caused by a defect in the low-density lipoprotein (LDL) receptor with subsequent buildup of LDL, the main carrier form for cholesterol.

39. The answer is A. *(Biochemistry)*
In coconut and palm oils, 85% to 95% of the total fat is saturated; in lard and butter, 41% to 66% of the total fat is saturated.

Both linoleic and linolenic acids are essential polyunsaturated fatty acids, and both are required in the diet. They have different metabolic functions and dietary distributions. Both of these essential fatty acids are required for membrane fluidity, and thus one can probably substitute for the other. However, linoleic is a precursor of thromboxanes and prostaglandins of the two series, whereas only linolenic acid is a precursor of thromboxanes and prostaglandins of the three series. Moreover, the distribution of linolenic acid is more limited than that of linoleic, making a subclinical deficiency more likely. Some unsaturated oils (e.g., olive oil) have little of either essential fatty acid.

Although margarine is made from polyunsaturated oils, it is also partially hydrogenated. The final product is a mixture of saturated and unsaturated fatty acids that contain various amounts of *trans* fatty acids and other breakdown products.

Polyunsaturated fatty acids are susceptible to destruction by oxygenation, particularly at high temperatures. The polyunsaturated oils used in frying potatoes contain various peroxides and other breakdown products, depending upon the length of time the oil is used. Monounsaturated oils (e.g., olive oil) should be used for these processes, because they have cholesterol-lowering propensities but also are relatively stable. Although saturated fats raise cholesterol levels, if consumed in moderation, they are probably less of a health hazard than overheated polyunsaturated fats.

According to the recommended dietary goal, only 30% of an individual's caloric intake should be fat calories. Reporting by weight is misleading: Fat has twice as many calories per gram than either carbohydrate or protein, and food may have components, such as water or fiber, that yield no calories.

40. The answer is C. *(Pathology)*
Apoptosis is individual cell necrosis. It is typically operative in the normal turnover of cells (e.g., hormone-dependent involution in female menstrual cycle); programmed cell death in embryogenesis; toxin-induced injury (e.g., diphtheria); viral cell death (e.g., Councilman bodies in yellow fever); cell death via cytotoxic T cells, natural killer cells, and antibody-dependent cytotoxicity (type II); atrophy of tissue (e.g., red neurons in ischemic atrophy in the brain); and cell death in tumors.

An acute myocardial infarction is an example of coagulation necrosis, which involves more extensive cell necrosis. Acute appendicitis is an example of liquefactive necrosis. Type III hypersensitivity reactions are usually associated with fibrinoid necrosis. The formation of a venous thrombus is most commonly caused by venous stasis.

41. The answer is D. *(Behavioral science)*
The stage of the sexual response cycle that is most different between men and women is resolution. This is because, during the resolution stage, men have a refractory or resting period when restimulation is not possible. Women are less likely than men to have a refractory period after orgasm.

42. The answer is E. *(Pathology)*
Alcohol induces elevated levels of liver cytochrome P_{450}, a heme protein located in the smooth endoplasmic reticulum. It is the major pathway for the hydroxylation of aliphatic and aromatic compounds, resulting in their water solubility and eventual excretion by the kidneys. An alcoholic taking theophylline as a bronchodilator for chronic obstructive pulmonary disease will increase the metabolism of the drug in the liver, resulting in suboptimal levels in the blood.

Although decreased uptake in the gastrointestinal tract, increased uptake in fat, and alcohol directly blocking the reabsorption of the drug are theoretically possible, induction of the cytochrome P_{450} system is the most correct answer. Decreased urine excretion of the drug would increase, not decrease, the drug concentration. The most common cause of a suboptimal response to any drug is the lack of patient compliance.

43. The answer is C. *(Microbiology)*
This patient's case is a typical presentation of ulceroglandular tularemia caused by *Francisella tularensis*. The ulceroglandular form of this disease, which is acquired by direct contact with tissues of infected animals (e.g., jackrabbits, muskrats, squirrels), represents approximately 75% of tularemia cases in the United States. Systemic symptoms appear abruptly, and an ulcerating papule at the entry site of the organisms develops within 2 to 6 days. Regional lymph nodes may become extremely large, painful, and necrotic. Convalescence from tularemia is slow, and lymphadenopathy often persists for several months.

F. tularensis is highly infectious. The organisms are very small, pleomorphic, intracellular gram-negative rods. Because of these characteristics, they are rarely observed in clinical specimens, and they require cysteine for growth. A 10-day course of streptomycin or gentamicin is effective treatment; however, relapses can occur.

44. The answer is A. *(Pathology)*
Cimetidine blocks the cytochrome P_{450} system in the liver, which decreases the metabolism of drugs typically handled by the liver. Therefore, a standard dose of a drug such as theophylline could potentially result in toxicity because it is not metabolized as quickly by

the liver. This potential situation underscores the importance of asking patients about the drugs they are taking to avoid adverse drug interactions.

45. The answer is B. *(Pharmacology)*
Several antibiotics are primarily excreted in the bile; therefore, patients with renal disease do not require dosage adjustments. These antibiotics include the macrolides (e.g., erythromycin, azithromycin), doxycycline, some β-lactam antibiotics (e.g., ceftriaxone, nafcillin), clindamycin, and chloramphenicol. Aminoglycosides (e.g., gentamicin) are completely dependent on renal function for elimination, and they require reduction in dosage and dosage interval during renal impairment. Many other antibiotics, including most β-lactams, require some dosage adjustment when renal impairment is moderately severe.

46. The answer is E. *(Microbiology)*
Group B streptococci (e.g., *Streptococcus agalactiae*) are members of the normal flora of the female genital tract, and they are the most important cause of neonatal sepsis and meningitis, and in the mother, of chorioaminonitis, causing spontaneous abortion. They are beta-hemolytic, positive in the CAMP test, positive in the sodium hippurate hydrolysis test, and they are unusually resistant bacteria. Infections in neonates need to be accurately and quickly diagnosed so that prompt antimicrobial treatment can be instituted. Although *S. pyogenes*, *S. pneumoniae*, *Listeria monocytogenes*, and *Staphylococcus aureus* may invade the central nervous system and cause meningitis, the Group B streptococci are the most significant organisms in neonatal meningitis.

47. The answer is A. *(Behavioral science)*
Premature ejaculation is a common male sexual dysfunction, comprising about 35% of male sexual disorders. Primary erectile disorder, in which the man has never had an erection sufficient for penetration, is seen in 1% of men. Male orgasmic disorder (i.e., delayed or absent orgasm) is relatively rare and is seen in only 5% of men. Dyspareunia, pain associated with intercourse, is rare in men.

48. The answer is E. *(Microbiology)*
Humans are the only natural host of *Neisseria meningitidis*. Organisms are transmitted by airborne droplets and are inhaled. They colonize the membranes of the posterior nasopharynx and are transient. While present, they are antigenic and antibodies (especially IgA) will protect against future encounters with the organism. Three organisms cause 80% of bacterial meningitis in children older than 2 months of age: *Haemophilus influenzae* (40% to 60%), *Streptococcus pneumoniae* (10% to 20%), and *N. meningitidis* (25% to 40%). *N. meningitidis* is most likely to cause epidemics. The principal laboratory diagnostic procedures for *N. meningitidis* are gram-staining of smears and culture of blood and spinal-fluid samples. The oxidase-positive organism enters the bloodstream from the nasopharynx and spreads to specific sites or is disseminated (i.e., meningococcemia). Culture requires the use of Thayer-Martin medium and 10% carbon dioxide atmosphere. Sugar fermentation tests distinguish between species. All of the other diseases listed in this question (i.e., *Staphylococcus* food poisoning, toxic shock syndrome, rheumatic fever, and infant botulism) involve toxins (e.g., enterotoxins, toxic shock syndrome test, botulinum toxin), and blood cultures from these are negative for the causative organism. Thayer-Martin is composed of chocolate agar plus antibiotics to suppress normal flora and is used to isolate gonococci from urethral exudates.

49. The answer is B. *(Biochemistry)*
A nick is a break in the backbone of a DNA strand. No nucleotides are missing, and a 5′ phosphate group and a 3′ hydroxyl group are present on the neighboring nucleotides at the site of the nick. DNA ligase seals the nick by covalently joining the phosphate and hydroxyl groups to form a phosphodiester linkage. This enzyme is used during DNA replication to join together the fragments of DNA synthesized on the lagging strand. It is also used during DNA repair and other processes involving the sealing of nicks. DNA polymerase I is used by bacteria for DNA repair and for the removal of RNA primers during DNA replication. DNA polymerase III synthesizes the bulk of the DNA during replication. Helicase is an enzyme used to separate the two strands of the parental DNA double helix during DNA replication. An endonuclease is an enzyme that can cut the backbone in the middle of a DNA strand.

50. The answer is B. *(Microbiology)*
Pasteurella multocida is probably the most common bacteria that is isolated from wounds inflicted by cat bites, and to a lesser extent, dog bites. It is found worldwide in the upper respiratory tract of many domestic and wild animals.

P. multocida causes a local cellulitis at the site of the bite, which evolves rapidly. Complications are common and include osteomyelitis of the underlying bone, necrotizing synovitis, and pyarthrosis. Penicillin is the drug of choice.

More than 90% of cellulitis cases that do not involve animal bites are caused by *Staphylococcus aureus* and group A streptococci. *Haemophilus influenzae* type B is an important cause of cellulitis in children.

51. The answer is B. *(Behavioral science)*
The tendency of a newborn infant to turn its head in the direction of stroking its cheek is an example of the rooting reflex. The rooting reflex is beneficial for nursing infants. The rooting reflex, as well as the Babinski reflex, the grasp reflex, and the Moro (startle) reflex, are all normal in a newborn infant. The Babinski reflex occurs when the sole of the neonate's foot is stroked; he spreads his toes (adults flex their toes). The grasp reflex occurs both with fingers and with toes. Upon placing an object in the neonate's palm or on the sole of the foot, the infant will grasp the object. The Babinski and grasp reflexes subside by the end of 3 months of life. The Moro reflex occurs when the infant is startled. The infant puts his fingers in a "C" position and adducts his legs, as if to protect himself. This reflex subsides around the end of the fourth or fifth month of life.

52. The answer is A. *(Microbiology)*
Spirochetes are the etiologic agents of relapsing fever, syphilis, Lyme disease, leptospirosis, yaws, and other diseases.

Spirochete	Disease
Treponema pallidum	Syphilis
T. subspecies *pertenue*	Yaws
T. subspecies *endemicum*	Bejel
Treponema carateum	Pinta
Borrelia recurrentis	Relapsing fever
Borrelia burgdorferi	Lyme disease
Leptospira interrogans	Leptospirosis

Spirochetes are spiral-shaped, long, flexible bacteria with thin walls and multiple axial filaments that give them an undulating, corkscrew-like motility. *Treponema* and *Leptospira* species are too thin to be seen with an ordinary light microscope, whereas *Borrelia* species can be seen after staining with Giemsa or another blood stain; Borrelia is gram negative.

53. The answer is B. *(Pharmacology)*
Most β-lactam antibiotics (e.g., cephalexin) are relatively safe for pregnant women. They are classified in the Food and Drug Administration (FDA) pregnancy category B. Aminoglycosides (e.g., amikacin, streptomycin) pose a risk of ototoxicity in a fetus. Because of the demonstrated risk, aminoglycosides are in FDA pregnancy category D. Tetracycline may stain fetal teeth and they also are potentially toxic to pregnant women. Griseofulvin, an antifungal agent, may cause birth defects or rare conjoined twins when administered to women during the first trimester of pregnancy.

54. The answer is A. *(Microbiology)*
A single intramuscular injection of benzathine penicillin G maintains treponemacidal levels in the body for approximately 2 weeks. This treatment is effective in eradicating *Treponema pallidum* infection that is of less than 1-year duration. If the patient has been infected for longer than 1 year, the treatment is usually administered 3 times during a 3-week period. Immunity is short-lived if the patient is treated early, and an individual can be infected repeatedly with the organisms.

Hypersensitivity reactions to penicillin may occur, particularly in promiscuous individuals who require repeated treatments with the drug. Tetracycline, erythromycin, and chloramphenicol are alternative drugs for patients who are allergic to penicillin.

If large numbers of spirochetes are present at the time of treatment, a Jarisch-Herxheimer reaction (intensification of the maculopapular rash) may occur within hours. This reaction is apparently caused by the release of toxic materials from the dying spirochetes and is not an allergic reaction.

The incidence of syphilis in the United States has increased steadily since the mid-1980s. This increase is attributed in large part to the increase in drug addiction and the exchange of drugs for sex (i.e., prostitution to support a drug habit). However, syphilis is not considered to be a highly contagious disease. The incidence of transmission after one sexual encounter is estimated to be approximately 30%. High-risk individuals are those who have multiple partners, newborn infants of infected mothers, and individuals with AIDS. The organisms die rapidly when dried and are killed by numerous disinfectants.

55. The answer is C. *(Behavioral science)*
Gender identity, the sense of oneself as male or female, is established by 2 to 3 years of age.

56. The answer is A. *(Microbiology)*
Mycoplasma consists of a distinct group of extremely small, flexible bacteria that do not have a cell wall. They are the smallest organisms that can replicate in cell-free media. The smallest reproductive forms are 125 to 250 nm in diameter.

Mycoplasmas are highly pleomorphic. They are bound by a triple-layered "unit membrane" that contains sterol. The membrane allows the organisms to survive in nature (e.g., in high-temperature springs and acid outflows of mining wastes). Humans can harbor several species (e.g., *Mycoplasma salivarium*, *Mycoplasma orale*) as part of the normal flora of the oropharyx. *Mycoplasma pneumoniae* is the etiologic agent of primary atypical pneumonia, which occurs primarily in individuals 5 to 20 years of age.

Mycoplasmas are not derived from, nor can they revert back to, any parental cell that has a wall. They are different from L-forms, which are wall-defective microbial forms that are derived from well-known organisms. L-forms are resistant to penicillin and other wall-inhibiting drugs.

57. The answer is D. *(Pharmacology)*
Methotrexate is a competitive inhibitor of mammalian dihydrofolate reductase, and it prevents the formation of active folate derivatives that are required for thymidylate and purine synthesis. Methotrexate also forms polyglutamate derivatives that have long-acting effects on folate metabolism. Unlike most antineoplastic agents, methotrexate does not require metabolic activation. Leucovorin is an active form of folic acid that bypasses the inhibition of dihydrofolate reductase produced by methotrexate. Leucovorin rescue is the process of using leucovorin to treat methotrexate toxicity.

58. The answer is C. *(Microbiology)*
Legionella pneumophila, first identified as the causative agent of Legionnaire disease in 1978, is an oxidase-positive, poorly staining, gram-negative rod that is associated with severe pneumonia. It is a ubiquitous organism in warm, moist environments, including air-conditioning systems and shower heads. It is resistant to chlorine.

Subclinical infections with *L. pneumophila* are common in all age groups. However, in men who are older than 55 years of age and who have certain risk factors (e.g., smoking, chronic bronchitis, emphysema, immunosuppressive therapy, cancer chemotherapy, and diabetes mellitus), it can cause pneumonia. The pneumonia is often severe, bilateral, and results in the loss of the alveolar epithelium. Treatment includes administration of erythromycin, rifampin, or both; ventilation assistance; and management of shock.

Acinetobacter, formerly known as *Mimeae/Herellae*, is an aerobic, gram-negative coccobacillus. It is a ubiquitous organism found in soil and water, including the water of humidifiers and vaporizers. It is an occasional cause of nosocomial infections (e.g., septicemia, meningitis, urethritis/vaginitis). It may be confused with *Neisseria meningitidis* or *Neisseria gonorrhoeae*, except that it is oxidase negative.

Calymmatobacterium granulomatis, the cause of granuloma inguinale, is a gram-negative rod related to *Klebsiella*.

Afipia felis, a small gram-negative rod, causes cat-scratch disease.

Streptobacillus moniliformis, one of the agents of rat-bite fever, is a gram-negative, pleomorphic rod.

59. The answer is E. *(Behavioral science)*
In a cohort study, the relative risk measures the ratio of incidence in one group (e.g., miscarriage among women exposed to oral contraceptives) in relation to incidence in another group (e.g., miscarriage among women not exposed to oral contraceptives). An example of attributable risk is the incidence rate of miscarriage among women exposed to oral contraceptives minus the incidence rate of miscarriage among women not exposed to oral contraceptives. The odds-risk ratio is a measure of relative risk for a case-control study. The incidence rate is the number of new individuals who develop an illness in a given time period, whereas the prevalence rate is the number of individuals in

the population who have an illness at a specific point in time or during a specific time period.

60. The answer is D. *(Microbiology)*
Pseudomonas aeruginosa is an aerobic, gram-negative rod that does not ferment glucose or any other sugar; thus, it is known as a "nonfermenter." The organisms colonize within the respiratory tract of patients with cystic fibrosis and other chronic respiratory tract diseases. Respiratory diseases caused by the organisms range from relatively benign tracheobronchitis to severe necrotizing bronchopneumonia.

P. aeruginosa is a ubiquitous, opportunistic pathogen. In addition to its involvement in the respiratory tract, it is associated with other nosocomial infections. In debilitated individuals, it can cause bacteremia, particularly in patients with diabetes, extensive burns, hematologic malignancies, or neutropenia; endocarditis; and urinary tract infections. Ear infections caused by the organisms include external otitis ("swimmer's ear") and malignant external otitis.

P. aeruginosa is hardy and can grow in environments that are often hostile to other bacteria. It has few nutritional requirements and survives extremes of temperature. In hospitals, it can often be isolated from respiratory therapy equipment, sinks, water, bed pans, and floors.

Escherichia coli and *Klebsiella pneumoniae* ferment glucose, and *Mycoplasma pneumoniae* and *Mycobacterium* species are not gram-negative rods.

61. The answer is C. *(Physiology)*
The symptom of menopause most likely to be seen cross culturally is hot flashes. Hot flashes are a physiologic symptom caused by vasomotor instability, which is caused by decreased ovarian estrogen production. Hot flashes can be treated effectively with estrogen replacement therapy. Dysphoria, memory problems, depression, and anxiety, which are seen in some women at menopause, are more likely than hot flashes to be related to psychosocial as well as to physiological factors.

62. The answer is B. *(Microbiology)*
The *Mycobacterium avium-intracellulare* complex (sometimes referred to as the *Mycobacterium avium* complex or MAC) is the most common bacterial infection in AIDS patients in the United States. Historically, it was a relatively uncommon cause of human infection, and disease was usually restricted to the pulmonary region.

Mycobacterium avium-intracellulare is often widely disseminated in AIDS patients, especially when the CD4+ lymphocyte count falls below $100/\mu l$. In some patients, hundreds of thousands of organisms per milliliter of blood are present.

The organisms are present in birds (pigeon droppings) and other animals, water, and soil. Inhalation or ingestion of the organisms by a debilitated individual can result in its colonization of the respiratory or gastrointestinal tracts, respectively. After an initial episode of bacteremia and spread into tissues, persistent bacteremia and extensive tissue invasion may occur. Clinical manifestations include fever, night sweats, weight loss, diarrhea, and abdominal pain. Many organs can be involved, including the lungs, lymph nodes, bone, pericardium, skin, and brain.

Mycobacterium avium-intracellulare is almost always resistant to the first line of drugs used for tuberculosis. Unfortunately, there is no rapid or reliable method for testing drug susceptibility for these organisms. Clarithromycin or azithromycin combined with ethambutol is often used for initial therapy. Rifabutin may be used prophylactically to reduce the risk for bacteremia and decrease the severity of symptoms.

Mycobacterium kansasii is an opportunistic organism that causes pulmonary and systemic disease in debilitated individuals. *Mycobacterium bovis* is considered a pathogen. When inhaled, it causes disease that is virtually indistinguishable from tuberculosis. These organisms are no longer prevalent in the United States. An attenuated strain is used in the bacille Calmette-Guérin (BCG) vaccine for immunization against tuberculosis. *Mycobacterium fortuitum-chelonae* complex rarely causes disease in humans. The organisms have been occasionally isolated from porcine valves implanted during cardiac surgery. *Mycobacterium scrofulaceum* may cause cervical lymphadenitis in children and has been isolated from adults with chronic lung disease.

63. The answer is D. *(Behavioral science)*
The strength of an association between a factor and a disease is best measured by relative risk. Relative risk measures how much higher a patient's risk of disease is because of exposure to a specific risk factor. In contrast, attributable risk measures the impact that

the risk factor may have on the incidence of the disease in the population. Prevalence is the number of individuals with the disease in the total population, whereas incidence is the number of new cases occurring per year in the total population. Reliability measures the reproducibility of results.

64. The answer is D.   *(Microbiology)*
Corynebacterium diphtheriae secretes a protein of approximately 62,000 molecular weight that exhibits toxicity against mammalian cells. Therefore, it is called an exotoxin (i.e., a toxic protein that is secreted by bacterial cells). It is a single polypeptide chain held together by two disulfide bridges. Fragment A exhibits enzymatic activity, resulting in permanent inactivation of elongation factor 2 (EF-2), whereas fragment B binds to cells and mediates entry of the toxic portion.

The diphtheria toxin binds to epithelial cells of the pharynx and initially produces local damage. However, the toxin is absorbed into the body and blood circulation (toxemia) and can induce deleterious effects distant from its site of production. Paralysis of the soft palate, pharynx, larynx, and respiratory muscles may appear weeks after onset of symptoms. The toxin may also cause myocarditis. Electrocardiographic abnormalities correlate with the level of toxemia. In rare cases, hypotension, peripheral circulatory failure, and skin hemorrhages may occur.

65. The answer is B.   *(Behavioral science)*
Compared with males between the ages of 20 and 30 years, males between the ages of 70 and 80 years are more likely to have health insurance. Health insurance for people 65 years and older is provided to all Americans who are eligible for social security under Medicare.

66. The answer is E.   *(Microbiology)*
Watery diarrhea caused by *Vibrio cholerae* is the result of the action of a secreted enterotoxin that consists of a toxic A subunit and multiple-binding B subunits. The A subunit catalyzes the ribosylation of adenosine diphosphate, which results in persistent activation of adenylate cyclase. The adenylate cyclase enzyme converts adenosine triphosphate into cyclic adenosine monophosphate, which accumulates at the mammalian cell membrane and results in hypersecretion of water, chloride, potassium, and bicarbonate. In severe cases, as much as 15

to 20 liters of fluid is lost in 1 day. Flecks of mucous in the diarrheal fluid give the appearance of "rice-water" stools. The mechanism of action of the toxin is similar to the heat-labile enterotoxin of *Escherichia coli*.

Members of the Vibrionaceae family are curved, gram-negative rods that are commonly found in water. They have a single polar flagellum, are highly motile, and are facultatively anaerobic. *V. cholerae* is distinguished from other *Vibrio* species by using a battery of biochemical assays, by the structure of its O antigen, and by its secretion of the potent enterotoxin.

Campylobacter jejuni produces fever, abdominal pain, and diarrhea in which stools usually contain red blood cells and leukocytes. Acute mesenteric lymphadenitis is the most common clinical manifestation in humans infected with *Yersinia pseudotuberculosis*. *Salmonella typhi* causes enteric (typhoid) fever, which is characterized by high fever, constipation, and hepatosplenomegaly. *Shigella sonnei* causes dysentery.

67. The answer is D.   *(Behavioral science)*
Otherwise normal infants, who because of parental absence or neglect do not have a primary attachment figure, are at risk for anaclitic depression. Children with anaclitic depression become withdrawn and unresponsive, and they may show developmental retardation or poor health. Infantile autism and Asperger syndrome (which is a lesser form of autism) are pervasive developmental disorders of childhood that are characterized by failure to relate normally to others. These two disorders are believed to be neurologic in origin. Childhood schizophrenia and bipolar illness in childhood are similar to these illnesses in adults.

68. The answer is B.   *(Pathology)*
The patient who has no secondary sex characteristics or no menstruation but who has a short stature and a thick neck is probably suffering from Turner syndrome. Because Turner syndrome is characterized by an XO chromosome complement, the best way to diagnose it is by examining cells via a buccal smear to determine the presence or absence of Barr bodies. Although a gonadal hormone profile will show reduced levels of female hormones because the secretory gonads are absent, an abnormal hormone profile can occur with other conditions. Determination of gender identity, gender role, and sexual preference are not diagnostic of Turner syndrome.

69. The answer is C. *(Biochemistry)*
Enzymes increase the rate with which substrates are converted to products. They work by decreasing the free energy of the transition state. That is, they provide an alternate reaction pathway with a lower free energy of activation (i.e., the amount of energy required to form a high-energy intermediate that is involved in generating the product). The free energies of the substrates and the products are not altered. Because the energies of the initial state and the final state are not changed, the free energy change is not altered. The equilibrium of the reaction also remains unchanged.

70. The answer is B. *(Biochemistry)*
Cytosine is a pyrimidine base. The other commonly occurring pyrimidines are thymine and uracil. Adenine and guanine are the commonly found purine bases. A base becomes linked to a sugar molecule to form a nucleoside. The addition of a phosphate group to a nucleoside forms a nucleotide. Nucleic acids are polymers created by joining nucleotides.

71. The answer is D. *(Biochemistry)*
Protein synthesis is a complicated process during which the ribosome moves along the messenger RNA (mRNA), synthesizing a protein with an amino acid sequence that is specified by the message. In response to the chain initiation codon UAG, the initiator transfer RNA (tRNA) enters the P site on the ribosome. In prokaryotes, this first tRNA carries formylmethionine (fmet), whereas methionine is used in eukaryotes.

Peptidyl transferase is a ribosome-associated enzyme that links amino acids together during the elongation stage of translation. The same enzymatic activity also is used during termination to cleave the completed polypeptide from the tRNA to which it is covalently linked. The 28S rRNA is a structural component of the ribosome and is not translated.

72. The answer is C. *(Biochemistry)*
The *uvr*ABC endonuclease is an enzyme that is involved in the repair of DNA that has been damaged by thymine dimer formation. It cuts a DNA strand on both sides of the thymine dimer, which allows the damaged region of DNA to be removed. DNA repair is completed by the action of DNA polymerase I,

which fills in the gap with new DNA, and DNA ligase, which seals the remaining nick at the repaired area.

73. The answer is B. *(Physiology)*
Both histamine and serotonin act to stimulate sensory nerve endings to cause intense itching. Both histamine and serotonin may contribute to these symptoms during allergic reactions and after insect stings. Only histamine causes gastric acid secretion and relaxation of vascular smooth muscle, whereas serotonin causes vasoconstriction in most vascular beds, except the skeletal muscle and heart.

74. The answer is D. *(Pharmacology)*
Losartan is a new nonpeptide angiotensin II antagonist. Unlike the peptide antagonist saralasin, losartan is orally effective and lacks agonist activity. Angiotensin converting enzyme (ACE) inhibitors (e.g., captopril) also inhibit the degradation of bradykinin. Adrenergic β-receptor antagonists (e.g., propranolol) inhibit the release of renin from renal juxtaglomerular cells.

75. The answer is B. *(Behavioral science)*
Secondary prevention involves the early identification of a disorder to reduce its occurrence or duration. Thus, early intervention programs for children with emotional disorders can reduce the likelihood that the problems will persist into adulthood.

76. The answer is D. *(Pathology)*
Desmin is the intermediate filament of muscle, and it is used as a marker for rhabdomyosarcoma tumors. Keratin is the intermediate filament of epithelium, and it is used as a marker for carcinoma tumors. Actinin is an actin-associated protein, present along bundles of microfilaments. It is considered a bundling protein. Desmoplakin is the protein found in the dense plaques of desmosomes.

77. The answer is C. *(Microbiology)*
Giardia lamblia cysts are found in approximately 5% of the stool specimens in the United States, with about half coming from asymptomatic carriers. Although water contamination is the usual mechanism of transmission, the incidence is high among children in day care centers, as well as among patients in mental hospitals. *Enterobius vermicularis* causes pinworm infection.

The infection is acquired by ingesting the embryonated eggs. Although autoreinfection is quite common, fingers become contaminated with eggs after the person has scratched the itching, perianal skin. *Enterobius* is the most common helminth found in the U.S. Sampling the perianal skin with cellophane tape and observing the eggs is the primary method for diagnosis. Both organisms are easily transmitted from child-to-child or child-to-fomite by means of contaminated fingers. No means of prevention exists for *Enterobius*.

Isospora causes human gastroenteritis and usually occurs when fecally contaminated food or water is ingested. The life cycle in humans is poorly understood. Similarly, *Entamoeba histolytica* usually is spread by fecal contamination of water containing cysts rather than by direct transmission from individuals. *Balantidium coli* are also transmitted by cyst ingestion, usually in contaminated water. *Dientamoeba fragilis* lacks a cyst stage and differs from true amoeba. The method of transmission is unknown, but it has been suggested that ingested trophozoites is the most likely procedure. *Necatur americanus*, a helminth, is transmitted by a free-living filariform larva that penetrates the skin. *Taenia saginata*, the beef tapeworm, is transmitted in raw or poorly cooked meat.

78. The answer is C. *(Biochemistry)*
Type II granular pneumocytes in the lung synthesize dipalmitoylphosphatidylcholine, which is the major lipid component of lung surfactant. This phosphatidylcholine (lecithin) is characterized by having the 1 and 2 positions of glycerol esterified by palmitic acid. Surfactant decreases the surface tension of the fluid layer between the alveoli and the chest wall, which allows the alveoli to freely expand upon inspiration. Respiratory distress syndrome (i.e., hyaline membrane disease) in infants is associated with delayed synthesis of dipalmitoylphosphatidylcholine and an insufficiency of surfactant. De novo synthesis of choline does occur, so choline is not an essential nutrient. The synthesis of choline from phosphatidylserine is an energy-consuming process. Therefore, choline in the diet may be of value for individuals who are on a low-calorie or protein-deficient diet. Because the phosphatidylcholines play an important role in the formation

of very low-density lipoprotein (VLDL) particles, choline may be particularly beneficial in the diet of alcoholics who not only eat poorly, but also are prone to developing fatty livers.

The quaternary amine formed by putting three methyl groups on what was the α-amino group of serine has a positive, not a negative charge.

Sphingomyelin is formed by putting a phosphocholine group onto a ceramide. However, ceramides do not contain choline. The inability to remove the phosphocholine group from sphingomyelin is caused by a deficiency of the enzyme sphingomyelinase and causes Niemann-Pick disease.

Cardiolipin is composed of two molecules of phosphatidic acid connected by a molecule of glycerol and contains no choline. Cardiolipin is an important constituent of the inner membrane of the mitochondrion and is the only antigenic phospholipid.

79. The answer is B. *(Biochemistry)*
Hexokinase, phosphofructokinase-1, and pyruvate kinase are the three enzymes involved in the irreversible reactions of glycolysis. The reversal of these steps during gluconeogenesis requires different enzymes. Each of these glycolytic enzymes must be regulated because the products of the gluconeogenic process are glycolytic substrates, and a futile cycle would be created if the glycolytic enzymes were active. To prevent such energy-consuming cycles, mechanisms exist to inhibit the irreversible glycolytic steps under gluconeogenic conditions, and conversely, to inhibit the irreversible gluconeogenic enzymes when glycolysis predominates.

Gluconeogenesis occurs only when the blood glucose level and consequently the insulin-glucagon ratio are low. Under these conditions, phosphofructokinase-2 and pyruvate kinase are phosphorylated. Phosphofructokinase-2 breaks down fructose 2, 6-bisphosphate, which causes the levels of fructose 2, 6-bisphosphate to decrease and deactivates phosphofructokinase-1. The resulting decrease in the level of fructose 1,6-biphosphate and the phosphorylation of pyruvate kinase inhibits this enzyme. In the liver, the activity of these two key glycolytic enzymes are coordinated.

80. The answer is C. *(Biochemistry)*
The glycosphingolipids and the phosphosphingolipids are basically very similar. Both require ceramide as

the basic building block. Phosphosphingolipids are synthesized by adding phosphocholine to ceramide, which forms sphingomyelin. Glycosphingolipids add a variety of sugars to the ceramide. Therefore, phosphosphingolipids are classified as phospholipids, and glycosphingolipids are classified as glycolipids. Despite the fact they fall into different categories when defined chemically, they have similar structures, distribution, and clinical manifestations. Both groups are found in high concentration in the membranes of the nervous system, and both groups cause aberrations when they accumulate. The generic term for these diseases is the sphingolipidoses. Specific lysosomal enzyme deficiencies that cause the accumulation of glycolipids include Tay Sachs disease, Gaucher disease, and Fabry disease. Niemann-Pick disease is caused by an accumulation of sphingomyelin, which is a phospholipid, whereas Farber disease is caused by an accumulation of ceramide.

81. The answer is C. *(Behavioral science)*
Approximately 40 health care workers have been infected with HIV during the past 14 years. Fewer than 5 of these workers have been physicians; most have been laboratory personnel.

82. The answer is D. *(Physiology)*
In a female adolescent, the time from the appearance of breast buds (10.5 years) to first menstruation (12.5 years) is most typically about 24 months.

83. The answer is B. *(Behavioral science)*
Middle adolescents (14 to 16 years) are more likely than older or younger adolescents to follow a peer group that appears to dictate their dress and behavior. They also are more likely to be disruptive in school than younger or older adolescents.

84. The answer is B. *(Biochemistry)*
In eukaryotes, DNA replication occurs in the S phase of the cell cycle. Cells undergo mitosis or cell division in the M phase. The G_1 phase follows mitosis, but precedes DNA replication. The G_2 phase follows replication and precedes mitosis. Non-dividing cells are said to have entered the G_0 phase.

85. The answer is C. *(Pharmacology)*
Captopril is an angiotensin-converting enzyme (ACE) inhibitor that inhibits the conversion of angiotensin I to angiotensin II. Because angiotensin II acts directly on the adrenal cortex to stimulate the synthesis and release of aldosterone, ACE inhibitors lower both serum angiotensin II and aldosterone levels. The reduction in aldosterone causes a secondary elevation of serum potassium, because aldosterone increases renal sodium retention potassium excretion. Renin levels increase after ACE inhibitors, diuretics, or vasodilators are administered because these agents lower blood pressure, which activates renin secretion. β-blockers (e.g., propranolol) block the sympathetic component of renin secretion and lower plasma renin levels. Thiazide diuretics often decrease serum potassium. Spironolactone antagonizes aldosterone and may increase serum potassium, but it does not decrease aldosterone serum levels.

86. The answer is A. *(Anatomy)*
The tight junction at (1) seals the membranes of the two adjoining cells. The outer leaflets of the cell membrane fuse, creating a barrier to penetration across the junctional space. This junctional complex extends around the apex of the cell, thus it is also called the zonula occludens.

The zonula adherens is the next junctional complex (2), and it encircles the cell. Microfilaments insert into this junction, giving it and the cell apex rigidity.

The next junction is the macula adherens (3) or desmosome, which is a spot or disc-shaped junction braced by intermediate filaments. These filaments wrap through the dense cytoplasmic plaque of the macula adherens.

Hemidesmosomes are junctions that bind the cell to the basal lamina. Seen on the cytoplasmic basal surface, they appear as only one-half of a desmosome.

87. The answer is B. *(Microbiology)*
The herpesvirus has double-stranded linear DNA, which is unusual because it has terminal and internal repeated sequences. The DNA of some of its members (e.g., herpes simplex viruses) can undergo genetic rearrangement, which results in four different genomic isomers. In an isomer, there is the same molecular formula but different arrangement.

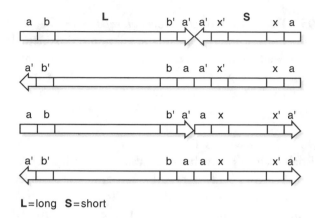

L=long S=short

The DNA of herpesviruses is large (molecular weight = $90–150 \times 10^6$), encoding at least 100 proteins. There is little sequence homology in the DNA among the various members of the family (30% to 50%), except between herpes simplex virus types 1 and 2 and between human herpes 6 and 7. Morphologically, however, they are indistinguishable.

The nucleocapsid of herpesviruses has icosahedral symmetry. The lipid envelope, which is derived from the nuclear membrane of the infected cell during budding, contains viral glycoproteins. The area between the capsid and the envelope is the tegument, and it contains several viral proteins.

Poxviruses have double-stranded, linear DNA.

Rabiesviruses, orthomyxoviruses (influenza), and retroviruses have single-stranded, linear RNA.

88. The answer is E. *(Biochemistry)*
Neighboring amino acids in a protein molecule are covalently linked by the formation of peptide bonds between the α-carboxyl group of one amino acid and the α-amino group of another. Peptide bonds have partial double-bond character and are not broken by ordinary handling. Although chemical groups on amino acid side chains can interact as the molecule folds into its three-dimensional configuration, none of them are involved in the formation of peptide bonds.

89. The answer is E. *(Microbiology)*
Cyclosporin A, a cyclic product of a fungus, blocks the synthesis of interleukin-2 (IL-2) and IL-2 receptors in T-helper lymphocytes. Specifically, it inhibits signal transduction to the nucleus by binding to cyclophilin (peptide-prolyl *cis-trans* isomerase, or PPlase, which

is an enzyme that catalyzes the folding of protein). Therefore, the transcription of messenger RNA for IL-2 and IL-2 receptors is limited. The ability of cyclosporin A to form a complex with cyclophilin may account, at least partly, for the toxicity associated with the drug.

Cyclosporin A does not directly inhibit cytotoxic T-cell activity. Its action on cytotoxic T cells is indirect—i.e., lack of IL-2 limits clonal expansion of cytotoxic T lymphocytes as well as T helpers.

Cyclosporin A does not have a direct effect on DNA synthesis.

Cyclosporin A has little or no effect on immature lymphocytes, and bone marrow toxicity is not a major problem associated with the use of this drug.

FK-506 is a new drug currently being tested in transplant patients. Its mechanism of action is similar to that of cyclosporin A, and it may be more immunosuppressive and less toxic. Clinical trials are in progress.

90. The answer is E. *(Pathology)*
Tumors derived from all three cell layers are called teratomas. In a newborn infant, the most common location is the sacrococcygeal area. Overall, however, a hemangioma is the most common tumor in infancy, and the majority of these regress over time.

91-93. The answers are: 91-C, 92-A, 93-B. *(Biochemistry)*
The substrates and enzymes are as follows:

> **A** Phenylalanine
> ↓   **1** Phenylalanine hydroxylase
> **B** Tyrosine
> ↓
> 4-Hydroxyphenylpyruvate
> ↓
> **C** Homogentisate
> ↓   **2** Homogentisate oxidase
> Maleylacetoacetate
> ↓
> Fumarylacetoacetate
> ↓   **3** Fumarylacetoacetate hydrolase
> **D** Fumarate (Tricarboxylic acid cycle) +
> **E** Acetoacetate

Substrate C, or homogentisate, turns black in urine when exposed to light and deposits in cartilage to produce a crippling degenerative joint disease called alcaptonuria. When it binds to collagen in connective tissue, tendons, and cartilage, it also imparts a black color to these tissues. The intervertebral disc is a prime target for deposition of homogentisate.

The enzyme deficiency that results in the buildup of a substrate leading to mental retardation and the formation of intermediate compounds that give an individual's sweat a mousy odor is phenylalanine hydroxylase (enzyme 1), the cause of phenylketonuria (PKU). In classic PKU, babies are normal at birth; the defect is uncovered when they are exposed to milk containing phenylalanine, which underscores the need to collect blood 3 days after birth rather than at delivery. Rising phenylalanine concentrations and its abnormal catabolic products impair development of the brain, causing severe mental retardation by 6 months of age if left untreated. Treatment involves strict adherence to a phenylalanine-free diet. Clinically, the patients present with projective vomiting, resembling congenital pyloric stenosis. Patients are hypopigmented and have blonde hair because of tyrosine deficiency (tyrosine is the substrate that forms dopamine, which is required for melanin synthesis). Buildup of minor shunt pathways with an increase in phenylpyruvic acid, phenyllactic acids, and phenylacetic acid imparts a mousy odor to the sweat.

Tyrosine (compound B) is the substrate that can be used to synthesize hormones derived from the adrenal medulla, mainly, norepinephrine and epinephrine.

94. The answer is E.   *(Microbiology)*
There are two types of bacteriophages—"lytic" and "temperate." The distinction is made according to the life cycle of the bacteriophage. Upon entering a bacterium, lytic phages produce phage nucleic acids and proteins, assemble many new phage particles, lyse the cell, and release the progeny phage. Temperate phages, on the other hand, can penetrate the bacterium and enter a dormant state called "lysogeny" in which most viral genes are repressed. Bacterial functions remain active and the bacterium is not harmed. Some dormant phages replicate as plasmids, while others, such as phage lambda, become integrated into the host genome as "prophages." The prophage DNA is replicated along with the host DNA as the bacterium grows and divides.

95. The answer is D.   *(Behavioral science)*
Functions of the ego include regulation of instinctual drives, adaptation to reality, reality testing and sustaining interpersonal relationships. Representing moral values and conscience are functions of the superego.

96. The answer is E.   *(Microbiology)*
Rhabdoviruses, which cause rabies, are helical, enveloped viruses with a negative-sense, single-stranded linear RNA genome. (Negative-sense RNA has a base composition opposite that of messenger RNA.) Within the virion, there is an RNA-dependent RNA polymerase for viral mRNA production. Polioviruses and rhinoviruses are nonenveloped icosahedral viruses with a positive-sense, single-stranded linear RNA genome. Flaviviruses and retroviruses have the same type of genome and are enveloped. By definition, all genomes from these viruses can function directly as mRNA.

97. The answer is E.   *(Biochemistry)*
Glycosaminoglycans, or mucopolysaccharides, are negatively charged polysaccharides (usually linear) that have a small amount of protein. They are composed of repeating disaccharide units, consisting of an acidic sugar (D-glucuronic acid or L-iduronic acid) and an amino sugar (D-glucosamine or D-galactosamine). Examples of glycosaminoglycans include heparin, heparan sulfate, chondroitin sulfate, keratin sulfate, and hyaluronic acid.

Glycosaminoglycans are used in the formation of the gel matrix of the ground substance in the interstitial tissue; the formation of the glomerular basement membrane, in which they provide the negative charge (polyanions) to repel negatively charged proteins; the lubrication of joints (hyaluronic acid); and in the matrix of bone, skin, tendons, and cartilage.

Glycosaminoglycans are degraded in lysosomes. Deficiencies of the enzymes cause an accumulation of glycosaminoglycans in the lysosomes, producing lysosomal storage diseases such as Hurler and Hunter syndromes. These patients have mental retardation, coarse facial features, joint abnormalities, corneal clouding, and coronary artery disease.

Blood group antigens are glycoproteins, which are proteins attached to oligosaccharides. The carbohydrate chains are usually short and branched.

98. The answer is C. *(Pathology)*
Hypertrophy is an increase in the size of a cell, whereas hyperplasia is an increase in the number of cells. Increased expression of cellular oncogenes responsible for the growth of cells leads to cellular hypertrophy, hyperplasia, or both, depending on the tissue type, the type of growth factors involved, and the type of growth factor inhibitors that are operative in the tissue. The same stimulus (e.g., growth factor) can lead to either hypertrophy, hyperplasia, or both.

There are three types of cells: labile, stable, and permanent. Permanent cells cannot divide because they are terminally differentiated. Only labile cells (e.g., squamous cells in the skin, hematopoietic cells in the bone marrow and lymphoid tissue) and stable cells (e.g., hepatocytes, endocrine cells, mesechymal cells, smooth muscle cells, renal tubular cells) can undergo both hypertrophy and hyperplasia, whereas permanent cells, such as those in skeletal and cardiac muscle, undergo only hypertrophy.

99. The answer is D. *(Biochemistry)*
Acetyl coenzyme A (acetyl CoA) is not involved in the formation of pyruvate. Rather, pyruvate dehydrogenase catalyzes the conversion of pyruvate to acetyl CoA. Acetyl CoA is used in the synthesis of ketone bodies:

Acetoacetyl-CoA thiolase   HMG CoA synthase   HMG CoA lyase
                                         (mitochondrial)

(2) Acetyl CoA → Acetoacetyl CoA ⟶ HMG -CoA ⟶ Acetoacetate ⟶ 3-hydroxybutyrate

The abbreviated schematic below shows how acetyl CoA is used in the synthesis of fatty acids:

←⟶ Mitochondrial reaction ⟶   ←⟶ Cytosol reactions ⟶

Acetyl CoA + Oxaloacetate ⟶ Citrate ⟶ Citrate ⟶ **Acetyl CoA** ⟶ Fatty acids

Acetyl CoA is used in the synthesis of cholesterol. Note how the first two steps are the same as in ketogenesis, except for the type of β-hydroxy-β-methylglutaryl coenzyme A (HMG CoA) synthase catalyzing the second reaction.

Acetyl-CoA thiolase   HMG CoA synthase   HMG CoA reductase

(2) Acetyl CoA → Acetoacetyl CoA ⟶ HMG CoA ⟶ Mevalonic acid ⟶ Cholesterol

Acetyl CoA is also used in the formation of citrate:

Citrate synthase   Cytosol ⟶ Acetyl CoA ⟶ Fatty acids

Acetyl CoA + Oxaloacetate ⟶ Citrate
        Mitochondria ⟶ Tricarboxylic acid (TCA) cycle

100. The answer is E. *(Microbiology)*
Entamoeba histolytica causes amoebiasis, which is primarily a disease of humans that is frequently complicated by liver abscess. The recommended treatment for both conditions is metronidazole (Flagyl). Asymptomatic cyst carriers should be treated with iodoquinol. The life cycle of *E. histolytica* has two stages: the motile amoeba (trophozoite) and the nonmotile cyst. The cysts are passed in feces. They can be killed by boiling but not by water chlorination. A typical "teardrop" or flask-shaped ulcer in the cecum is characteristic. The most frequent site of systemic disease is the liver. Once in the liver, the organisms can directly invade the diaphragm and pass into the lung cavity. Diagnosis and differentiation from other amoebas utilize the fact that the *E. histolytica* trophozoites contain ingested red blood cells.

101. The answer is E.   *(Biochemistry)*

The substrates and enzymes in the schematic are as follows:

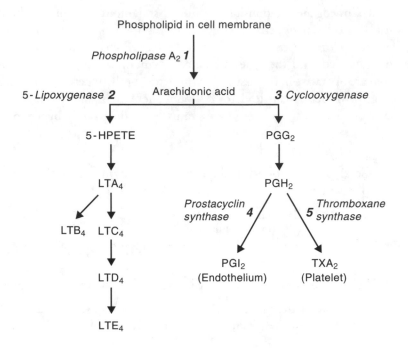

Although liberated prior to utilization in a reaction catalyzed by enzyme 1 (phospholipase A_2), compound A (arachidonic acid) is synthesized from linoleic acid, an essential fatty acid. Liberation of arachidonic acid can be blocked by corticosteroids because they inhibit phospholipase A_2. Phospholipase A_2 activity is enhanced by calcium. Compound B (leukotriene B_4[LTB_4]) is a potent chemotactic agent and increases adhesion molecule synthesis in leukocytes. It plays a pivotal role in inflammation. Leukotreines C_4, D_4, and E_4 (LTC_4, LTD_4, LTE_4), the slow-reacting substance of anaphylaxis, play a key role in bronchial asthma and asthma associated with aspirin sensitivity. These leukotrienes are potent vasoconstrictors and bronchoconstrictors and also increase vessel permeability. In asthma related to aspirin sensitivity, aspirin blocks cyclooxygenase activity and leaves the leukotriene pathway open for activation. The increase in these leukotrienes is responsible for the bronchoconstriction. Compounds F and G, representing prostaglandin I_2 (PGI_2, prostacyclin) and thromboxane A_2

(TXA_2), respectively, inhibit and enhance platelet aggregation and vasodilate and vasoconstrict vessels, respectively. Low-dose aspirin blocks enzyme 3 (the platelet cyclooxygenase) and, therefore, the generation of thromboxane A_2 more than it blocks enzyme 4 (prostacyclin synthase) and its production of prostacyclin, thus inhibiting platelet aggregation and reducing the potential for a coronary thrombosis. Cyclooxygenase, not enzyme 5 (thromboxane synthase), is blocked irreversibly by aspirin and reversibly by nonsteroidal agents.

102. The answer is E.   *(Pathology)*

The hemoglobin concentration, although the most important variable in the oxygen-carrying capacity of the blood, is least likely to influence whether an infarct will occur in tissue. Reduction in the hemoglobin concentration, or anemia, produces tissue hypoxia, which ultimately causes a decrease in adenosine triphosphate synthesis; atrophy or organ dysfunction is more likely occur than a localized area of infarction.

Coagulation necrosis, or infarction, is most commonly caused by ischemia, which, in turn, is most commonly the result of atherosclerosis. Factors influencing the development of infarcts include the size of the vessel that is obstructed (e.g., medium-size muscular artery is most likely to cause an infarction), the preexisting state of development of the collateral circulation (e.g., the circle of Willis, the arcade system in the mesentery), the presence or absence of a dual blood supply (e.g., the liver is least likely to infarct because it has a blood supply from the portal vein and hepatic artery), the presence or absence of preexisting disease in the tissue (e.g., a pulmonary infarct is more likely to occur in the presence of chronic obstructive pulmonary disease), the oxygen requirements of the tissue (e.g., the brain is the organ that is most sensitive to oxygen deprivation), and how quickly the vessel is occluded (e.g., acute occlusion is more likely to infarct than chronic ischemia).

103. The answer is A.   *(Biochemistry)*
The substrates and enzymes involved in alcohol metabolism are as follows:

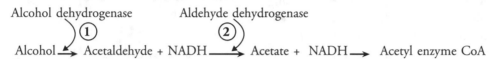

Enzyme 1 (alcohol dehydrogenase) also catalyzes reactions involving the metabolism of methyl alcohol and ethylene glycol, an example of competitive enzyme inhibition. The Vmax of an enzyme is the maximum velocity of the reaction when all of the enzyme sites are saturated. The Km of an enzyme is the substrate concentration at one-half the Vmax. A decreased Km represents an increased affinity of the enzyme for substrate, whereas an increased Km indicates decreased affinity of the enzyme for substrate. The Vmax of alcohol dehydrogenase would remain the same (an adequate amount of substrate is present), but the apparent Km would be increased (decreased affinity for ethanol), because the enzyme is also reacting with other substrates (e.g., methanol or ethylene glycol). Increasing the substrate, ethanol, would correct this enzyme inhibition. Enzyme 2 (aldehyde dehydrogenase) is in the cytosol and in the mitochondria of the hepatocytes. A variant found in high frequency in Asians is less active, causing the effects of drinking ethanol to be more pronounced in people with the variant enzyme due to the accumulation of acetaldehyde (compound A). Disulfiram blocks aldehyde dehydrogenase in the mitochondria so acetaldehyde builds up in the blood and produces a similar unpleasant reaction. Acetaldehyde is also toxic to hepatocytes and is partially responsible for the liver disease associated with alcoholism. An increase in compound B [reduced nicotinamide adenine dinucleotide (NADH)] drives the reversible pyruvate reaction in the direction of lactate, resulting in lactic acidosis. In addition, the accumulation of compound C (acetyl coenzyme A) is used by the liver to generate ketone bodies.

104. The answer is A.   *(Behavioral science)*
Sexual interest is less likely to be affected than other aspects of sexuality in aging patients. Sexuality in aging men is characterized by decreased ejaculation intensity, increased refractory period, delayed ejaculation, and decreased opportunity for sexual expression because of loss of sexual partners.

105. The answer is E.   *(Pathology)*
Free radicals primarily injure the cell membrane (via lipid peroxidation) and the nucleotides in DNA. They are produced by radiant energy or redox reactions; or, they are derived from parent chemicals, such as oxygen, acetaminophen, or carbon tetrachloride, the latter of which is derived by the cytochrome oxidase system in the liver. Because free radicals have a single, unpaired electron in their outer orbit, they are very unstable and capable of damaging tissue. Examples of oxygen free radicals include superoxide, peroxide, and hydroxyl ions generated from neutrophils and xanthine oxidase in tissue. Iron enhances free radical production, which is the primary mechanism of injury in the iron overload diseases (e.g., hemochromatosis, hemosiderosis).

The cell counteracts free radicals through many mechanisms. Superoxide free radicals undergo a dismutation reaction with superoxide dismutase and are converted into peroxide and oxygen. Peroxide is reduced to water by catalase and glutathione peroxidase via glutathione (GSH); the latter is generated in the hexose monophosphate shunt catalyzed by glucose-6-phosphate dehydrogenase. Antioxidants, such as vitamins C and E, neutralize free radicals, particularly oxidized low-density lipoprotein (LDL) and LDL free radicals that are more atherogenic than native LDL.

106. The answer is A. *(Microbiology)*
The exotoxins of enteric bacteria consist primarily of proteins that, following secretion into the surrounding milieu, exert their effects by binding to specific receptor molecules on the surface of mammalian cells.

Exotoxins often consist of an A subunit and one or more B subunits that are linked together by disulfide bonds. The effects of the toxins are mediated by the A subunit in a dose-dependent manner, whereas the B subunits bind to cells and facilitate entry of the A subunit. The genes encoding the exotoxins are often on plasmids rather than on chromosomes (i.e., they are extrachromosomal).

107. The answer is D. *(Pathology)*
The term *stat* usually infers that a life-threatening situation is present. Stat tests account for 10% to 30% of all laboratory requests, most of which come from the emergency room and intensive care units. The most frequently ordered stat tests are a complete blood cell count, which may be used assess hemoglobin and hematocrit or look for a left shift in the neutrophil series; serum glucose, which may rule out hypoglycemia or hyperglycemia; serum electrolytes, which may rule out significant acid–base disturbances, such as metabolic alkalosis and hypokalemia; arterial blood gases, which may rule out significant acid–base disturbances and problems with oxygenation; urinalysis, which may rule out a urinary tract infection or renal stone; Gram stain of spinal fluid or sputum, which may rule out a bacterial infection; serum amylase, which may rule out acute pancreatitis; and drug screens, which may rule out drug overdose.

The erythrocyte sedimentation rate (ESR) is a stat test in only one situation—when used to screen for temporal arteritis associated with visual disturbances. Although an increased ESR is not specific for temporal arteritis because it has a low specificity, a normal value

essentially excludes the disease because it has a high sensitivity. Serum transaminases used to rule out hepatitis are never indicated as a stat test.

108. The answer is A. *(Physiology)*
Endothelin is a potent vasoconstrictor peptide produced by vascular endothelial cells. Other vasoconstrictor peptides include angiotensin II, neuropeptide Y, and vasopressin. Bradykinin, vasoactive intestinal peptide, calcitonin gene-related peptide, and substance P cause vasodilation in most vascular beds. Other vasodilator peptides include atrial natriuretic peptide and neurotensin.

109. The answer is C. *(Microbiology)*
Echinococcus granulosus (dog tapeworm) larvae cause unilocular hydatid cyst disease. Dogs are the most important definitive hosts (contain adult worm). Humans are almost always dead-end intermediate hosts that can contain the larval forms of this tapeworm, which is one of the smallest. Worms in the dog's intestine liberate thousands of eggs, which are ingested by sheep (or humans). The embryos emerge in the small intestine, penetrate the intestinal wall, and migrate primarily to the liver (but also to the lungs, bones and brain). The embryos develop in one, large fluid-filled hydatid cyst (unilocular). The inner germinal layer of the cyst generates many protoscoleces within "brood capsules." Hydatid sand is a term applied to the individual scolices in hydatid cyst fluid. The life cycle is completed when sheep entrails are eaten by dogs. Rupture of the cyst can produce anaphylactic shock.

110. The answer is B. *(Behavioral science)*
The least effective treatment for enuresis in a 6-year-old child is punishment. Restriction of fluid before bedtime, bed-wetting alarms, midsleep awakenings for voiding, and antidepressant medication have all been shown to be useful in treating enuresis.

111. The answer is D. *(Microbiology)*
Corynebacterium species (diphtheroids), *Neisseria sicca* (commensal), streptococci (primarily alpha-hemolytic) and staphylococci (*S. epidermidis*, primarily) are all normal flora in the oral cavity and the nasopharyngeal areas of humans. Because they are part of the

normal flora, they are seldom involved in disease, but they are routinely recovered from clinical specimens collected from these areas. The laboratory technologists and physician should recognize these organisms as part of the normal flora and weigh their presence accordingly in relation to an existing disease. All *Treponema* organisms are harmless saprophytes under ordinary conditions, but they are difficult to grow under normal laboratory conditions. Most are strict anaerobes that must be cultured accordingly.

112. The answer is B.   *(Physiology)*

A genetic male with androgen-insensitivity (testicular feminization) syndrome has the sexual phenotype of a female. Because there is a genetic defect, the somatic cells do not respond to androgen, and masculinization does not take place prenatally. In adults with androgen-insensitivity syndrome, breast development occurs as a result of testicular estrogen secretion. However, menstruation does not occur because there is no uterus. Individuals with androgen-insensitivity syndrome are usually heterosexual with respect to their sexual phenotype (i.e., they have sexual interest in men).

113. The answer is B.   *(Microbiology)*

Bacteroides organisms are the most common cause of serious anaerobic infections, which include sepsis, peritonitis, and abscesses. *B. fragilis* is the most frequent pathogen, but it also is seen frequently in mixed cultures. Infections involving *B. melaninogenicus* (new name is *Prevotella melaninogenica*) occur mainly in the oral cavity, and the organism is involved in periodontal and endodontal infections, as well as lung abscesses because of aspiration of oropharyngeal contents. *B. fragilis* is the predominant organism in the human colon. Being part of the normal flora, infections are endogenous. These organisms are opportunists, causing disease once they leave their usual etiologic niches. Abscesses are the typical lesions, and they are often accompanied by a foul odor. Because abcesses are often resistant to penicillin and aminoglycosides, metronidazole is the treatment of choice. Endotoxin (gram-negative cell wall) and enzymes (e.g., collagenase, proteases) contribute to tissue destruction. They stain faintly with Gram stains. No significant exotoxins have been described.

114. The answer is C.   *(Biochemistry)*

Arachidonic acid metabolism proceeds via three pathways. The cyclooxygenase pathway, which is inhibited by aspirin and other nonsteroidal antiinflammatory drugs, leads to the formation of prostaglandins, prostacyclin, and thromboxanes. The lipooxygenase pathway leads to the formation of leukotrienes, whereas the cytochrome P_{450} monooxygenase pathway produces lipoxins and other products. Endothelin is a 21 amino-acid peptide that is produced by vascular endothelium and has potent vasoconstrictive properties.

115. The answer is D.   *(Microbiology)*

The quellung reaction (capsular swelling) is a diagnostic feature of *Streptococcus pneumoniae* (the pneumococcus). Before antibiotic availability, patients with pneumococcal pneumonia were treated by passive immunization. The virulence of a pneumococcus is determined by the polysaccharide capsule that surrounds the organism. There are currently more than 85 known antigenic types. When specific antibody and pneumococcus organisms are mixed, the capsule literally swells and can be observed under a microscope. Treatment then consisted of giving the patient specific, pre-made antibodies to opsonize the encapsulated pathogens. Even today, opsonizing antibodies exist and will allow efficient phagocytosis of the organisms, which are then killed intracellularly. The CAMP test (named for originators Christie, Atkins and Munch-Peterson) is based on the observation that beta-hemolytic group B streptococci produce a protein-like factor that acts synergistically with the beta toxin of *Staphylococcus aureus* to produce even more potent hemolysis. Suspect streptococci are streaked on a blood agar plate at right angles to a previous inoculation of *S. aureus*. An arrowhead zone of enhanced hemolysis at the junction of the two organisms is a positive test. Approximately 95% of the group B streptococci are CAMP positive. Sodium hippurate hydrolysis has largely replaced this test.

116. The answer is C.   *(Physiology)*

Prostaglandins of the E series and prostacyclin inhibit platelet aggregation, whereas thromboxane strongly facilitates aggregation. The E prostaglandins and prostacyclin relax bronchial and vascular smooth muscle, which causes bronchodilation and vasodilation.

Thromboxane and prostaglandin $F_{2\alpha}$ cause vasoconstriction and bronchoconstriction. Only the E prostaglandins have gastric cytoprotective effects and gastric-acid inhibitory secretion effects. Both prostaglandin E_2 and $F_{2\alpha}$ have oxytocic effects and may induce labor or abortion.

117. The answer is B.   *(Behavioral science)*
Immigrants to the United States have an increased risk for psychiatric problems, and they show a higher incidence of paranoid symptoms than the general population. Young immigrant men appear to be at greater risk for psychiatric problems than young immigrant women. However, paranoid symptoms in immigrants have a relatively good prognosis.

118. The answer is E.   *(Microbiology)*
There are two phases in the *Plasmodium* life cycle: the sexual cycle in the mosquito host (sporogony) and the asexual cycle in humans (schizogony). In humans, schizogony starts with the introduction of sporozoites into the blood from the bite of a mosquito. Hepatocytes take up sporozoites within 30 minutes. The exoerythrocyte phase consists of multiplication and differentiation of merozoites. Hepatocyte-released merozoites infect the red blood cells (RBCs). During the erythrocytic phase, the organism differentiates into a ring-shaped trophozoite. The ring form differentiates into a schizont filled with merozoites. The periodic release of merozoites causes the typical recurrent symptoms of chills and sweats seen in malaria patients. In *P. malariae*, the disease has a quartan fever pattern with temperature spikes every 3 days. For diagnosis, ring-shaped trophozoites can be seen within the infected RBCs. Sporozoites are introduced into the blood, but they are taken up by hepatocytes rather than RBCs. Therefore, sporozoites would not be present within the RBCs in a thin-smear preparation.

119. The answer is E.   *(Behavioral science)*
Parallel play (playing along side each other rather than cooperatively) occurs between 2 and 4 years of age. By the age of 4 years, children have learned to play cooperatively. A 5-year-old girl can hop on one foot, has a preference for using one hand over the other, uses the future tense in speech, and can follow a three-step command.

120. The answer is A.   *(Pharmacology)*
The class of drugs that is least likely to cause sexual dysfunction (e.g., erectile disorder) are antiparkinson drugs, such as L-dopa. Dopamine has a stimulatory effect on sexuality. Drugs like L-dopa, which increase dopamine levels, may stimulate sexuality. Similarly, antidopaminergic agents (i.e., antipsychotics) decrease sexuality. Because serotonin has negative effects on sexuality, MAO inhibitors, tricyclic antidepressants, and selective serotonin reuptake inhibitors (SSRIs) are all more likely than antiparkinson drugs to cause sexual dysfunction.

121. The answer is B.   *(Microbiology)*
The gram-positive bacterial cell wall is much thicker than the cell wall found in gram-negative organisms. The gram-positive wall consists of backbones of two alternating amino sugars, *N*-acetyl glucosamine and *N*-acetyl muramic acid. Polypeptide chains attached to the muramic acid residue crosslink with other polypeptide chains, forming a single molecular structure around the organism. Teichoic acids or lipoteichoic acid chains are polymers of glycerol phosphate or ribitol phosphate, which are located in the outer layer of the peptidoglycan cell wall. Teichoic acids are antigenic, inducing specific antibodies, and they are thought to attach microorganisms to tissue to impede phagocytosis and assist colonization. Lipid A is a component of the gram-negative cell wall and is responsible for the toxic effects of endotoxin.

Comparison of the Cell Walls of Gram-Positive and Gram-Negative Bacteria

Component	Gram-negative cells	Gram-positive cells
Peptidoglycan	Thick, many layers	Thin, one layer
Lipopolysaccharide (e.g., endotoxin, lipid A)	Yes	No
Teichoic acids	No	Yes

122. The answer is B. *(Pathology)*

Ras oncogenes are involved in the generation of signal-transducing proteins, or second messengers, via the guanosine triphosphate (GTP) system. When a growth factor attaches to its growth factor receptor in a cell, a signal is sent that activates the *ras* oncogene, which, in turn, exchanges guanosine diphosphate (GDP) for GTP. The activated *ras* further activates cytoplasmic kinases, which, in turn, activates transcription factors that are involved in cell division.

123. The answer is D. *(Biochemistry)*

The substrates and enzymes are as follows:

Methionine → *S*-adenosylmethionine (**A**) → *S*-adenosylhomocysteine →

Cystathionine synthase (**1**)

Homocysteine (**B**) ⟶ Cystathionine → Cysteine (**C**)

Substrate A is a high-energy compound called *S*-adenosylmethionine (SAM). Unlike adenosine triphosphate, it does not contain phosphate. SAM is involved in the transfer of methyl groups (1-carbon transfer), formation of methionine, synthesis of choline, synthesis of creatine, and synthesis of epinephrine.

Substrate B represents homocysteine, which accepts methyl groups from vitamin B_{12} and transfers them to methionine:

Methyl-B_{12} + Homocysteine → B_{12} + Methionine

Homocysteine, when it accumulates from a deficiency of cystathionine synthase, produces the autosomal recessive disease homocystinuria, not alkaptonuria.

Substrate C represents cysteine, which is a sulfur-containing amino acid that is a major component of α-keratin. In cystinuria, which is the most common genetic error in amino acid transport, there is a defect in the intestinal and renal reabsorption of cysteine as well as the basic amino acids, arginine, ornithine, and lysine. Cysteine is converted into cystine, which is an hexagonal crystal that can precipitate into cystine stones in the urine. These stones are usually the presenting symptom. The disease can be successfully treated by limiting protein in the diet and providing large volumes of water to prevent stone formation.

124. The answer is E. *(Microbiology)*

The steps in the growth cycle of a virus are as follows:

1. Attachment. A viral receptor specifically interacts with a cellular receptor.

2. Penetration (engulfment). Some systems accomplish penetration by receptor-mediated endocytosis; in other systems, direct penetration occurs by an unclear mechanism.

3. Uncoating. The genome is released from the viral capsid.

4. Synthesis. Growth occurs at the molecular level. Genome replication and protein production (for both enzymes and structural proteins) occur.

5. Maturation. Assembly of mature virions takes place within the cell.

6. Release. The virions are released from the cell by cell lysis or budding.

The attachment, penetration, uncoating, and synthesis stages are referred to as the eclipse phase. These stages obviously result in a loss of infectivity, because incomplete virions are present or growth is occurring at a molecular level.

125-128. The answers are: 125-A, 126-C, 127-D, 128-E. *(Behavioral science)*

The smell of pizza baking in the oven at lunchtime is an unconditioned stimulus because it automatically produces an instinctive response (i.e., salivation). The response of salivating upon smelling pizza baking is unconditioned because it is instinctive; that is, it does not have to be learned. Salivating in response to hearing the lunch bell at 12 P.M. is a conditioned response because it has been learned; that is, the bell has always been rung in conjunction with the presentation of food. Extinction is the disappearance of a learned behavior (e.g., salivation in response to the bell) when the conditioned stimulus is no longer followed by the unconditioned stimulus (e.g., when the 12 P.M. bell is no longer followed by lunch).

129-134. The answers are: 129-B, 130-A, 131-E, 132-C, 133-D, 134-B.   *(Pharmacology)*

First-generation cephalosporins (e.g., cefazolin) have greater activity against gram-positive cocci such as *Staphylococcus aureus*, whereas second-generation cephalosporins (e.g., cefaclor) have more activity against gram-negative organisms such as *Haemophilus influenzae*. Third-generation drugs (e.g., ceftazidime, ceftriaxone) have even greater activity against gram-negative organisms. Ceftriaxone is used to treat infections caused by *Neisseria gonorrhoeae* and *H. influenzae*; however, it is inactive against *Pseudomonas aeruginosa*. Ceftazidime has antipseudomonal activity. Monobactams such as aztreonam are highly active against gram-negative organisms, including *Pseudomonas*, but have little activity against gram-positive organisms. Imipenem is a carbapenem that has the broadest spectrum of any β-lactam antibiotic. It is particularly indicated for the treatment of infections caused by *Acinetobacter, Citrobacter, Enterobacter,* and *Morganella* species.

135-137. The answers are: 135-G, 136-L, 137-C.   *(Biochemistry)*

Progesterone is the precursor of the gluco- or mineral corticosteroids in the adrenals, of testosterone in the testis, and of estradiol in the ovaries. However, it is not further metabolized, and it is the major end product in the corpus luteum. During a woman's monthly cycle, it helps prepare the uterine endometrium for implantation of the fertilized egg.

Cortisol is the primary glucosteroid. It enhances gluconeogenesis and promotes protein catabolism to generate gluconeogenic precursors. Cortisol also has an anti-inflammatory action, which is achieved by inhibiting phospholipase A_2.

Cholesterol is a 27-carbon molecule. Six carbons are cleaved from the side chain, which is the first step in steroid hormone synthesis. The remaining two carbons of the side chain are removed when progesterone (C21) is converted to testosterone (C19). Carbon number 19, the methyl group between the A and B ring, is removed when testosterone is converted to estradiol (C18).

138-140. The answers are: 138-C, 139-A, 140-D.   *(Pharmacology)*

Alprostadil is a preparation of prostaglandin E_1 that maintains patency of a neonate's ductus arteriosus until surgical correction can be performed. Misoprostil is an orally active synthetic analogue of PGE_1 that is used to prevent stomach ulcers caused by nonsteroidal antiinflammatory drugs. Dinoprostone is a synthetic PGE_2 derivative, whereas carboprost is 15-methyl prostaglandin F_{2a}. Both dinoprostone and carboprost are used for the induction of labor or abortion. Carboprost has also been used to control postpartum hemorrhage.

141-142. The answers are: 141-A, 142-D.   *(Biochemistry)*

Chemical reactions have an energy barrier that separates the reactants from the products. In this graph, the peak of the *solid line* represents the energy level of the high-energy intermediate, or transition state, for the uncatalyzed reaction. Enzymes increase the speed of chemical reactions by providing an alternate reaction pathway with a lower-energy transition state (*dotted line*).

The free energy of activation is the difference between the energy levels of the transition state and the reactant. This energy change for the catalyzed reaction is represented by *D*, whereas the larger change for the uncatalyzed reaction is represented by *B*.

143-147. The answers are: 143-C, 144-C, 145-E, 146-A, 147-D.   *(Behavioral science)*

Most commonly, sitting unassisted and stranger anxiety (i.e., fear of unfamiliar people) first occur between 6 and 8 months. Rapproachment, which is the tendency to run away from and then return to the mother for comfort, first occurs between 16 and 24 months. The social smile is first seen between 1 and 2 months. Walking unassisted first occurs at approximately 12 months in most children.

148-150. The answers are: 148-H, 149-E, 150-F.   *(Microbiology)*

Entamoeba histolytica is a common parasite in the large intestine of humans. The active amoeba is found in fluid feces during amoebic dysentery. It is large (15 to 30 μm) and may contain ingested red blood cells. Disease results when trophozoites invade the intestinal epithelium and submucosa. Cysts, which are the form of transmission, are formed in the lumen of the colon and in mushy or formed feces. Diagnosis is usually by microscopic examination and detection of typical cysts, which contain one to four nuclei. Metronidazole (Flagyl) is the drug of choice for symptomatic amoebiasis.

Onchocerca volvulus causes onchocerciasis. Blackflies *(Simulium)* ingest microfilariae when they ingest blood from an infected human. Within this vector, metamorphosis to the infective larval stage occurs in 6 to 8 days. Humans are infected when the female blackfly *(Simulium)* deposits infective larvae when biting. The larvae enter the wound and migrate to the subcutaneous tissue, where they differentiate into adults (located within dermal nodules) and are called calabar swellings. The females produce microfilariae, which migrate through subcutaneous tissue and ultimately concentrate in the eyes. There, they can cause lesions that can lead to blindness. Millions of people in Africa and Central America are infected. Called "river blindness," the blackfly vector develops in the river and can cause infection rates as high as 80%. Dimethylcarbamazine is effective only for microfilariae, and suramin, which is quite toxic, kills adults involved in eye disease.

Strongyloides stercoralis has two distinct life cycles. One is within the human body and the other is free-living in the soil. In the human body, the life cycle begins with penetration of the skin (usually the feet). Infectious larvae (filariform) migrate to the lungs, enter the alveoli, travel up the bronchi and trachea, and are swallowed. Adults form in the small intestine and produce eggs within the mucosa. Hatching larvae are passed in the feces, but some penetrate the intestinal wall or perianal skin and migrate to the lungs (autoinfection), where they can produce a pneumonitis. As with all migratory nematode infections, eosinophilia is present. Thiabendazole is the drug of choice.

151-155. The answers are: 151-A, 152-H, 153-G, 154-I, 155-B. *(Biochemistry)*
Linoleic acid, a precursor of series 1 and 2 prostaglandins, is one of the two essential fatty acids. The other is α-linolenic acid, a precursor of series 3 prostaglandins. A deficiency of these fatty acids leads to dry skin,

thrombopenia, and eczema, and eventually leads to more serious health problems, including behavioral and cardiovascular abnormalities. These symptoms not only are related to their role as prostaglandin precursors, but also to the role the essential fatty acids play in maintaining the fluidity of membranes. They are found in particularly high concentrations in nerve membranes.

Unsaturated fatty acids having the trans configuration are formed when oils are partially hydrogenated to enhance their shelf life or to lower their melting points (e.g., in the manufacture of margarine and other spreads). A growing body of evidence suggests that these are unhealthy.

The long-chain ω-3 fatty acids, such as eicosapentaenoic acid and docosahexaenoic acid, are found in high concentration in the lipids of cold-water fish. These fatty acids are thought to provide protection from cardiovascular disease, by inhibiting platelet aggregation.

Arachidonic acid is a precursor of series 2 prostaglandins and an important membrane constituent. It is synthesized from linoleic acid. Therefore, if there is sufficient linoleic acid in the diet, arachidonic acid is not essential. However, arachidonic acid is the preferred fatty acid esterified on carbon 2 of glycerol on the membrane-bound phosphatidylinositol and phosphatidylcholine molecules. This is the position cleaved by phospholipase A_2, freeing arachidonic acid for conversion to eicosanoids.

Phospholipase A_2 is inhibited by corticosteroids blocking further synthesis of all series 1 and 2 prostaglandins, thomboxanes, and leukotrienes. This accounts for the anti-inflammatory effect of corticosteroids.

Long-chain saturated fatty acids such as palmitic acid increase serum cholesterol levels. These are found in meats and dairy products, as well as coconut and palm oils. Stearic acid does not raise or lower serum cholesterol levels.

156-157. The answers are: 156-D, 157-E. *(Microbiology)*
Borrelia recurrentis causes relapsing fever, a disease characterized by several episodes of fever. After an incubation period of 3 to 10 days, there is a sudden onset of chills and a rise in body temperature (103°F to 105°F). The organisms are present in the blood

during the fever. Antibodies bind, agglutinate, and lyse most of the bacteria, and the fever falls. However, a few antigenic variants escape the attack and continue to multiply. As the number of variant organisms increase in the blood, the fever rises, and a new wave of antibodies attack. The rise and fall of the fever and the selection of new variants usually continue for 3 to 10 episodes.

Infection with *Borrelia burgdorferi* causes Lyme disease, and a unique "bulls-eye" skin lesion, known as erythema chronica migrans, develops. The lesion can appear anywhere from 3 days to 4 weeks after the organisms are introduced by a tick bite. The lesion begins as a flat red area near the tick bite. As it slowly migrates outward, the central portion clears.

B. burgdorferi is present in the midgut of infected ticks. The reservoir for the spirochete is the white-tailed deer. For transmission to occur, the tick must bite and remain attached for at least 24 hours. After the organisms enter the body, they migrate outward, enter the blood and lymphatics, and become disseminated to virtually all organs of the body.

158-162. The answers are: 158-D, 159-E, 160-C, 161-B, 162-A. *(Behavioral science)*
Correlation is used to evaluate the relationship between two variables—in this case, medical students' scores on USMLE Step 1 and the parental income of those students.

Analysis of variance is used to evaluate differences among mean scores in more than two groups. This example uses board scores of medical students in three different age groups.

Chi-squared test, a nonparametric statistical test, is used to examine differences between frequencies in a sample—in this case, the percentage of medical students who pass USMLE Step 1 versus those who pass USMLE Step 2 on their first attempt.

A *t*-test is used to examine differences between means of two samples. In question 161, a paired *t*-test is used, because the scores evaluated are from the same medical students on two different examinations, USMLE Step 1 and USMLE Step 2. In contrast, an independent *t*-test is used to evaluate differences between scores of medical students from two different medical schools on USMLE Step 1, because two different groups of medical students are examined.

163-166. The answers are: 163-C, O; 164-I, P, Q; 165-H, 166-D. *(Biochemistry)*
Aspartate and glutamate are amino acids with acidic side chains. The carboxylic group on the side chain is ionized at neutral pH, providing an additional negative charge on the molecule.

Histidine tryptophan and phenylalanine are essential amino acids. Essential amino acids are those amino acids that must be ingested through a person's diet, because the human body cannot synthesize them.

Uric acid is the major degradation product derived from purines. Guanine is the only purine listed. Uric acid is excreted in the urine and may cause problems because of its relatively low solubility.

Cysteine is an amino acid with a sulfhydryl group on its side chain. The sulfhydryl group can form covalent disulfide bonds with other cysteine residues on polypeptide chains.

167-171. The answers are: 167-B, 168-E, 169-A, 170-C, 171-D. *(Pharmacology)*
Imipenem is inactivated by renal dehydropeptidase I, which causes low urinary concentrations. Cilastatin inhibits this enzyme and is combined with imipenem for clinical use.

Trimethoprim inhibits dihydrofolate reductase and is combined with sulfamethoxazole to sequentially inhibit two steps in bacterial folic acid synthesis.

Probenecid is a weak organic acid that competes with other acids for renal tubular secretory transport, thereby reducing the excretion and increasing serum levels of penicillin G and other penicillins.

Sulbactam is a β-lactamase inhibitor that is combined with ampicillin to prevent its inactivation. Other β-lactamase inhibitors include clavulanate, which is used with amoxicillin and ticarcillin, and tazobactam, which is used with piperacillin.

Drugs must be used in combination to prevent the emergence of bacterial resistance during the treatment of tuberculosis. The most commonly used drugs for acute tuberculosis are isoniazid and rifampin.

172-173. The answers are: 172-C, 173-A. *(Pathology)*
The sensitivity of a test defines how often the test returns positive in an individual with a disease.

Individuals with a disease have either a positive (true positive) or a negative (false negative) test result. The following is the formula for the sensitivity of a test:

$$\text{Sensitivity (\%)} = \frac{\text{True positives}}{\text{True positives + False negatives}} \times 100$$

Therefore, the higher the sensitivity of a test, the lower the false negative rate.

The specificity of a test defines how often the test returns negative in an individual without a disease. Individuals without a disease have either a negative (true negative) or positive (false positive) test result. The following is the formula for the specificity of a test:

$$\text{Specificity (\%)} = \frac{\text{True negatives}}{\text{True negatives + False positives}} \times 100$$

Therefore, the higher the specificity of the test, the lower the false positive rate.

Regarding the patient with a positive rapid plasma reagin (RPR) test and a negative fluorescent treponemal antibody absorbtion (FTA-ABS) test, because the FTA-ABS is a specific treponemal antibody test, a negative result indicates that the RPR test result is a false positive. The antigen in the RPR test is beef cardiolipin. Reagin antibodies in syphilis react with the antigen to produce a positive test. However, anticardiolipin antibodies are frequently seen in patients with systemic lupus erythematosus. These antibodies also react with the cardiolipin antigen to produce a positive test result. Because it is not a treponemal antibody, the FTA-ABS is negative. A biologic false-positive syphilis serology indicates the need for a serum antinuclear antibody test to rule out an autoimmune disease.

Enzyme-linked immunosorbent assay (ELISA) primarily detects antibodies against glycoprotein (gp) 120 and has a sensitivity of 97% to 99% and a specificity of 90% to 99%. The Western blot detects more than one antibody, thus increasing the overall specificity of the test. For example, the assay is considered positive if antibodies are present against gp 41 and protein (p) 24 or gp 120 and gp 160. Because the Western blot is the confirmatory test for the human immunodeficiency antibody, a positive test indicates that the ELISA screen is a true, rather than a false, positive.

174-175. The answers are: 174-E, 175-B. *(Biochemistry)*
The carboxyl group of an amino acid becomes covalently linked to the 3' end of a transfer RNA (tRNA) molecule. tRNA contains the sequence CCA at the 3' end, which is added as a post-transcriptional modification. Amino acids are attached to the tRNA molecule by enzymes called aminoacyl-tRNA synthetases, which derive their energy from adenosine triphosphate (ATP). Each aminoacyl-tRNA synthetase is specific for a single amino acid.

The anticodon of a tRNA molecule binds to a codon on a messenger RNA (mRNA) molecule by forming complementary base pairs, with the strands oriented in antiparallel fashion. tRNA molecules can recognize more than one codon for a specific amino acid because nontraditional base pairing is allowed at the "wobble" position, which corresponds to the 3' base of the codon and the 5' base of the anticodon. In the diagram, points B, C, and D are the three bases of the anticodon, with point B being the 5', or wobble, base.

176-180. The answers are: 176-A, 177-E, 178-D, 179-C, 180-B. *(Microbiology)*
Hepatitis B virus has a circular, double-stranded DNA genome with an unusual configuration. It has one complete negative strand that is nicked and a second strand that is one-half to two-thirds complete. The virion contains a virally coded DNA-dependent DNA polymerase. This enzyme, in a host cell, ligates the nicked strand and completes the second strand, producing a covalently closed circular double-stranded DNA genome. This circular DNA serves as a template for all viral messenger RNA (mRNA) transcripts, including a 3.5-kilobase pregenome RNA. The pregenome RNA becomes encapsulated with newly synthesized hepatitis B core antigen (HBcAg). Within the cores, the viral polymerase synthesizes, by reverse transcription, a negative-stranded DNA copy. A positive DNA strand is also started, but not completed. Cores may bud from the cell, acquiring hepatitis B surface antigen (HBsAg).

Coxsackieviruses are picornaviruses, possessing a single-stranded, positive-sense RNA genome. (Positive-sense genomes have the same base sequence as mRNA.) Polioviruses, echoviruses, and hepatitis A virus are also picornaviruses. These viruses have no lipid envelopes and grow entirely within the cytoplasm of the host cell. An unusual biochemical feature of this growth cycle is that the entire RNA genome acts directly as mRNA and is translated into a single polypeptide. This protein is later divided into structural proteins and enzymes by protease activity (post-translational maturation of proteins). The mature viruses are released by cell lysis.

Adenoviruses are DNA-containing, medium-sized viruses (70–90 nm in diameter), which contain a linear, double-stranded genome. They are icosahedral and have no envelope. They replicate in the nucleus of the host cell. At least 41 types infect humans, especially in the mucous membranes. Some human infections caused by adenoviruses include acute respiratory disease, pharyngitis, conjunctivitis, and gastroenteritis. Some strains can induce tumors in newborn hamsters.

Mumps virus is a paramyxovirus. Like respiratory syncytial virus (RSV) and rubeola virus, mumps virus contains a linear, single-stranded RNA genome. The genome is contained within a helical capsid, which in turn is surrounded by a lipid envelope containing hemagglutinin-neuraminidase and fusion glucoproteins. In order for paramyxoviruses to grow in the host cell cytoplasm, they must carry an RNA-dependent RNA polymerase within their virions. This enzyme produces mRNA and is responsible for genome replication.

Influenza viruses are orthomyxoviruses. These viruses contain a segmented, single-stranded RNA genome with a negative polarity (i.e., a base composition opposite that of mRNA). The virion contains an RNA-dependent RNA polymerase that transcribes ten mRNA transcripts from the eight viral RNA segments. Most RNA viruses grow in the cytoplasm of the host cells, but influenza viruses have a special need for capped and methylated 5′ termini for the viral mRNA transcripts. Cellular transcripts newly synthesized by cellular RNA polymerase II are ligated to the viral mRNA transcripts, which can then be translated into proteins. Influenza viruses are assembled and mature in the nucleus of the host cell and then are released by a budding process.

Papillomaviruses contain double-stranded, circular DNA genomes in a super-coiled configuration within the virions.

Rotaviruses have segmented double-stranded RNA genomes. The virions contain an RNA-dependent RNA polymerase to produce mRNA within the host cell's cytoplasm.

Test 3

QUESTIONS

DIRECTIONS:

Each of the numbered items or incomplete statements in this section is followed by answers or by completions of the statement. Select the ONE lettered answer or completion that is BEST in each case.

1. Compliance with medical advice is most closely associated with

(A) intelligence
(B) race
(C) religion
(D) educational level
(E) a good doctor–patient relationship

2. A 21-year-old male visits a sexually transmitted disease (STD) clinic with complaints of a purulent urethral discharge and dysuria. Pus cells, but no bacteria, are noted on the Gram stain examination of the exudate. Which of the following organisms are the most likely cause of this infection?

(A) *Neisseria gonorrhoeae* and *Gardnerella vaginalis*
(B) *Neisseria gonorrhoeae* and *Treponema pallidum*
(C) *Haemophilus ducreyi* and *Neisseria gonorrhoeae*
(D) *Ureaplasma urealyticum* and *Chlamydia trachomatis*
(E) *Mycoplasma hominis* and *Neisseria gonorrhoeae*

3. A man presents himself at a police station in Texas claiming that he does not know who he is. A fingerprint check reveals that he has been reported as a missing person by a family in Ohio. The most accurate diagnosis for this man is

(A) dissociative identity disorder
(B) dissociative fugue
(C) dissociative amnesia
(D) derealization
(E) depersonalization

4. Kwashiorkor is similar to marasmus in that both diseases have

(A) a normal total caloric intake
(B) a fatty liver
(C) an apathetic affect
(D) pitting edema
(E) anemia

5. Which of the following is most characteristic of sleep in a 45-year-old woman with major depressive disorder?

(A) Sleeping too many hours at night
(B) Falling asleep suddenly during the daytime
(C) Waking up too early in the morning
(D) Having difficulty coming fully awake after sleep
(E) Cessation of breathing during sleep

6. In yellow fever infections, death most often results from necrotic lesions observed in which of the following organs?

(A) Liver
(B) Spleen
(C) Brain
(D) Blood vessels
(E) Skin

7. A 50-year-old happily married male patient tells you that, prior to having sex with his wife of 15 years, he often enjoys watching videos of women getting undressed. This man is

(A) a voyeur
(B) an exhibitionist
(C) a fetishist
(D) a frotteur
(E) normal

8. Induration in the rectal pouch on a rectal examination in a 65-year-old woman with bilateral ovarian masses is an example of

(A) lymphatic spread of tumor
(B) seeding of tumor
(C) hematogenous spread of tumor
(D) discontinuous spread of tumor
(E) an inflammatory response to the presence of tumor

9. A primary care physician should use which of the following personality tests to evaluate the level of depression in a 50-year-old patient?

(A) Rorschach (ink blot) test
(B) Thematic apperception test (TAT)
(C) Sentence completion test (SCT)
(D) Minnesota multiphasic personality inventory (MMPI)
(E) Draw-a-person test

10. All live, attenuated viral vaccines now available have been developed by which of the following methods or mechanisms?

(A) Temperature-sensitive mutants
(B) Host range mutants
(C) Chemical inactivation
(D) Recombinant DNA technology
(E) Monoclonal antibody production

11. Which set of fatty acids is most effective in increasing cholesterol levels?

(A) Linoleic and linolenic
(B) Myristic and palmitic
(C) Butyric and stearic
(D) Oleic and palmitic
(E) Oleic and stearic

12. Which of the following is an example of an amine precursor uptake and decarboxylation (APUD) type of tumor in the lung?

(A) Squamous cell carcinoma
(B) Adenocarcinoma
(C) Bronchial hamartoma
(D) Bronchial carcinoid
(E) Bronchioloalveolar carcinoma

13. Arrange the following steps in collagen synthesis into the proper sequence.

1. Glycosylation
2. Post-translational modification of proline and lysine residues
3. Cross-linking of collagen fibrils using lysyl oxidase
4. N-terminal and C-terminal propeptides cleaved by peptidases
5. Assembly of three pro-α chains and formation of disulfide bonds

(A) 1–2–4–5–3
(B) 2–1–5–4–3
(C) 1–2–4–3–5
(D) 1–2–5–3–4
(E) 2–1–5–3–4

14. Quinolone antibiotics inhibit bacterial growth by affecting

(A) reverse transcriptase
(B) RNA polymerase
(C) DNA polymerase
(D) DNA gyrase
(E) transpeptidase

15. Which of the following DNA segments in the lactose operon of *Escherichia coli* is a *trans*-acting regulatory element?

(A) β-galactosidase gene
(B) Operator
(C) Promoter
(D) CAP binding site
(E) i gene

16. Which of the following clinical disorders is primarily associated with coagulation necrosis?

(A) Embolic stroke in a patient with infective endocarditis
(B) Acute tubular necrosis in a patient with hypovolemic shock
(C) Vasculitis associated with Henoch Schoenlein's purpura
(D) Clostridia infection of a gangrenous toe in a diabetic
(E) Intracerebral bleed in a patient with hypertension

17. Which of the following nutrients is more likely to promote coronary artery disease?

(A) Polyunsaturated fatty acids
(B) Dipalmitoylphosphatidylcholine (a lecithin)
(C) Monounsaturated fatty acids
(D) Megadoses of vitamin E
(E) Moderate consumption of alcohol (no more than two drinks per day)

18. In which of the following combinations are both conditions more likely to have pale infarctions than hemorrhagic infarctions?

(A) Atherosclerotic stroke and liver infarction
(B) Small bowel infarction and splenic infarction
(C) Torsion of the testicle and torsion of a cystic teratoma of the ovary
(D) Pulmonary infarction and embolic stroke
(E) Adrenal glands in Waterhouse-Friderichsen syndrome and an acute myocardial infarction

19. Steroid hormones exert their effects by binding to

(A) cell surface receptors
(B) G proteins
(C) transcription factors
(D) cyclic adenosine monophosphate (AMP)
(E) calcium ions

20. Which of the following statements about male homosexuality is true?

(A) Homosexual individuals cannot be sexually aroused by a member of the opposite sex
(B) Homosexuality is statistically more common in brothers than in unrelated men
(C) Intensive psychotherapy can often reverse homosexual orientation
(D) Testosterone levels in homosexual men commonly are below normal values
(E) Homosexuality is more common in the United States than in European countries

21. Ehlers-Danlos syndrome is a group of disorders that result from inherited defects in

(A) cell membranes
(B) gangliosides
(C) hemoglobin
(D) collagen
(E) elastin

22. In which one of the following situations is the affected tissue histologically normal?

(A) Thyroid gland in a patient with hypopituitarism
(B) Cerebral cortex in a patient with severe carotid artery atherosclerosis
(C) Leg muscle after a cast is removed 2 months after injury
(D) Hypoplastic adrenal gland removed at autopsy from a child who died in a car accident
(E) Hepatocytes surrounding the central vein in a patient with right heart failure

23. Which of the following statements concerning the relationship between diet and cancer is most accurate?

(A) Women who have a high intake of animal fat have a greater risk of developing breast and colon cancer

(B) β-carotene has anticancer properties because it is a precursor of vitamin A

(C) Vitamins C and E are antioxidants and have almost identical protective effects against cancer

(D) Organically grown foods are free of carcinogens

(E) Fiber in the diet decreases the incidence of stomach cancer

24. In which of the following combinations do both entities involve a different cell accumulation or pigment?

(A) Coal worker's pneumoconiosis; dust cells in the sputum of a person who lives in Los Angeles

(B) Ringed sideroblast in the bone marrow; heart failure cells in the sputum of a patient with mitral stenosis

(C) Lip pigmentation in a patient with Peutz-Jeghers syndrome; melanosis coli in a patient with chronic constipation

(D) Scleral icterus in a patient with viral hepatitis; kernicterus in a child with hemolytic disease of the newborn

(E) Radiologic densities in the pancreas of an alcoholic; nephrocalcinosis in a patient with primary hyperparathyroidism

25. The gamma proteins generated during herpesvirus multiplication are products of

(A) immediate early viral genes

(B) cell genes that are activated late after infection

(C) early viral genes

(D) cell genes that are activated early after infection

(E) late viral genes

26. Which of the following is more a feature of coagulation necrosis than apoptosis?

(A) An inflammatory infiltrate

(B) Nuclear condensation

(C) Cells with a dense eosinophilic cytoplasm

(D) Single-cell necrosis

(E) Gene activation

27. Ingestion of which of the following has been shown to have the greatest potential for inducing coronary artery disease?

(A) Cholesterol

(B) Olive oil

(C) Corn oil

(D) Animal fat

(E) Trans fatty acids

28. Which of the following disorders has a different mechanism of injury from the other disorders listed?

(A) Retrolental fibroplasia

(B) Bronchopulmonary dysplasia

(C) Hepatitis B

(D) Acetaminophen toxicity

(E) Carbon tetrachloride toxicity

29. Cytarabine and 5-fluorouracil (5-FU) are both effective in

(A) inhibiting DNA polymerase

(B) producing dose-limiting bone marrow depression

(C) inhibiting thymidylate synthetase

(D) treating acute myelocytic leukemia

(E) treating basal cell carcinoma

30. The gross (A) and microscopic (B) findings from the study of this lung removed at autopsy from a 45-year-old man demonstrate which of the following types of necrosis?

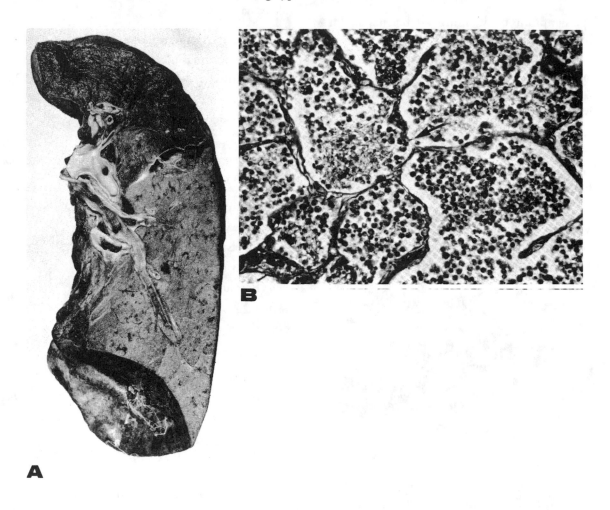

(A) Fibrinoid necrosis
(B) Coagulation necrosis
(C) Caseous necrosis
(D) Gummatous necrosis
(E) Liquefactive necrosis

31. Which of the following statements concerning vitamin B_{12} is most accurate?

(A) The symptoms of vitamin B_{12} deficiency are limited to problems with hematopoiesis

(B) Vitamin B_{12} is widely distributed in the plant and animal kingdom

(C) Vitamin B_{12} deficiency can lead to a functional folate deficiency

(D) Vitamin B_{12} deficiency is most commonly due to inadequate consumption

(E) Vitamin B_{12} contains a molybdenum atom in the center of four pyrolle rings

32. Which of the following would most likely cause the abnormality shown in this cross-section of spleen removed at autopsy?

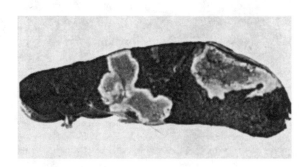

(A) Long-standing mitral stenosis

(B) Stage IV Hodgkin disease

(C) Carcinoid heart disease

(D) Atrial septal defect

(E) Primary cancer in the lung or breast

33. A 27-year-old patient, who just returned from St. Petersburg, has cramps and diarrhea. The motile organism noted on an Enterotest capsule string test is mostly

(A) *Cryptosporidium* species

(B) *Isospora belli*

(C) *Balantidium coli*

(D) *Giardia lamblia*

(E) *Strongyloides stercoralis*

34. A 3-year-old child with recurrent *Staphylococcus aureus* infections and an absent respiratory burst most likely has

(A) a defect in microtubule polymerization

(B) an autosomal recessive disease

(C) a deficiency of complement component C3

(D) a deficiency of NADPH oxidase

(E) a deficiency of myeloperoxidase

35. In which of the following stages of the sexual response cycle does erection first occur?

(A) Excitement

(B) Plateau

(C) Orgasm

(D) Emission

(E) Resolution

36. Fever associated with infection

(A) accelerates bacterial and viral replication

(B) left shifts the oxygen dissociation curve

(C) is due to interleukin-1 released from CD4 T-helper cells

(D) increases oxygen release to tissue

(E) inhibits wound healing

37. β-Lactamases cause resistance to penicillins and cephalosporins by

(A) breaking one chemical bond

(B) breaking two chemical bonds

(C) adding amino (NH_2) groups to a molecule

(D) inhibiting transpeptidase enzymes

(E) altering receptor attachment sites

38. Arrange the following events in wound healing by primary intention in the proper sequence.
1. Granulation tissue peaks
2. 75% to 80% tensile strength attained
3. Blood clot in the wound
4. Neutrophil influx into the wound

(A) 3-1-4-2
(B) 3-4-1-2
(C) 4-3-2-1
(D) 3-4-2-1
(E) 4-3-1-2

39. The Shine-Delgarno sequence is most closely associated with

(A) initiation of replication
(B) initiation of transcription
(C) initiation of translation
(D) termination of transcription
(E) termination of translation

40. In which of the following patients would you expect a normal to low erythrocyte sedimentation rate?

(A) 7-year-old child with sickle cell disease
(B) 72-year-old man with temporal arteritis
(C) 23-year-old woman with iron deficiency anemia
(D) 26-year-old man with lobar pneumonia
(E) 4-year-old child with cystic fibrosis

41. Which of the following antibiotics has excellent selective toxicity, is bactericidal, but depends on actively growing cells?

(A) Polymyxins
(B) Quinolones
(C) Rifampin
(D) Cephalosporins
(E) Aminoglycosides

42. Which of the following characterizes a secondary intention wound rather than a primary intention wound?

(A) Wound edges are approximated
(B) Less granulation tissue
(C) Less chance for infection
(D) Shorter time to heal
(E) Presence of myofibroblasts

43. Allopurinol therapy necessitates a reduction in the concurrent dosage of

(A) 6-thioguanine
(B) 6-mercaptopurine
(C) cytarabine
(D) 5-fluorouracil
(E) methotrexate

44. In which of the following combinations of chemical mediators of inflammation do both mediators have the same function?

(A) Histamine and Hageman factor
(B) C3a and C5a
(C) C3b and platelet-activating factor
(D) Leukotriene LTB4 and bradykinin
(E) Leukotrienes LTC4, -D4, -E4, and plasmin

45. Polyenes and polymyxins inhibit, respectively, which of the following groups of organisms?

(A) Gram positives and gram negatives
(B) Gram negatives and fungi
(C) Gram positives and protozoa
(D) Fungi and gram negatives
(E) Protozoa and fungi

46. Arrange the following neutrophil-related events in acute inflammation into the proper sequence.
1. Adhesion (pavementing)
2. Margination
3. Respiratory burst
4. Emigration
5. Chemotaxis

(A) 1-2-4-5-3
(B) 4-2-1-3-5
(C) 2-1-4-5-3
(D) 4-2-1-5-3
(E) 2-1-4-3-5

47. IQ is normally distributed with a mean of 100 and a standard deviation of 15. What percentage of people have an IQ of 145 or higher?

(A) 0.15%
(B) 2.35%
(C) 2.5%
(D) 13.5%
(E) 27%

48. Which of the following combinations contains one factor that is beneficial rather than detrimental to wound healing?

(A) Infection and ultraviolet light
(B) Zinc deficiency and corticosteroids
(C) Scurvy and radiation
(D) Absolute neutropenia and foreign body
(E) Diabetes mellitus and fibrinogen deficiency

49. An otherwise healthy 65-year-old man was in a car accident and broke ribs 4 through 8 on the left side. Approximately 12 days later he developed a painful, well-demarcated vesicular rash over the left rib cage that persisted for several weeks. Of the following, the rash is most likely due to

(A) primary infection with herpes simplex virus type 1
(B) primary infection with herpes simplex virus type 2
(C) reactivation of latent varicella-zoster virus (VZV)
(D) reactivation of latent Epstein-Barr virus
(E) primary infection with cytomegalovirus

50. The diagram of a serum protein electrophoresis performed on cellulose acetate has arrows depicting alterations under some of the protein components. This electrophoresis pattern would be expected in a

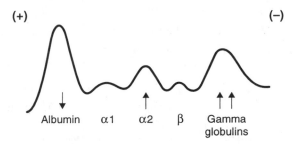

(A) 65-year-old man with multiple myeloma
(B) 23-year-old woman with acute appendicitis
(C) 6-year-old boy with a pure B-cell deficiency state
(D) 22-year-old, nonsmoking man with panacinar emphysema involving the lower lobes
(E) 36-year-old black man with sarcoidosis

51. Which of the following statements about a hydrophobic "signal sequence" is correct? It

(A) facilitates binding of polysomes to the endoplasmic reticulum
(B) is located at the carboxyl terminus of secretory proteins
(C) is found in most mature protein molecules
(D) is attached to protein molecules after translation by the ribosome
(E) is not found on any precursors of collagen

52. A newborn is diagnosed by biopsy as having encephalitis due to herpes simplex virus. Which of the following drugs is most likely to be administered?

(A) Idoxuridine
(B) Acyclovir
(C) Foscarnet
(D) Ganciclovir
(E) Vidarabine

53. In the United States, suicide rates are higher in

(A) the western mountain states than in northeastern states
(B) urban than in rural areas
(C) African Americans than in European Americans
(D) European Americans than in native Americans
(E) People under age 45 than in people over age 45

54. The human diploid cell vaccine (HDCV) for rabies

(A) is a live attenuated vaccine
(B) is made from virus grown in nervous tissue of animals
(C) should be administered only if symptoms develop
(D) is associated with development of encephalomyelitis
(E) is effective when given after infection with the virus

55. In the process of protein synthesis, the "P" site is a binding site that is part of the

(A) messenger RNA
(B) ribosome
(C) transfer RNA
(D) codon
(E) endoplasmic reticulum

56. An encephalitis characterized by an intense immune response which results in infiltration of lymphocytes and plasma cells into the brain is

(A) subacute sclerosing panencephalitis (SSPE)
(B) Creutzfeldt-Jakob disease
(C) progressive multifocal leukoencephalopathy
(D) kuru
(E) Whitlow's infection

57. In a group of 52-year-old men and women, which individual is most likely to commit suicide?

(A) A married man
(B) A married woman
(C) A divorced man
(D) A divorced woman
(E) A single woman

58. Which of the following best describes prions?

(A) They are defective viruses.
(B) They consist only of DNA or RNA.
(C) They are pseudovirions.
(D) They are proteinaceous particles.
(E) They are viroids.

59. Which of the following events causes a frameshift mutation?

(A) Substitution of adenine for guanine
(B) Substitution of thymine for adenine
(C) Transversion
(D) Transition
(E) Insertion of a single base

60. Creutzfeldt-Jakob disease can be transmitted by

(A) urine or feces of mice
(B) medical instruments
(C) inhalation of aerosols
(D) cannibalism
(E) arthropods

61. Neoplastic cells lacking hypoxanthine-guanine phosphoribosyl transferase (HGPRTase) are unresponsive to treatment with

(A) methotrexate
(B) 5-fluorouracil
(C) 6-mercaptopurine
(D) cytarabine
(E) doxorubicin

62. A cell that is transformed by a virus

(A) is always malignant
(B) never produces progeny virus
(C) exhibits normal growth patterns
(D) expresses one or more viral genes
(E) induces little or no immune response

63. A newborn infant who extends its large toe upward in response to stroking the lateral surface of the sole of its foot is demonstrating which reflex?

(A) Babinski reflex
(B) Rooting reflex
(C) Grasp reflex
(D) Startle reflex
(E) Moro reflex

64. Which of the following applies to oncogenic DNA viruses?

(A) Their early gene expression induces cell transformation
(B) Their oncogenes induce tumor by a common mechanism
(C) Their oncogenes are very similar to those of RNA tumor viruses
(D) They are associated only with tumors found in animals
(E) They induce expression of the p53 gene

65. A 54-year-old diabetic has questions concerning his sexual functioning. Which of the following statements provides the most correct information for this man?

(A) Five to 10% of diabetic men eventually have erectile dysfunction
(B) The major problem for diabetic men is delayed ejaculation
(C) The major cause of sexual problems in diabetic men is psychological
(D) Poor metabolic control of diabetes is associated with sexual problems
(E) The impotence associated with diabetes does not respond to treatment of any kind

66. A boy whose dog died suddenly expects that his pet will wake up and come back to life. This child is most likely to be age

(A) 4 years
(B) 8 years
(C) 10 years
(D) 12 years
(E) 14 years

Questions 67-69

In 1990, 1200 deaths occurred within a population of 1,000,000. At the beginning of the year, this population was known to include 900 individuals with lung cancer. During the year, 300 new cases of lung cancer were diagnosed, and by the end of 1990, 60 people had died of the disease.

67. The incidence rate for lung cancer per 100,000 population in 1990 was:

(A) 0.3
(B) 6
(C) 30
(D) 90
(E) 120

68. The crude mortality rate per 100,000 population in 1990 was

(A) 0.2
(B) 6
(C) 30
(D) 90
(E) 120

69. The cause-specific mortality rate for lung cancer per 100,000 population in 1990 was

(A) 0.2
(B) 6
(C) 30
(D) 90
(E) 120

70. Which of the following physical problems is more common in a competitive, driving (type A) individual?

(A) Prostate cancer
(B) Obesity
(C) Coronary artery disease
(D) Pruritus (itching)
(E) Bronchial asthma

71. Cells that secrete product into the extracellular matrix, influencing other nearby cells without the product entering the circulation, are called

(A) exocrine cells
(B) endocrine cells
(C) paracrine cells
(D) neurocrine cells
(E) second messenger cells

72. Antimicrobial agents that exert their primary action on the synthesis of bacterial cell walls include

(A) erythromycin and chloramphenicol
(B) nalidixic acid and penicillin
(C) bacitracin and vancomycin
(D) polymyxins and erythromycin
(E) erythromycin and clindamycin

73. Which of the following statements concerning cholesterol consumed in the diet is correct? It

(A) decreases the rate of endogenous cholesterol synthesis by inhibiting 3-hydroxy-3-methylglutaryl CoA (HMG-CoA) reductase
(B) is first carried to the liver, where it is packaged into a very low-density lipoprotein (VLDL) particle
(C) generally is not absorbed from the digestive tract and is excreted in the feces as free cholesterol
(D) is not as readily esterified as endogenous cholesterol and, therefore, it is more prone to cause arteriosclerosis
(E) can be used to synthesize choline, one of the bile acids

74. Pharmacotherapy for premature ejaculation most likely includes

(A) fluoxetine
(B) opioid antagonists (e.g., naloxone)
(C) α-adrenergic antagonists
(D) nitroglycerine ointment applied to the penis
(E) intracorporeal administration of vasoactive drugs

Questions 75-77

To determine the relationship between chronic bronchitis in children and the history of such infections in their parents, a pediatrician reviewed the records of a large pediatrics practice. She identified 100 children between the ages of 5 and 7 years, 50 of whom had chronic bronchitis and 50 of whom had other health problems. The pediatrician then interviewed the parents of each child to determine their history of bronchitis in childhood. Thirty parents of children with recurrent bronchitis had a history of bronchitis. Twenty parents of the other children had such a positive history.

75. Which of the following labels best describes this type of study?

(A) Clinical trial
(B) Case control
(C) Cohort
(D) Prospective
(E) Cross-sectional

76. What is the odds ratio of chronic bronchitis in children ages 5 to 7 years?

(A) $30 \times 30 \div 20 \times 20$
(B) $20 \times 30 \div 20 \times 30$
(C) $20 \times 20 \div 30 \times 30$
(D) $20 \div 30 \times 20$
(E) Cannot be calculated from data given

77. What is the relative risk of chronic bronchitis in children ages 5 to 7 years?

(A) $30 \times 30 \div 20 \times 20$
(B) $20 \times 30 \div 20 \times 30$
(C) $20 \times 20 \div 30 \times 30$
(D) $20 \div 30 \times 20$
(E) Cannot be calculated from data given

78. Identify the structure denoted by the arrow in the figure below.

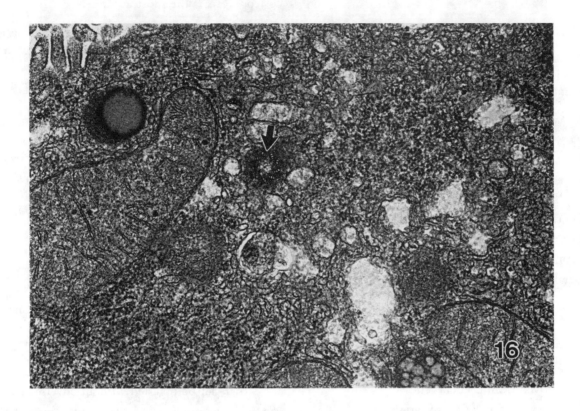

(A) Glycogen

(B) Centriole

(C) Basal body

(D) Mitochondrion

(E) Ciliary axoneme

79. Fatty acid synthesis and degradation are similar in that both processes

(A) take place in the mitochondrion

(B) use acyl CoA-thioesters

(C) use NADPH or NADP as a cofactor

(D) have malonyl CoA as an intermediate

(E) use acyl carrier protein

80. Which of the following antimicrobials inhibits function of the 50S ribosomal subunit?

(A) Sulfonamides

(B) Erythromycins

(C) Aminoglycosides

(D) Tetracyclines

(E) Rifampin

81. The "postage stamp test" is used in the diagnosis of

(A) female orgasmic disorder
(B) erectile disorder
(C) vaginismus
(D) premature ejaculation
(E) dyspareunia

82. The Epstein-Barr virus (EBV) belongs in which of the following subfamilies?

(A) Alphaherpesvirinae
(B) Lentivirinae
(C) Oncovirinae
(D) Gammaherpesvirinae
(E) Betaherpesvirinae

83. The oncogenes of RNA tumor viruses

(A) exist in several RNA virus families
(B) have low oncogenic potential
(C) are derived from cellular genes
(D) are necessary for their replication
(E) are not expressed at any time in normal cells

84. Which of the following statements concerning the consumption of carbohydrate is true?

(A) Individuals must ingest at least 20% of their caloric intake in the form of carbohydrate
(B) Complex carbohydrates provide no calories but are an important dietary component because they enhance bowel motility
(C) There is a direct correlation between sucrose consumption and dental caries
(D) There is a direct correlation between sucrose consumption and obesity
(E) A national dietary goal is to reduce carbohydrate consumption in the diet of Americans from the present value of 46% of the total calories in the diet to 30% of total calories.

85. Which of the following statements concerning osteoporosis is the most accurate?

(A) Although estrogen replacement therapy is an effective treatment for preventing bone loss in postmenopausal women, available data strongly suggest that testosterone therapy accelerates the development of osteoporosis in men
(B) Long-term ingestion of low levels of fluoride increases the rate of bone dissolution
(C) The tendency of many young women to follow a vegetarian diet reduces the incidence of osteoporosis among them as they age
(D) Intranasal administration of calcitonin has been effective in the treatment of osteoporosis
(E) Running is an effective means of reducing osteoporosis in all of the bones of the body

86. Which of the following statements concerning proteins is most accurate?

(A) Provided all the other dietary factors are supplied, there is no upper limit to the amount of protein that can be ingested without adverse effects
(B) The amount of protein required is inversely related to the biologic value of the protein
(C) Use of complementary protein foods, ingested simultaneously or many hours apart, permits vegetarians to get adequate protein intake from foods with low biologic value
(D) An individual suffering from marasmus requires less protein than does a well-fed individual
(E) Kwashiorkor is most commonly observed in elderly individuals

87. In which of the following combinations do both carcinogens predispose to different cancers?

(A) Asbestos (smoker)—uranium
(B) Cyclophosphamide—aniline dyes
(C) Aflatoxins—vinyl chloride
(D) Benzene—alkylating agents
(E) Chewing tobacco—alcohol

88. The toxic effect of an increased amount of ammonium (NH_4^+) in the body due to disease is most effectively reduced by

(A) converting it into ammonia (NH_3), which is non-diffusible
(B) combining it with alpha ketoglutarate to form glutamate
(C) anti-oxidants in the body, such as glutathione (GSH)
(D) converting it into glutamine
(E) increasing its elimination in the stool

89. Which laboratory test below readily distinguishes *Escherichia coli* from *Salmonella paratyphi* organisms?

(A) Gram stain
(B) Glucose fermentation
(C) Lactose fermentation
(D) Glucose oxidation
(E) Hemolysis on blood agar

90. Which of the following statements best characterizes natural killer cells?

(A) They are a subset of T cells
(B) They are involved in type III hypersensitivity reactions
(C) They require prior sensitization in order to kill virally infected cells or tumor cells
(D) They participate in antibody-dependent cellular cytotoxicity reactions
(E) They cannot be differentiated morphologically from small B cells

91. Which of the following is most likely to cause death in a 35-year-old woman?

(A) An abortion
(B) An intrauterine device
(C) Pregnancy
(D) An oral contraceptive
(E) A barrier contraceptive

DIRECTIONS:

Each of the numbered items or incomplete statements in this section is negatively phrased, as indicated by a capitalized word such as NOT, LEAST, or EXCEPT. Select the ONE lettered answer or completion that is BEST in each case.

92. A 64-year-old man has become ill. In this society, he now assumes the "sick role," which includes all of the following EXCEPT

(A) acceptance of responsibility for becoming ill
(B) exemption from usual responsibilities
(C) working toward becoming well
(D) cooperation with health care personnel
(E) expectation of care by others

93. Which of the following is NOT correct concerning a high-protein diet?

(A) Primary treatment for raising the serum albumin concentration in cirrhotics
(B) Produces an increase in the serum blood urea nitrogen level
(C) Produces excess carbon skeletons from amino acid metabolism that can be converted into glucose
(D) Produces excess carbon skeletons from amino acid metabolism that can be converted into fat
(E) Contraindicated in patients with chronic renal disease

94. Which of the following is LEAST likely to be seen in an 8-year-old child with attention deficit hyperactivity disorder (ADHD):

(A) Mental retardation
(B) Distractibility
(C) Impulsiveness
(D) Restlessness
(E) Frustration

95. Fatty change in the liver would LEAST likely be associated with

(A) alcoholism
(B) kwashiorkor
(C) carbon tetrachloride poisoning
(D) patient taking methotrexate
(E) acute viral hepatitis

96. Which of the following is NOT correct concerning the urea cycle?

(A) There is increased production of urea in starvation (prolonged fasting) due to an increase in amino acid metabolism
(B) N-Acetylglutamate is required to activate carbamoyl phosphate synthase I, the rate-limiting enzyme of the cycle
(C) It supplies intermediates for the tricarboxylic acid cycle
(D) It is defective in cirrhosis of the liver, resulting in a low serum blood urea nitrogen level and increased serum ammonia level
(E) Enzyme deficiencies earlier in the cycle are more likely to produce elevation in ammonia than deficiencies of enzymes that are operative later in the cycle

97. Antimicrobials that inhibit bacterial cell wall formation include all the following EXCEPT

(A) cycloserine
(B) vancomycin
(C) cephalosporin
(D) penicillin
(E) polymyxin

98. Ammonia derives from all of the following sources EXCEPT

(A) bacterial ureases in the stomach, colon, and urine
(B) reaction of glutamate dehydrogenase on glutamine in the renal tubules
(C) glutamate derived from transamination reactions
(D) amino acids such as histidine, asparagine, serine, and threonine
(E) amino group in nucleic acids

99. Which of the following does NOT contribute to the anti-inflammatory activity of corticosteroids?

(A) Increase of leukocyte adhesion to endothelial cells
(B) Inhibition of phospholipase A_2
(C) Inhibition of production of prostaglandins
(D) Inhibition of production of leukotrienes
(E) Suppression of antibody synthesis

100. The nucleotide that is LEAST likely to serve as a substrate for the enzyme primase is

(A) cytidine triphosphate (CTP)
(B) adenosine triphosphate (ATP)
(C) thymidine triphosphate (TTP)
(D) uridine triphosphate (UTP)
(E) guanosine triphosphate (GTP)

101. Which of the following is LEAST likely to contribute to normal wound healing?

(A) Fibronectin
(B) Integrins
(C) Growth factors
(D) Type IV collagen
(E) Endothelial cells

102. Which of the following is LEAST likely to be a complication of obesity?

(A) Essential hypertension
(B) Increased risk for breast and endometrial cancer
(C) Osteoarthritis
(D) Reduction in insulin receptors
(E) Hypothyroidism

103. All of the following statements concerning the bacterium *Chlamydia trachomatis* or its life cycle are correct EXCEPT that

(A) they are susceptible to tetracyclines
(B) the extracellular stage consists of elementary bodies
(C) α-hemolytic colonies form on blood agar
(D) they depend on the host cells' energy production
(E) they primarily infect epithelial cells

104. Which of the following amino acid relationships is NOT correct?

(A) Arginine and histidine are required for growth
(B) Leucine and lysine are the only exclusive ketogenic amino acids
(C) Isoleucine, leucine, and valine can be used by skeletal muscle for fuel in the fasting state
(D) Tyrosine is an essential amino acid that can be used for the synthesis of catecholamines, thyroid hormone, fumarate, and melanin
(E) Tryptophan is an essential amino acid that can be used for the synthesis of serotonin, melatonin, and the nicotinamide moiety of NAD^+ and $NADP^+$

105. Which of the following is NOT a function of interleukin-1?

(A) Inhibits the release of the postmitotic neutrophil pool in the bone marrow
(B) Increases the liver synthesis of fibrinogen, C-reactive protein, and coagulation factors
(C) Stimulates prostaglandin synthesis in the hypothalamus, which initiates fever
(D) Stimulates the synthesis of adhesion molecules on leukocytes and endothelial cells
(E) Decreases the liver synthesis of albumin and transferrin

106. Which of the following amino acids is NOT a neurotransmitter or involved in the synthesis of a neurotransmitter?

(A) Glycine
(B) Tryptophan
(C) Histidine
(D) Glutamine
(E) Lysine

107. All of the following statements about suicide are true EXCEPT that

(A) most suicides can be prevented
(B) many individuals seek medical care in the week preceding suicide
(C) patients usually know that their method of suicide is lethal
(D) marriage is associated with a reduced risk of suicide
(E) professional women are at greater risk for suicide than are nonprofessional women

108. Which of the following statements regarding the F factor is NOT correct?

(A) The F factor usually exists as a linear, double-stranded DNA molecule
(B) The F factor codes for the synthesis of the F pilus
(C) Cells containing the F factor act as donors during conjugation
(D) Only one strand of F factor DNA moves through the pilus to the recipient cell
(E) The 5′ end of an F factor DNA strand moves across the pilus to the recipient cell before the 3′ end moves

109. Which of the following relationships is NOT a cardinal sign of inflammation and pathogenesis?

(A) Rubor—vasodilatation
(B) Calor—vasodilatation
(C) Tumor—neurogenic response
(D) Dolor—prostaglandin D and bradykinin
(E) Functio laesa—swelling and pain

110. All of the following statements regarding transposons are true EXCEPT

(A) transposons sometimes carry genes that code for antibiotic resistance
(B) transposons are only found in bacteria
(C) the target sites for transposons appear to be randomly selected
(D) insertion of a transposon causes the duplication of nucleotides at the target site
(E) insertion of a transposon into the coding region of a gene often destroys the function of that gene

111. All of the following statements concerning Rocky Mountain spotted fever are true EXCEPT that

(A) rash, fever, and a history of tick exposure are classic diagnostic features
(B) the disease is more common in western states than in eastern states
(C) the rash is a vasculitis resulting from rickettsial invasion of capillary endothelial cells
(D) the microimmunofluorescent antibody (IFA) serologic test yields positive results
(E) tetracycline is used for treatment

112. Which of the following cells would LEAST likely be involved in chronic inflammation?

(A) Endothelial cells
(B) Platelets
(C) Macrophages
(D) Lymphocytes
(E) Neutrophils

113. A particular stretch of DNA in *Escherichia coli* is transcribed into messenger RNA, which in turn is translated to form a protein molecule. Which of the following statements is NOT true?

(A) If you know the DNA sequence, you can predict the corresponding RNA sequence
(B) If you know the DNA sequence, you can predict the corresponding protein sequence
(C) If you know the RNA sequence, you can predict the corresponding DNA sequence
(D) If you know the protein sequence, you can predict the corresponding RNA sequence
(E) If you know the RNA sequence, you can predict the corresponding protein sequence

114. Which of the following inflammatory cell relationships is NOT matched correctly?

(A) Plasma cells—vasculitis in syphilis
(B) Basophils—type I hypersensitivity reactions
(C) T lymphocytes—antibody-dependent cytotoxicity
(D) Eosinophils—Charcot-Leyden crystals in sputum
(E) Monocytes—chronic inflammation

115. All of the following autacoids are classified as cytokines EXCEPT

(A) tumor necrosis factor
(B) granulocyte colony-stimulating factor
(C) interferon-α
(D) platelet-activating factor
(E) interleukin-2

116. Mature mammalian messenger RNA (mRNA) molecules would be LEAST likely to contain

(A) a 5' cap structure
(B) a 3' tail structure
(C) an exon
(D) an intron
(E) amino acid sequence codes

117. All of the following statements about homicide in the United States are true EXCEPT that

(A) it is the second-to-third most common cause of death in people aged 15 to 24 years
(B) it is more common in low socioeconomic populations
(C) it is more likely committed by males than by females
(D) at least one half are accomplished with guns
(E) homicide rates are decreasing

118. All of the following agents are used in the treatment of prostate cancer EXCEPT

(A) diethylstilbestrol (DES)
(B) leuprolide
(C) flutamide
(D) tamoxifen
(E) goserelin

119. A 35-year-old man has been living with another man in a stable sexual and love relationship for 6 years. All of the following statements about this man are likely to be true EXCEPT that he

(A) has a normal gender identity
(B) has normal testosterone levels
(C) has a sexual dysfunction according to the DSM-IV
(D) has a homosexual relative
(E) showed cross-gender behavior during childhood

120. Antibiotic therapy is appropriate for people experiencing infections caused by all of the following EXCEPT

(A) *Clostridium difficile*
(B) *Clostridium botulinum*
(C) *Listeria monocytogenes*
(D) *Bacillus anthracis*
(E) *Clostridium perfringens*

121. N-acetylneuramic acid (NANA) is a nine-carbon sugar derivative belonging to the family of sialic acids that is an integral component of all the following structures EXCEPT

(A) glycoproteins
(B) glycolipids
(C) glycosaminoglycans
(D) gangliosides
(E) phospholipids

122. The herpes simplex viruses (HSV) are known to cause all of the following EXCEPT

(A) oropharyngeal disease
(B) keratoconjunctivitis
(C) encephalitis
(D) neonatal disease
(E) Ramsay-Hunt syndrome

123. Which of the following is LEAST likely to be involved in the pathogenesis of the lesion (arrow) noted in the lung of this 45-year-old patient with fever?

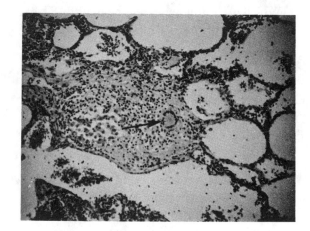

(A) CD4 T-helper cells
(B) Macrophages
(C) γ interferon
(D) Macrophage inhibitory factor
(E) Antibodies and complement

124. The cytochrome P-450 system is LEAST likely to be involved in the

(A) synthesis of steroids in the adrenal cortex
(B) conversion of drugs into lipid-soluble compounds
(C) conversion of testosterone to estradiol
(D) oxidation of lipophilic substrates (xenobiotics)
(E) generation of free radicals from drugs and chemicals

Questions 125-126

The following questions pertain to grief reactions in a 62-year-old woman whose husband died 6 months previously.

125. This woman would be LEAST likely to show which of the following symptoms?

(A) Mild anxiety
(B) Mild insomnia
(C) Intermittent crying spells
(D) Illusions
(E) Severe weight loss

126. For the patient experiencing a normal grief reaction, proper treatment by the physician should NOT include

(A) reassurance
(B) increased frequency of medical appointments
(C) antidepressants
(D) benzodiazepines for insomnia
(E) advice

DIRECTIONS:

Each set of matching questions in this section consists of a list of four to twenty-six lettered options (some of which may be in figures) followed by several numbered items. For each numbered item, select the ONE lettered option that is most closely associated with it. To avoid spending too much time on matching sets with large numbers of options, it is generally advisable to begin each set by reading the list of options. Then for each item in the set, try to generate the correct answer and locate it in the option list, rather than evaluating each option individually. Each lettered option may be selected once, more than once, or not at all.

Questions 127-131

For each characteristic, select the appropriate cell type.

(A) Skeletal muscle cells
(B) Hepatocyte
(C) Brain neuron
(D) Adipocyte
(E) Erythrocyte
(F) Heart muscle cells

127. Has glucose 6-phosphatase activity

128. Uses phosphocreatine kinase activity to form MB (CK-2) creatine kinase

129. Possesses mitochondria, but glucose is the primary fuel source

130. Relies on glycolysis as the only energy-producing metabolic sequence

131. Has glycerol kinase activity in humans

Questions 132-134

For each clinical goal, select the appropriate form of behavior modification therapy.

(A) Extinction
(B) Token economy
(C) Biofeedback
(D) Aversive conditioning
(E) Stimulus generalization

132. Alleviate the symptoms of Raynaud disease

133. Stop a child from raising his hand excessively in the classroom by not calling on him when he raises his hand

134. Aid in treating pedophilia using electric shock paired with photographs of undressed children

Questions 135-136

The diagram below shows Lineweaver-Burke plots for an enzyme-catalyzed reaction in the absence and presence of two different inhibitors. Which point in the diagram is described by each of the following?

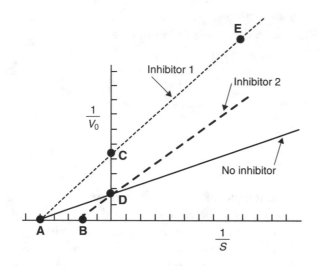

135. $-1/K_m$ in the presence of the competitive inhibitor

136. $1/V_{max}$ in the presence of a noncompetitive inhibitor

Questions 137-141

Select the agent that is used in the treatment of each of the following disorders.

(A) Interferon-α
(B) Erythropoietin
(C) Interleukin-2
(D) Cyclosporine
(E) Granulocyte colony-stimulating factor

137. Anemia in renal failure patients

138. "Graft-versus-host" syndrome

139. Leukopenia secondary to cancer chemotherapy

140. Metastatic renal cell carcinoma

141. Hairy cell leukemia

Questions 142-143

The diagram shows the effect of substrate concentration on the initial velocity of an enzyme-catalyzed reaction. Which point on this diagram is described by each of the following?

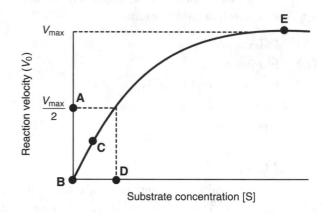

142. The K_m of the enzyme for the substrate

143. The point at which the rate of reaction is zero order with respect to the substrate

Questions 144-148

For each of the following descriptions, select the appropriate type of study.

(A) Cross-sectional study
(B) Case-control study
(C) Nonconcurrent cohort study
(D) Concurrent cohort study
(E) Randomized clinical treatment trial

144. A study is designed to see whether ninth-grade girls who attend sex education lectures will have a lower rate of teenage pregnancy by their sixteenth birthdays than girls who do not attend these lectures.

145. A study shows that a significantly higher percentage of 300 women with fibrocystic breast disease report a history of birth control pill use than 800 women who do not have fibrocystic breast disease.

146. A random telephone sample of people 20 years of age or older living in Los Angeles reveals that those respondents who are smokers are more likely than nonsmokers to have a current upper respiratory infection.

147. A study is designed to determine whether chemical exposure 30 years ago is associated with an increased incidence of testicular cancer in 1000 men who worked in a chemical plant.

148. A study is designed to compare the utility of a high-fiber diet versus surgery in the treatment of hemorrhoids. Fifty patients follow a high-fiber diet and 50 other hemorrhoid patients are treated surgically. All 100 patients report the persistence of their symptoms 1 year later.

Questions 149-153

For each of the following descriptions, select the appropriate neurotransmitter substance.

(A) Adenosine triphosphate
(B) Vasoactive intestinal peptide
(C) Enkephalins
(D) Nitric oxide
(E) Dopamine
(F) Neuropeptide Y

149. Released with norepinephrine from sympathetic nerves, it causes vasoconstriction

150. Released from vascular endothelium and pelvic and gastric nerves, it causes vasodilation, inhibition of platelet aggregation, gastric emptying, and penile erection

151. Closely related to the structure of secretin and glucagon, it is a powerful vasodilator that also stimulates intestinal water and electrolyte secretion

152. A postganglionic sympathetic neurotransmitter in renal blood vessels, it produces vasodilation

153. Present in secretomotor and interneurons in the enteric nervous system, it inhibits acetylcholine release and peristalsis, except in the presence of naloxone

Questions 154-157

For each clinical description, select the most appropriate hormone.

(A) Estradiol
(B) Testosterone
(C) Progesterone
(D) Dihydrotestosterone
(E) Cortisone

154. Involved in masculinization of male external genitalia

155. Exerts the strongest positive influence on sex drive in women

156. Plays a role in the development of the adrenogenital syndrome

157. Exerts the strongest negative influence on sex drive in women

Questions 158-162

Select the drug that inhibits the following enzyme or synthetic reactions.

(A) Etoposide
(B) Finasteride
(C) Hydroxyurea
(D) Aminoglutethimide
(E) Methotrexate

158. Adrenal steroid and extra-adrenal estrogen synthesis

159. Dihydrofolate reductase

160. Ribonucleotide reductase

161. Dihydrotestosterone synthesis

162. Topoisomerase II

Questions 163-165

For each set of physical findings, select the most likely causal virus.

(A) Herpes simplex virus type 1
(B) Herpes simplex virus type 2
(C) Varicella-zoster virus (VZV)
(D) Epstein-Barr virus (EBV)
(E) Cytomegalovirus (CMV)
(F) Human herpes virus 6

163. A 5-year-old girl presents with a fever and a generalized macular rash that appears mostly on the scalp and the trunk of the body. Several waves of lesions appear, one after another, and evolve rapidly into vesicles and then pustules over a period of 2 to 4 days.

164. An 18-month-old child with microencephaly and hepatosplenomegaly is diagnosed with a hearing impairment and mental retardation. Laboratory tests indicate that cells in the urine have large intranuclear inclusion bodies.

165. During exam week, a fatigued freshman college student presents with low-grade fever, headache, exudative tonsillitis, and painful cervical adenopathy. The serum transaminase levels are elevated, and the total bilirubin level is normal.

Questions 166-170

Choose the antineoplastic drug most frequently associated with the following organ toxicities.

(A) Vincristine
(B) Doxorubicin
(C) Cisplatin
(D) Cyclophosphamide
(E) Bleomycin

166. Cardiac toxicity

167. Pulmonary fibrosis

168. Hemorrhagic cystitis

169. Peripheral neuropathy

170. Renal toxicity

Questions 171-174

All of the compounds in this list are nitrogen-containing compounds.

(A) Attenuator
(B) AUG
(C) CAAT
(D) CCA
(E) fMet
(F) GAATTC
(G) GU..........AG
(H) Hogness box
(I) 7-Methylguanosine
(J) Poly A
(K) Polyadenylation sequence
(L) Pribnow box
(M) Shine-Delgarno sequence
(N) TATA
(O) UAG

171. Part of the "cap" structure found at the 5' end of eukaryotic mRNA

172. Removed during processing of eukaryotic mRNA

173. Occurs at the 3' end of tRNA

174. Signals termination of translation

Questions 175-176

For each case description, select the most likely inflammation.

(A) Serous inflammation
(B) Phlegmonous inflammation
(C) Fibrinous inflammation
(D) Pseudomembranous inflammation
(E) Granulomatous inflammation
(F) Suppurative inflammation

175. Forty-five-year-old man with chronic renal failure and a pericardial friction rub

176. Eight-year-old child with dysphonia, a gray-white exudate in the oropharynx, and cervical lymphadenopathy

Questions 177-180

Match each of the following statements with the antimicrobial agent that it most closely describes.

(A) Rifampin
(B) Cephalosporins
(C) Quinolones
(D) Erythromycin
(E) Polymixins
(F) Sulfonamides

177. Antimicrobial agent affecting cell wall

178. Antimicrobial agent that interferes with DNA function

179. Antimicrobial agent that inhibits protein synthesis by inhibiting transcription

180. Antimicrobial agent that affects cell membranes

ANSWER KEY

1. E	31. C	61. C	91. C	121. E	151. B
2. D	32. A	62. D	92. A	122. E	152. E
3. B	33. D	63. A	93. A	123. E	153. C
4. E	34. D	64. A	94. A	124. B	154. D
5. C	35. A	65. D	95. E	125. E	155. B
6. A	36. D	66. A	96. A	126. C	156. E
7. E	37. A	67. C	97. E	127. B	157. C
8. B	38. B	68. E	98. B	128. F	158. D
9. D	39. C	69. B	99. A	129. C	159. E
10. B	40. A	70. C	100. C	130. E	160. C
11. B	41. D	71. C	101. D	131. B	161. B
12. D	42. E	72. C	102. E	132. C	162. A
13. B	43. B	73. A	103. C	133. A	163. C
14. D	44. B	74. A	104. D	134. D	164. E
15. E	45. D	75. B	105. A	135. B	165. D
16. B	46. C	76. A	106. E	136. C	166. B
17. B	47. A	77. E	107. C	137. B	167. E
18. A	48. A	78. B	108. A	138. D	168. D
19. C	49. C	79. B	109. C	139. E	169. A
20. B	50. E	80. B	110. B	140. C	170. C
21. D	51. A	81. B	111. B	141. A	171. I
22. D	52. B	82. D	112. E	142. D	172. G
23. A	53. B	83. C	113. D	143. E	173. D
24. C	54. E	84. C	114. C	144. D	174. O
25. E	55. B	85. D	115. D	145. B	175. C
26. A	56. A	86. B	116. D	146. A	176. D
27. D	57. C	87. C	117. E	147. C	177. B
28. C	58. D	88. D	118. D	148. E	178. C
29. B	59. E	89. C	119. C	149. F	179. A
30. E	60. B	90. D	120. B	150. D	180. E

ANSWERS AND EXPLANATIONS

1. The answer is E. *(Behavioral science)*
Patient compliance is greater with written rather than with verbal instructions. Compliance with medical advice is not associated with intelligence, race, religion, or educational level.

2. The answer is D. *(Microbiology)*
The condition described is nongonococcal urethritis (NGU). Although *Neisseria gonorrhoeae* routinely causes urethritis in males, the gram-negative diplococci would be readily observed in a Gram stain examination of the exudate. The organisms are often found within white blood cells. Such observation would be sufficient to assume gonococcal infection and treatment.

Gardnerella vaginalis is normally found in the female genitourinary tract and is associated with vaginitis. Gardnerella infection often yields "clue cells," which are vaginal epithelial cells covered with many tiny rods.

Ureaplasma urealyticum and *Chlamydae trachomatis* are the best choices for the described condition. The agents are quite small and would not be seen by microscopic examination. *Ureaplasma urealyticum* requires 10% urea for growth and is responsible for some cases of nongonococcal urethritis. *Chlamydae tranchomatis,* however, probably causes the majority of such cases. *Mycoplasma hominis,* like *Ureaplasma,* lacks a cell wall. It is considered to be a normal flora organism that may be opportunistic, and is more often associated with disease in women than men. *Haemophilus ducreyi* is a sexually transmitted pathogen that causes chancroid (soft chancre). It is a small gram-negative rod that can be obtained from the chancroid lesion, which is a ragged ulcer on the genitalia accompanied by marked swelling and tenderness.

3. The answer is B. *(Behavioral science)*
This man is suffering from dissociative fugue. In dissociative fugue, loss of personal identity is combined with wandering away from home. In dissociative amnesia, the individual has loss of memory and may also have a loss of personal identity. In dissociative identity disorder, the individual has multiple personalities. Derealization and depersonalization are lesser forms of dissociative disorder in which an individual feels separate from others or from the environment.

4. The answer is E. *(Pathology)*
Both marasmus and kwashiorkor are associated with anemia.

Marasmus is characterized by a low calorie intake. Dietary deficiencies are compensated for by the breakdown of protein and fats. Key findings include:

- growth failure
- alertness
- hunger
- monkey-like appearance
- broomstick extremities
- muscle wasting
- mild anemia

Kwashiorkor is characterized by a normal total caloric intake but a decreased intake of protein (minimum protein intake is 8% of the total calories). Key findings are as follows:

- growth failure
- apathy and irritability with difficulty in feeding
- hepatomegaly (fatty liver)--> apoprotein deficiency
- pitting edema
- flaky paint dermatitis (looks like paint coming off a building)
- areas of depigmentation
- diarrhea due to the loss of brush border enzymes ("use it or lose it") and parasitic diseases
- flag sign in hair (alternating dark and light areas)
- protuberant abdomen (fatty liver from decreased apoproteins, ascites, bowel distention with air)
- laboratory findings include hypoproteinemia with hypoalbuminemia, depressed immune response, lymphopenia, and anemia

5. The answer is C. *(Behavioral science)*
Although excessive sleeping may also occur, the sleep problem most characteristic of major depressive disorder is early morning awakening, commonly called "terminal insomnia." Falling asleep suddenly during the daytime is narcolepsy, and cessation of breathing during sleep is sleep apnea. "Sleep drunkenness" involves difficulty in coming fully awake after sleep.

6. The answer is A. *(Microbiology)*
Yellow fever is an acute, febrile, mosquito-borne disease. Severe cases are characterized by jaundice, proteinuria, and hemorrhage. It is caused by a flavivirus with a wide host range.

The virus enters through the skin and spreads to the local lymph nodes, where it multiplies. From the lymph nodes, it undergoes viremia and localizes in many organs, causing lesions to occur. Although the infection is truly systemic, with degenerative changes possible in the spleen, lymph nodes, and heart, the most serious damage occurs in the liver and kidney. Death most often results from necrotic lesions in the liver and kidney. Hemorrhage occurs most frequently in the mucosa of the pyloric end of the stomach. Nerve and glial cells of the brain may develop intranuclear inclusions, and mononuclear cells may occur as perivascular infiltrations.

The incubation period is 3 to 6 days, and illness starts with fever, chills, nausea, and vomiting. High fever and moderate jaundice ensue, and blood may color the vomitus black. At this stage, mortality may be high. There is no sequelae; patients either die or recover completely.

7. The answer is E. *(Behavioral science)*
Enjoying sexually provocative visual material is often a part of normal sexuality. This patient is not suffering from voyeurism, exhibitionism, fetishism, or frotteurism. Voyeurism involves observing people engage in sexual activity without them being aware that they are being watched. Exhibitionism involves exposing the genitals to unsuspecting people. Fetishism involves sexual interest in inanimate objects. Frotteurism involves rubbing the penis against an unsuspecting, clothed woman.

8. The answer is B. *(Pathology)*
Induration in the rectal pouch on a rectal exam in a 65-year-old woman with bilateral ovarian masses is an example of seeding most likely secondary to a serous cystadenocarcinoma of both ovaries.

The dissemination of tumor occurs by seeding within body cavities, lymphatic spread or hematogenous spread. Seeding is commonly seen with colorectal cancers and ovarian cancers. The rectal pouch of Douglas (anterior to the rectum and posterior to the

uterus) in women is a common site for seeding to occur. Tumor implants in the pouch are easily detected by rectal examination. Lymphatic invasion is more common in carcinomas than in sarcomas. Lymphatic spread initially goes to the regional lymph nodes (subcapsular sinus is the first site) and from there into the systemic circulation via the thoracic duct. Hematogenous spread is favored by sarcomas (not exclusively), with spread to the lungs and liver as a common finding.

9. The answer is D. *(Behavioral science)*
Because it is easily administered and objectively scored, the MMPI can be used by a primary care physician to evaluate the level of depression in a patient. The Rorschach test, thematic apperception test, sentence completion test, and draw-a-person test are all projective tests that require special training to administer and score, and are usually used by clinical psychologists.

10. The answer is B. *(Microbiology)*
There are three main mechanisms currently employed to develop viral vaccines. All of the licensed viral vaccines that are currently available for use as live, attenuated products have been developed as **host range mutants.** By growing a human pathogenic virus in an unusual host (e.g., cell culture, lab animal host), eventually a strain develops that loses pathogenicity for humans. It retains the same antigenic properties as the wild-type virus and is capable of growing in the body in a similar manner. However, the new strain has lost its virulence and pathogenicity, and does not cause disease. Because it grows like the wild-type virus, it is able to stimulate both the humoral and the cell-mediated arms of the immune system. One disadvantage, however, is that such vaccines should not be used on immunocompromised individuals.

Temperature-sensitive mutants have been developed for respiratory viruses. They are capable of growing at 33°C, the temperature in the upper respiratory tract, but not at 37°C, the temperature of the lower respiratory tract. These are live viruses, and unfortunately, they have shown a strong tendency to backmutate to the fully virulent wild-type virus. These are not considered to be successful vaccine preparations.

Chemically inactivated, or killed, vaccines, and vaccines developed as a result of recombinant DNA technology, are not live, attenuated viral vaccines. Monoclonal antibodies could, theoretically, be used as a passive immune therapy for some viral diseases. Again, this would not represent a live, attenuated viral vaccine preparation.

11. The answer is B. *(Biochemistry)*

Lauric (12:0), myristic (14:0), and palmitic (16:0) acids raise cholesterol levels and are found primarily in animal fat and dairy products. Palmitic acid, the fatty acid that most effectively raises serum cholesterol levels, is also the major fatty acid found in palm and coconut oils. Stearic acid and fatty acids that have fewer than 10 carbon atoms tend not to raise cholesterol levels. Polyunsaturated fatty acids such as linoleic and linolenic and oleic acid (an ω-9 monounsaturated fatty acid found as approximately 70% of the total fatty acid in olive oil and 55% in canola oil) tend to lower cholesterol levels.

12. The answer is D. *(Pathology)*

A bronchial carcinoid is an example of an amine precursor uptake and decarboxylation (APUD) tumor, or neuroendocrine tumor. This name is applied to certain cells of the endocrine organs (e.g., anterior pituitary, pancreatic islets, C-cells in the thyroid, adrenal medulla, paraganglia) as well as single cells in various tissues (e.g., Kulchitsky's cells in the bronchial epithelium, argentaffin cells in the gut). APUD tumors are thought to have a common derivation from neural crest and neuroectoderm, thus the appellation, neuroendocrine tumors. However, there are some APUD tumors of endodermal origin. These tumors have dense core neurosecretory granules present on electron microscopy.

Tumors involving these cells can be adenomas or carcinomas. They are characterized by the production of various polypeptide hormones that have either a local, paracrine effect (e.g., bombesin, vasointestinal peptide) or a more generalized effect (e.g., insulin, glucagon).

Squamous cell carcinoma and adenocarcinoma are of epithelial origin. Bronchial hamartomas are not neoplastic and are an exaggerated overgrowth of tissue normally present in that organ. Bronchioloalveolar carcinomas are derived from mucin-secreting bronchiolar cells, Clara cells, or type II pneumocytes.

13. The answer is B. *(Biochemistry)*

Collagen synthesis begins within the fibroblast and is completed in the extracellular matrix. The correct sequence of events for the synthesis of collagen is as follows:

Post-translational modification of proline and lysine residues is the hydroxylation of proline and lysine using ascorbic acid as a cofactor. This occurs after the pre–pro-α polypeptide chains have been synthesized by translation of messenger RNA, which is located on the ribosomes of the rough endoplasmic reticulum.

Glycosylation of lysine residues by glucose and galactose occurs after hydroxylation.

Assembly of three pro-α chains, and formation of disulfide bonds at the C terminus, occurs in the Golgi apparatus. A triple helix begins to form by a zipper-like folding.

N-terminal and C-terminal propeptides are cleaved by peptidases once the procollagen molecule is secreted from the Golgi vacuoles into the extracellular matrix.

Cross-linking of collagen fibrils using lysyl oxidase (with copper as a cofactor) produces a strong collagen.

14. The answer is D. *(Microbiology)*

Quinolones block bacterial DNA synthesis by inhibiting DNA gyrase. This introduces negative superhelical turns into duplex DNA, thereby maintaining the negative superhelical tension of the bacterial chromosome during DNA replication. Ciprofloxacin and norfloxacin are active against a broad range of organisms that cause infections of the lower respiratory tract, intestinal tract, urinary tract and soft tissues. The original form, nalidixic acid, is useful only for urinary tract infections.

Rifampin directly inhibits bacterial RNA polymerase. The reverse transcriptase of human immunodeficiency virus is inhibited by azidothymidine (AZT). Penicillins and cephalosporins are transpeptidase enzymes that function in the final stages of cell wall synthesis. They are inactivated by β-lactamase enzymes, which break a single bond in the β-lactam ring of these antibiotics. Nonclinically useful drugs such as mitomycin C and actinomycin D can directly interfere with DNA polymerase activity, but they are useful only as biochemical tools in experiments.

15. The answer is E. *(Biochemistry)*
Regulatory sequences in DNA are classified as *cis-* or *trans-*acting elements, depending on the mechanism of action. *Cis-*acting elements function only when located on the strand of DNA being regulated, relatively close to the regulated gene. The operator (O), the promoter (P), and the CAP binding site all are located just upstream from the regulated structural genes of the operon, and do not function if placed at other locations. The β-galactosidase gene is one of the regulated structural genes of this operon. *Trans-*acting elements can function from long distances, and can even be on a different DNA molecule in the cell. The i gene, which encodes the repressor protein, is an example of a *trans-*acting regulatory element. Because the i gene encodes a diffusible product, it doesn't matter where it is placed relative to the regulated genes.

16. The answer is B. *(Pathology)*
Coagulation necrosis (infarction) is most commonly caused by ischemia secondary to atherosclerosis. It also occurs in heavy metal poisoning, where the heavy metal denatures proteins (e.g., lead denaturing ferrochelatase) and in radiation. In ischemia, the intracellular accumulation of lactic acid from anaerobic metabolism denatures cytoplasmic and lysosomal enzymes, which renders the latter incapable of liquefying the tissue. Therefore, vague cellular outlines remain on histologic examination of the tissue. Cytoplasmic eosinophilia is present on hematoxylin-eosin staining. The positively charged denatured proteins in ischemic tissue bind to the negative charge of eosin.

The term infarction refers to a localized area of coagulation necrosis secondary to a reduction in blood flow to the tissue. In vessels with dichotomous branching, the infarcts have a wedge-shaped appearance (e.g., lung, kidney, spleen). Dry gangrene is a variant of coagulation necrosis wherein the tissue appears to be mummified (e.g., diabetic foot).

Acute tubular necrosis in a patient with hypovolemic shock produces coagulation of the renal tubular epithelium. The epithelial cells slough off the basement membrane and block the flow of urine. Renal tubular casts are formed in the urine.

An embolic stroke in a patient with infective endocarditis is an example of liquefactive necrosis. The cells in the brain contain more lysosomes than do most other tissues; therefore, when brain tissue infarcts, the enzymes are released and liquefy the tissue leaving a cystic cavity. This is an exception, because an infarction is usually coagulation necrosis. Liquefactive necrosis most commonly implies an inflammation in which the enzymes from neutrophils and monocyte/macrophages digest the tissue and produce an exudate.

Vasculitis associated with Henoch-Schoenlein purpura is a type III hypersensitivity, which produces a fibrinoid necrosis with the deposition of immune complexes in the vessels and attraction of neutrophils from complement activation.

Clostridia infection of a gangrenous toe in a patient with diabetes is an example of liquefactive necrosis. Clostridia produce a myositis with subsequent liquefaction of the tissue.

An intracerebral bleed in a patient with hypertension is secondary to rupture of a Charcot-Bouchard microaneurysm involving the lenticulostriate vessels supplying the globus pallidus, putamen, and internal capsule area. The localized bleed into this area is a blood clot rather than a type of necrosis.

17. The answer is B. *(Biochemistry)*
Lecithin is widely touted by food faddists as a highly beneficial food supplement. However, some lecithins are rich sources of saturated fatty acids. Dipalmitoylphosphatidylcholine provides two palmitic acids per molecule. Palmitic acid is the most potent cholesterol-raising fatty acid. However, lecithin does have nutritional value: It aids in emulsification of lipid in the intestine, and it is a source of choline. In addition to its role in phospholipid metabolism, choline is needed to synthesize the neurotransmitter acetylcholine. Because de novo synthesis of choline is an expensive process requiring three methylations by S-adenosylmethionine, a dietary source of choline is beneficial. Soybean and other vegetable lecithins also are sources of essential fatty acids and accordingly contain less saturated fatty acid. However, if lecithin intake is abused, it may stimulate the development of obesity and coronary artery disease.

The polyunsaturated and monounsaturated fatty acids lower cholesterol levels.

Daily consumption of at least 100 IUs of vitamin E has been reported to reduce death from coronary heart disease by up to 40%, compared with diets with lower levels of the vitamin. This presumably relates to vitamin E's role in preventing the oxidation of low-density lipoproteins (LDL). Oxidized LDL is a potent stimulant in atherosclerosis.

Moderate consumption of alcohol also appears to lower the risk of death from coronary disease. Alcohol increases high-density lipoprotein (HDL) levels by inhibiting the activity of phosphotidylcholine:cholesterol acyltransferase (PCAT).

18. The answer is A. *(Pathology)*
Two morphologic types of coagulation necrosis are pale and hemorrhagic infarcts. Pale infarcts are most commonly found in solid organs, where the compactness of the surrounding tissue limits the spread of red blood cells released from necrotic vessels, thus giving the tissue a pale appearance. Pale infarcts are commonly seen in the heart, kidney, spleen, and liver.

Hemorrhagic infarcts occur in loose-textured organs, where the loose texture of the tissue allows the red blood cells released from damaged vessels to diffuse throughout the necrotic tissue. These infarcts are more commonly seen in lung, bowel, ovary, and testis. Hemorrhagic infarcts also occur with complete blockage of venous outflow from an organ (e.g., thrombosis of the superior mesenteric vein), which increases hydrostatic pressure in the venous system and decreases the inflow of arterial blood.

The only two conditions listed that both have pale infarctions are atherosclerotic stroke and infarction of the liver. Atherosclerotic strokes are caused by a thrombus overlying an atheromatous plaque in the carotid artery. The pale infarct usually occurs in the distribution of the middle cerebral artery. Because it is liquefactive necrosis, the brain tissue is dissolved by enzymes, and a cystic cavity remains after a few weeks. The liver is the least likely organ to infarct because it has a dual blood supply (portal vein and hepatic artery).

A small bowel infarction is a hemorrhagic infarction most commonly caused by thrombosis of the superior mesenteric artery, whereas a splenic infarction is usually a pale infarction, most commonly caused by systemic embolization from the left heart.

Torsion of the testicle and torsion of a cystic teratoma of the ovary both produce hemorrhagic infarctions.

A pulmonary infarction is a hemorrhagic infarction that is most commonly caused by a venous emboli from the deep saphenous vein of the lower leg. An embolic stroke from an embolus originating in the left heart is most commonly hemorrhagic because once the embolus is dissolved, the blood flow reperfuses the area of infarction causing blood to primarily leak out of the damaged gray matter vessels.

The adrenal glands in Waterhouse-Friderichsen syndrome display a hemorrhagic infarction. This syndrome is most commonly caused by a Neisseria meningitidis septicemia with an associated disseminated intravascular coagulation causing obstruction to blood flow in the adrenal glands. An acute myocardial infarction due to coronary artery thrombosis is an example of a pale infarct.

19. The answer is C. *(Biochemistry)*
Steroid hormones cross the cell membrane and bind to specific receptors within the cell. These receptors are transcription factors that are active only in the presence of particular hormones. The hormone–transcription factor complex binds to steroid hormone–responsive elements in DNA to influence transcription from steroid-sensitive genes. Thyroid hormone, retinoic acid, and 1,25-dihydroxycholecalciferol exert their effects in a similar way.

20. The answer is B. *(Behavioral science)*
Homosexuality is statistically more common in relatives than in unrelated men. This fact supports the theory of genetic influence in the etiology of homosexual behavior. Under some conditions, homosexual individuals can be sexually aroused by members of the opposite sex. Intensive psychotherapy has little or no effect on homosexual orientation. Testosterone levels in homosexual men are normal, and homosexuality is found in all countries and cultures to the same extent.

21. The answer is D. *(Biochemistry)*
Ehlers-Danlos syndrome is a group of disorders that result from inherited defects in collagen. These diseases prevent collagen from forming fibers properly. The skin is stretchy and the joints are loose. These diseases are also characterized by poor wound healing.

22. The answer is D. *(Pathology)*
The question contrasts two growth alterations, mainly atrophy and hypoplasia. Atrophy refers to a shrinkage

in cell size (organ size as well) with a loss of cell substance and a reduction in overall metabolic activity. There is a diminution in the number of cell organelles (e.g., mitochondria) and an increase in lipofuscin (pigment by-product of free radical damage) and autophagic vacuoles with a surplus in enzymes. There is an increased concentration of DNA per unit of tissue weight. Conditions associated with atrophy include

- decreased work load, such as a muscle in a cast
- loss of nerve innervation, as in lower motor neuron disease
- ischemia to tissue (e.g., cerebral atrophy)
- the normal aging process
- malnutrition associated with protein deprivation. Atrophy is greater in nonessential cells than in higher functional tissue. The order of atrophy is adipose, then muscle, then brain (least affected).
- hormone deficiency, such as the effect of hypopituitarism on producing atrophy in target organs (e.g., thyroid gland atrophy) or atrophy of parenchymal tissue surrounding a hormone secreting adenoma
- compression atrophy from an expanding mass, such as renal cortical atrophy in hydronephrosis (dilatation of renal pelvis by back-up of urine from ureter obstruction) or venous congestion in the central vein causing compression atrophy of neighboring hepatocytes

In aplasia (agenesis), there is nondevelopment of the primitive organ anlagen (e.g., aplasia of the adrenal cortex). Hypoplasia is a decrease in size of an organ with a corresponding decrease in cell number. It can be congenital (e.g., hypoplastic left heart syndrome) or acquired (e.g., intestinal enzymes disappear after prolonged by-pass or parenteral feeding). In congenital hypoplasia, the organ is structurally and histologically normal but does not have complete development of the organ anlagen (analogous to pituitary dwarf). Hypoplasia differs from atrophy in that atrophy begins with a normal organ that shrinks in size; whereas in hypoplasia, the organ never develops its full size.

23. The answer is A. *(Biochemistry)*
High-fat diets promote the formation of breast and colon cancer in women and of colon and prostate cancer in men. The probable mechanism is the oxidation of unsaturated fatty acids and the formation of free radicals and other carcinogens induced by the high temperatures associated with cooking. These effects are partially mitigated by the presence of the fat-soluble antioxidants, vitamin E and β-carotene. Another protective mechanism is the consumption of sufficient fiber (20–35 g per day). The fiber speeds the passage of the carcinogens through the colon, giving less exposure time to induce harmful mutation. Fiber also complexes some carcinogens and procarcinogens, preventing their absorption into the system, and helps suppress an appetite for fatty foods by filling the stomach.

β-Carotene is a vitamin A precursor, but it owes its anticancer effects to its antioxidant properties. Populations consuming carotene-rich foods have a lower incidence of lung, stomach, esophageal, and oral cavity cancer. β-carotene, however, does not protect cigarette smokers from lung cancer.

Along with β-carotene, vitamins E and C also help protect against certain types of cancer. Vitamin C is water soluble and has a different spectrum of activity than do vitamin E or β-carotene, which are fat soluble. The spectrum of activity of vitamin E and β-carotene also differs, but there is no clear rationale for these differences.

Organically grown foods may have fewer carcinogens, but all foods have some carcinogenic activity.

Fiber in the diet lowers the incidence of colon, not stomach, cancer. It also lowers the incidence of breast, endometrial, and ovarian cancer.

24. The answer is C. *(Pathology)*
The only combination of disorders involving different accumulations is Peutz-Jeghers syndrome, an autosomal dominant disease with melanin pigmentation of the lips and hamartomatous polyps in the gastrointestinal tract, and melanosis coli, which is a black colon caused by deposition of phenanthracene pigment in the macrophages of the lamina propria from laxative abuse.

Coal worker's pneumoconiosis (black lung) and dust cells in the sputum both are associated with an accumulation of anthracotic pigment from coal dust. Dust cells are alveolar macrophages containing the pigment.

Ringed sideroblasts in the bone marrow and heart failure cells in the sputum of a patient with mitral stenosis both have an accumulation of hemosiderin. Ringed sideroblasts are nucleated red blood cells with a defect in heme synthesis, which occurs partly in the cytoplasm and partly in the mitochondria. Heme is the combination of iron and protoporphyrin. A defect in heme synthesis (e.g., in lead poisoning or pyridoxine deficiency) results in an excess of iron in the mitochondria, which are normally located around the nucleus. A Prussian blue stain for iron identifies these iron-laden mitochondria in a perinuclear location, thus the term ringed sideroblasts. Heart failure cells are alveolar macrophages that have phagocytized red blood cells. A stenotic mitral valve results in a back-up of blood into the lungs with subsequent pulmonary congestion and hemorrhage of red blood cells into the alveoli. These macrophages with hemosiderin are the cause of the "rusty colored" sputum associated with mitral stenosis.

Scleral icterus in a patient with viral hepatitis and kernicterus in a child with hemolytic disease of the newborn both show an increase in bilirubin. Bilirubin is a breakdown product of hemoglobin after it has been phagocytized by a fixed macrophage in the spleen. The macrophage produces a lipid-soluble, indirect bilirubin, which when released into the blood combines with albumin. It is then taken up by the liver by ligands and conjugated into a water-soluble direct bilirubin. In viral hepatitis, scleral icterus is caused by a combination of direct and indirect hyperbilirubinemia from liver cell necrosis. In hemolytic disease of the newborn due to Rh incompatibility, the jaundice (icterus) is primarily due to indirect bilirubin from excessive extravascular hemolysis by macrophages of anti-D–coated fetal red blood cells. If all of the binding sites on albumin are occupied, unbound (free) indirect bilirubin accumulates in the plasma. This lipid-soluble,

toxic pigment crosses the blood–brain barrier and deposits in the brain, a condition called kernicterus.

Radiologic densities in the pancreas of an alcoholic and nephrocalcinosis in a patient with primary hyperparathyroidism are both associated with abnormal calcification. In the pancreas, the calcium deposits are associated with enzymatic fat necrosis from acute pancreatitis. Calcification of damaged tissue in the presence of a normal serum calcium level is called dystrophic calcification. Nephrocalcinosis refers to the deposition of calcium in the basement membranes of the kidney due to hypercalcemia. When calcium is elevated and deposits into normal tissue, it is called metastatic calcification. A high serum phosphate level can also produce metastatic calcification, since phosphorus normally drives calcium into tissue. Primary hyperparathyroidism is the most common cause of hypercalcemia in the ambulatory population and malignancy in the hospitalized patient.

25. The answer is E. *(Microbiology)*
The gamma proteins are the products of herpesvirus genes that are expressed late after infection of the cell. They are mostly structural proteins. More than 35 structural proteins are present in the mature virion.

The replication of herpesviruses takes place in the nucleus. It proceeds in a highly organized and tightly controlled manner.

The viral envelope glycoprotein attaches to the cell receptor; the virus enters by fusion of its envelope with the cytoplasmic membrane. The virus envelope is transported through the cytoplasm to a nuclear pore and is uncoated; viral DNA enters the nucleus. Transcription of viral DNA is accomplished by cellular RNA polymerase II plus viral factors.

Gene Stage	Protein	Description
Immediate	Alpha	Mostly enzymes needed for further steps in the growth cycle
Early	Beta	Mostly enzymes needed for further steps in the growth cycle
Late	Gamma	Mostly structural proteins

New viral DNA is packaged into preformed empty nucleocapsids. Nucleocapsids bud through the inner nuclear membrane and acquire an envelope.

Spontaneous deletions in parts of the DNA are common during multiplication, and defective particles frequently are found. The herpesviruses are unusual among nuclear DNA viruses in that they carry the genetic information for so many different enzymes.

A productive infection with herpesviruses often results in early shutdown of cell macromolecular synthesis, cytopathic effects, and cell death.

26. The answer is A. *(Pathology)*
Apoptosis refers to individual cell necrosis. It is normally operative in

- the normal turnover of cells (hormone-dependent involution in female menstrual cycle)
- programmed cell death in embryogenesis (e.g., Mullerian and Wolffian duct involution; formation of lumens in organs)
- toxin-induced injury (e.g., diphtheria)
- viral cell death (e.g., Councilman bodies in yellow fever)
- cell death via cytotoxic T cells, natural killer cells, antibody-dependent cytotoxicity (type II)
- atrophy of tissue (e.g., red neurons in ischemic atrophy in the brain)
- cell death in tumors
- clonal deletion of lymphocytes that would react against self

Unlike coagulation necrosis, apoptosis

- involves single cells rather than sheets of cells
- has densely stained eosinophilic cytoplasm and pyknotic nuclei (Councilman bodies), whereas coagulation necrosis has cells with less intense eosinophilia
- lacks inflammation, whereas coagulation necrosis is associated with eventual removal of necrotic tissue by neutrophils and macrophages
- has intact organelles in the cell, whereas the cells in coagulation necrosis have abnormal organelles (giant mitochondria with calcium deposits)
- has programmed death that is controlled by apoptosis genes, whereas coagulation necrosis is more commonly associated with ischemia due to atherosclerosis rather than programmed death

27. The answer is D. *(Biochemistry)*
The intake of excess quantities of saturated fatty acids with chain lengths from 12 to 16 carbons increases both serum cholesterol levels and the risk of coronary artery disease. Palmitic acid (16:0) is particularly abundant in most animal fats as well as in palm and coconut oils and is most efficient in this respect. The mode of action of these saturated fatty acids is at least twofold: They are readily broken down to acetyl-CoA, which is the building block for cholesterol synthesis, and they also exclude cholesterol from cell membranes. The fluidity of membranes must be maintained within narrow limits. If the membrane is too rigid, membrane proteins, such as transporters and receptors, cannot change their conformations. If the membrane is too fluid, the proteins fall out. The fluidity level is maintained by balancing the content of polyunsaturated and saturated fatty acid in the phospholipid core and by adjusting the cholesterol content. Polyunsaturated fatty acids promote fluidity because of their shape; the *cis* configuration of the double bonds produces a kink in the acyl chain, prohibiting tight packing. This raises their melting points (creating oils rather than fats) and increases the fluidity of membranes of which they are a part. Cholesterol acts as a space filler in membranes, but gets "pushed out" if unsaturated fatty acids are partially replaced by saturated ones. Therefore, diets high in saturated fatty acids that can get into membranes, such as palmitic, push cholesterol out of membranes and raise serum levels, whereas diets high in polyunsaturated fatty acids induce cholesterol to enter into the membrane and lower serum levels.

There is a clear correlation between risk of coronary artery disease and serum cholesterol levels, but there is ambiguity concerning the correlation between cholesterol consumption and serum levels. This is because β-hydroxy-βmethylglutaryl CoA reductase (HMG CoA reductase), the rate-limiting step in cholesterol synthesis, is inhibited by cholesterol. Thus, most individuals make less cholesterol if they eat more, within reason.

Trans fatty acids are produced when oils are partially hydrogenated. These have the "kink" removed and therefore should behave like saturated fatty acids; however, few clinical studies on their effects have been conducted.

28. The answer is C. *(Pathology)*
The mechanism of cell death in hepatitis B is that viral neoantigens alter the class I antigens on the hepatocyte. Cytotoxic CD8 T cells recognize these altered class I antigens and release perforin, which drills a hole through the cell membrane and kills the cell. The other disorders listed involve free radical injury as their primary mechanism of injury. Free radicals (FRs) primarily injure the cell membrane (via lipid peroxidation) and the nucleotides in DNA. They are produced by radiant energy, redox reactions, or are derived from parent chemicals, such as oxygen, acetaminophen, and carbon tetrachloride. Because they have a single, unpaired electron in their outer orbit, they are very unstable and damage tissue. Examples of oxygen FRs include superoxide, hydrogen peroxide, and hydroxyl ions generated from neutrophils and xanthine oxidase in tissue. Superoxide FRs are responsible for retrolental fibroplasia and bronchopulmonary dysplasia in newborns with the respiratory distress syndrome who are receiving 100% oxygen. Other FRs include chemicals and drugs, like carbon tetrachloride (CCl_4) and acetaminophen, respectively. Exposure to carbon tetrachloride results in the generation of CCl_3 FRs by the cytochrome P450 system in the liver smooth endoplasmic reticulum. Similarly, acetaminophen is converted into FRs, which damage hepatocytes.

29. The answer is B. *(Pharmacology)*
As with other antimetabolites such as methotrexate and 6-mercaptopurine, the pyrimidine analogs (5-FU, cytarabine, and others) inhibit DNA synthesis in bone marrow cells, causing delayed leukopenia (anemia and thrombocytopenia may also occur). Only activated cytarabine inhibits DNA polymerase, whereas activated 5-FU inhibits thymidylate synthetase and deoxythymidine monophosphate formation. Cytarabine is used in treating acute myelocytic leukemia whereas 5-FU is a component of the therapy for various carcinomas (gastric, colon, breast, and ovarian), including superficial basal cell carcinoma of the skin.

30. The answer is E. *(Pathology)*
The gross findings of the lung study reveal a lower lobe lobar pneumonia exhibiting gray hepatization. The microscopic findings show numerous neutrophils in the alveoli, which is consistent with liquefactive necrosis. Liquefactive necrosis is caused by the destructive effect of proteolytic enzymes generated from neutrophils, monocytes, and macrophages in infected tissue (e.g., abscess, cellulitis) or is caused by the release of endogenous enzymes in infarcted brain tissue. Wet gangrene refers to an initial event with coagulation necrosis followed by a superimposed bacterial infection (usually anaerobic), which produces a liquefactive necrosis of the infarcted tissue.

Coagulation necrosis, or infarction, is most commonly caused by ischemia. The intracellular build-up of lactic acid denatures cytoplasmic and lysosomal enzymes, rendering the latter unable to liquefy the tissue. Vague cellular outlines remain on histologic examination of the tissue.

Caseous (cheese-like) necrosis is a combination of coagulation and liquefactive necrosis and is commonly associated with tuberculosis and certain systemic fungal infections (e.g., histoplasmosis, coccidioidomycosis). Caseous necrosis is a type IV hypersensitivity reaction, which involves an interaction between CD4 T-helper cells and macrophages. Granulomas are the key histologic feature of caseous necrosis.

Fibrinoid (fibrin-like) necrosis is an alteration in injured blood vessels/tissue characterized by an increase in eosinophilic-staining plasma proteins in the vessel wall/tissue. Fibrinoid necrosis is most often associated with immune complexes consisting of immunoglobulins and/or complement deposited in vessel walls, synovial tissue, and connective tissue in disorders such as systemic lupus erythematosus and rheumatic fever.

Gummatous necrosis is seen in tertiary syphilis and is a variant of granulomatous inflammation. The lesions of gummatous necrosis are destructive, have a rubbery consistency, and are called gummas.

31. The answer is C. *(Biochemistry)*
A functional deficiency of vitamin B_{12} causes a megaloblastic anemia and neurologic lesions that can eventually lead to death.

The cause of the megaloblastic anemia is a secondary functional folate deficiency that leads to diminished synthesis of purines and thymidine and a failure of DNA replication. This replication failure leads to a disproportionate increase in the nuclear–cytoplasmic ratio and megaloblastic cells. The functional folate deficiency is due to inhibition of the reaction illustrated.

$$\text{homocysteine} + \text{N}^5\text{-methyltetrahydrofolate} \xrightarrow{B_{12}} \text{methionine} + \text{tetrahydrofolate}$$

In this reaction, catalyzed by homocysteine methyltransferase, a methyl group is transferred from tetrahydrofolate (THF) to homocysteine to form methionine. The vitamin B_{12} is used as the methyl cobalamin cofactor.

Without vitamin B_{12}, N^5-methyltetrahydrofolate accumulates, thus depriving the cell of free THF and eventually inhibiting all the other one-carbon transfer reactions in which folate is normally involved. Although this is most clearly manifested by the megaloblastic anemia, there are also effects associated with the turnover of epithelial cells in the digestive system. In fact, the earliest presenting symptom of vitamin B_{12} or folate deficiency is often a soreness of the tongue, with intermittent inflammation and papillary atrophy.

In addition to its effects on hematopoiesis, vitamin B_{12} deficiency has severe neurologic effects, including demyelination of posterior columns and the lateral corticospinal tract (subacute combined degeneration). It is believed that these are caused by inhibition of the reaction illustrated.

$$\text{propionyl CoA} \rightarrow \text{methylmalonyl CoA} \xrightarrow{B_{12}} \text{succinyl CoA (TCA cycle)}$$

In this series of reactions propionyl CoA is converted to succinyl CoA via methylmalonyl CoA. The vitamin, as the deoxyadenosyl cobalamin cofactor of methylmalonyl CoA mutase, is required for the rearrangement of methylmalonyl CoA to form succinyl CoA.

The inhibition of this reaction increases propionate levels, which causes a concomitant accumulation of fatty acids with an odd number of carbons. It is thought that these odd numbered fatty acids find their way into the phospholipid constituent of membranes, thus deranging myelin formation. A decrease in vibratory sensation is the first neurologic manifestation of the deficiency.

A deficiency of the vitamin also induces an accumulation of methylmalonate, which is a useful test to confirm cases of B_{12} deficiency.

Plants have essentially no vitamin B_{12}. The vitamin finds its way into the mammalian food chain due to the action of bacteria in the stomachs of ruminants and from shellfish. Human bacterial flora do manufacture the vitamin, but it cannot be absorbed from the gut without intrinsic factor. Therefore, the natural sources of vitamin B_{12} are primarily of animal origin. Rich sources include liver, whole milk, eggs, oysters, fresh shrimp, pork, and chicken. Persons who live exclusively on vegetable products, and exclude eggs and dairy products, have a difficult time obtaining sufficient vitamin B_{12} in their diet. Such persons may not develop full-blown symptoms of vitamin B_{12} deficiency, but often develop neurologic problems without signs of anemia. Anemia is probably absent because the individuals are getting sufficient folate in the diet to overcome the trapping effect of vitamin B_{12} deficiency. Unfortunately, the neurologic symptoms are largely irreversible, even with massive doses of the vitamin.

Pernicious anemia, an autoimmune disease, is the most common cause of vitamin B_{12} deficiency. The formation of antibodies against parietal cells in the stomach inhibits the synthesis of a glycoprotein, called intrinsic factor. Normally intrinsic factor binds to ingested vitamin B_{12} in the stomach, and the complex travels to the small intestine. There it is dissociated by the releasing (R) factor. In the ileum the intrinsic factor–vitamin B_{12} complex is recognized by specific receptors. The vitamin is absorbed, bound to transcolbamin, and transported into the general circulation to be used by the cells or stored in the liver. Due to abundant liver stores of the vitamin, it takes years after a precipitating event before an anemia is manifested.

Individuals who have had a partial or total gastrectomy also lack intrinsic factor and will develop pernicious anemia unless treated. In the absence of intrinsic factor, vitamin B_{12} must be furnished by injection.

Vitamin B_{12} is a cobalt, not a molybdenum-containing molecule.

32. The answer is A. *(Pathology)*
The spleen exhibits multiple areas of roughly wedge-shaped pale infarctions most likely associated with systemic embolization from the left side of the heart. A patient with long-standing mitral stenosis would be expected to have left atrial dilatation and the potential for forming clots in the left atrium. Atrial fibrillation commonly occurs in this setting, which further increases the risk for systemic embolization by acting like a vibrator to break off pieces of clot material. Organs with a solid consistency most commonly develop pale infarcts.

A patient with stage IV Hodgkin disease is very likely to have spleen involvement, but the metastatic nodules would be either large, bulky masses or millet-seed–sized foci unlike the pale, wedge-shaped appearance of this spleen.

A patient with carcinoid heart disease should have right-sided heart lesions, mainly tricuspid insufficiency and pulmonic stenosis from the fibrogenic effect of serotonin. This condition would not be expected to produce systemic embolization.

A patient with an atrial septal defect uncommonly will suffer paradoxic embolization after the shunt reversed itself from an initial left-to-right flow to a right-to-left flow after development of pulmonary hypertension.

A patient's primary cancer in the lung or breast could potentially metastasize to the spleen, but this organ is a very infrequent site of metastasis. In addition, metastatic foci do not have the wedge-shaped appearance noted in this spleen.

33. The answer is D. *(Microbiology)*
Giardia lamblia infection is associated with non-bloody, foul-smelling diarrhea accompanied by nausea, anorexia, flatulence, and abdominal cramps for weeks or months. Patients typically are afebrile. The organism is found worldwide; approximately 5% of stool specimens tested in the United States contain the organism. Hikers who drink untreated water are frequently infected.

The clinical diagnosis is confirmed by finding trophozoites or cysts in stools. The trophozoite is pear-shaped with two nuclei, four pairs of flagella and a suction disc. The oval cyst is thick-walled with four nuclei. If the results of a microscopic examination are negative, the string test (Enterotest) is performed. A weighted piece of string is swallowed until it reaches the duodenum. The trophozoites (as well as *Cryptosporidium* and *Strongyloides*) adhere to the string and are visualized after string withdrawal. *Giardia* is treated with metronidazole (Flagyl).

34. The answer is D. *(Pathology)*
The patient most likely has chronic granulomatous disease of childhood, which is a sex-linked recessive disease characterized by absence of NADPH oxidase. In the destruction of bacteria, neutrophils and monocytes are armed with both oxygen-dependent and independent mechanisms for killing bacteria. The oxygen-dependent mechanisms include 1) the myeloperoxidase (MPO) system and 2) a system that involves the generation of oxygen-derived free radicals. Oxygen-independent systems use free radicals, pH changes in the phagolysosomes, and lysosomal enzymes to destroy pathogens. Overall, the MPO system is the most potent of all the bactericidal mechanisms. After phagocytosis has occurred, NADPH oxidase, located in the leukocyte cell membrane, converts molecular oxygen from the surrounding tissue into singlet oxygen, which is a free radical that generates the energy referred to as the respiratory burst. This event can be measured in the clinical laboratory (see below). The NADPH for the reaction is derived from the pentose phosphate shunt. Singlet oxygen is converted into hydrogen peroxide by superoxide dismutase. In the presence of MPO, a lysosomal enzyme present within the phagolysosome, peroxide plus chloride ions are converted into HOCl (bleach), which ultimately destroys the bacteria. The excess peroxide is either neutralized by catalase derived from peroxisomes (microbodies) in the cell or by glutathione in the pentose phosphate shunt.

The respiratory burst mechanism is evaluated with the nitroblue tetrazolium (NBT) dye test or the chemoluminescence assay. NBT is a colorless dye that is phagocytized and reduced to a visible blue compound only by neutrophils that possess a functioning respiratory burst mechanism. In the chemoluminescence assay, a beta scintillator detects the energy released in the production of singlet oxygen.

Because chronic granulomatous disease is characterized by the absence of NADPH oxidase, the respiratory burst mechanism is eliminated and peroxide is unavailable for the reaction with chloride ions to generate

HOCI. Patients who have the disease are unable to use the oxygen-dependent MPO system unless the bacterial pathogen supplies the peroxide during its own metabolism. Both the NBT and the chemoluminescence assays are negative, indicating absence of the respiratory burst. Because *S. aureus* is catalase positive, endogenously derived peroxide generated during its metabolism is quickly destroyed by its own catalase, thus evading destruction within the phagolysosome. Streptococci, however, are catalase negative; therefore, when they generate peroxide, the missing ingredient is now available to form HOCI, and the organisms are destroyed.

A defect in microtubule polymerization describes the autosomal recessive disease called Chediak-Higashi syndrome. Because microtubules are necessary for movement and phagocytosis, they are subject to bacterial infections.

A deficiency of complement component C3 would result in severe bacterial infections because C3b is an opsonin that aids in the phagocytosis of bacteria. However, there is a normal respiratory burst.

A deficiency of MPO does not result in any significant clinical problems except in patients with diabetes where it is associated with *Candida* infections. The MPO stain is negative on neutrophils and monocytes, but the respiratory burst is intact, albeit delayed.

35. The answer is A.   *(Behavioral science)*
Erection first occurs in the excitement phase, persists in the plateau phase, and decreases after orgasm and seminal emission. In the resolution phase of the cycle, the sex organs return to their nonstimulated condition.

36. The answer is D.   *(Pathology)*
Fever right shifts the oxygen dissociation curve, which allows for a greater release of oxygen to the tissue, making oxygen easily available to neutrophils and monocytes for use in the oxygen-dependent myeloperoxidase system of bactericidal killing. Having more oxygen available to tissue also enhances wound healing. In addition, fever interferes with bacterial and viral replication by providing a hostile environment for incubation. Fever is produced by the release of interleukin-1 from macrophages. Interleukin-1, in turn, stimulates the hypothalamus to synthesize prostaglandins, which interact with the thermoregulatory center to produce fever.

37. The answer is A.   *(Microbiology)*
Penicillins and cephalosporins are called beta-lactam (β-lactam) drugs because of the importance of the intact β-lactam ring for antimicrobial activity. β-Lactamases inactivate these drugs by breaking the single bond in their β-lactam ring. β-Lactamases are coded for by either a transferable plasmid or by the genome of the organism. Plasmids are extrachromosomal genetic elements that may be transferred among unrelated bacteria.

Penicillins and cephalosporins work by inhibiting transpeptidase enzymes. These enzymes do the final cross-linking in the cell wall production process, resulting in the peptidoglycan becoming a single molecular structure. The addition of amino groups to antibiotics (i.e., ampicillin) may actually improve the range of activity against gram-negative rods, such as *Escherichia coli*. Alteration of penicillin-binding proteins (PBP) may bring about a resistance to penicillin, but such resistance is not mediated by β-lactamase breakage of bonds.

38. The answer is B.   *(Pathology)*
Wound healing of the skin occurs by primary or secondary union (intention). In primary union, the wound edges are approximated by suture, staples, or an adhesive agent. The following sequence of events occurs in this type of wound healing.

1. The wound fills up with blood clot that dries to form a protective covering, or scab.
2. Neutrophils line the edge of the wound in 24 hours and act defensively against potential pathogens.
3. Within 24 to 48 hours, a thin, continuous epithelial covering derived from basal cells of the epithelium at the edge of the wound begins to develop beneath the blood clot in contact with living tissue.
4. Macrophages emigrate into the tissue and replace the neutrophils in 3 days. Granulation tissue begins to form in the wound site.
5. Granulation tissue fills the incision defect in 5 days. Fibroblasts begin to synthesize type III collagen fibers. Epithelium regeneration is complete. Skin appendages form if enough labile cells remain behind.
6. After 7 to 10 days, when sutures are usually removed, the tensile strength of the wound is only 10% of its original strength.

7. Collagenization progresses over the ensuing weeks and months. Type III collagen is eventually lysed by collagenases, which contain zinc as a cofactor and replaced by adult type I collagen.

8. Wound collagen is constantly degraded and remodeled in sigmoidal fashion until it plateaus at a tensile strength of 75% to 80% by the end of the third month.

Sutures or staples that hold a wound together constitute additional tissue injuries that also have their own healing and repair process, as well as their own predisposition to complications (a stitch abscess).

Mature scar tissue is avascular and does not contain skin appendages.

Entrapped squamous epithelium within scar tissue can form an epidermal inclusion cyst.

39. The answer is C. (Biochemistry)

The Shine-Delgarno sequence is found near the beginning of coding regions of bacterial messenger RNA molecules. This sequence binds to a portion of the 16S ribosomal RNA in the small ribosomal subunit. Binding of the small ribosomal subunit to this region helps the ribosome determine where to initiate translation, or protein synthesis. Polycistronic messages have Shine-Delgarno sequences just upstream from each coding region.

40. The answer is A. (Pathology)

The erythrocyte sedimentation rate (ESR) is increased in inflammation. The ESR is determined by measuring the rate of settling of red blood cells (RBCs) in a vertically oriented tube over 1 hour in mm/hr. The normal reference interval is 0 to 15 mm/hr in males and 0 to 20 mm/hr in females. Both RBC and plasma factors are responsible for these changes. RBC factors that increase the ESR do so by increasing the weight of the RBC aggregates. This increase occurs when RBCs approximate each other like a stack of coins (rouleaux) or stick together in large aggregates, as in IgM-related disease. Anemia and plasma factors, such as an increase in fibrinogen and/or γ globulins, enhance rouleaux formation, thus increasing the ESR.

RBC factors that decrease the ESR are abnormally shaped cells (sickle cells) or polycythemia (too many RBCs inhibit the settling of individual cells).

A 7-year-old child with sickle cell disease would have a low ESR because the RBCs cannot form aggregates.

A 72-year-old man with temporal arteritis would have an increase in fibrinogen as an acute phase reactant and increased γ globulins from chronic inflammation, both of which predispose to rouleaux and an increased ESR.

A 23-year-old woman with iron deficiency anemia would have an increased ESR because anemia increases rouleaux formation.

A 26-year-old man with lobar pneumonia and a 4-year-old child with cystic fibrosis would both have an increased ESR for the same reasons as listed for temporal arteritis.

41. The answer is D. (Microbiology)

Antibiotics that interfere with bacterial cell wall synthesis have excellent selective toxicity because eukaryotic cells do not have cell walls. Although penicillins and cephalosporins are bactericidal, they are most effective against actively growing organisms. Quinolones inhibit bacterial DNA gyrase and rifampin inhibits bacterial RNA polymerase. Polymyxins interfere with gram-negative cell membrane structure and function. Aminoglycosides interfere with bacterial protein synthesis.

42. The answer is E. (Pathology)

Wound healing of the skin occurs by primary or secondary union (intention). In primary union, the wound edges are approximated by suture, staples, or an adhesive agent. In healing by secondary union (intention), the wound edges are not approximated. Factors that differ from primary union include 1) it takes a longer time to heal; 2) more granulation tissue is formed; 3) myofibroblasts contribute to wound contraction and help approximate the edges of the wound; 4) there is more scar tissue formation; and 5) there is greater potential for complications (infections).

43. The answer is B. (Pharmacology)

Allopurinol inhibits xanthine oxidase, which catalyzes the formation of uric acid resulting from the breakdown of purines. It is used in cancer chemotherapy patients to prevent hyperuricemia that develops from the rapid catabolism of purines following cell lysis. Xanthine oxidase is also responsible for the catabolism of 6-mercaptopurine (6-MP) to 6-thiouric acid. When allopurinol and 6-mercaptopurine are used concurrently, the 6-MP dosage must be reduced to prevent toxicity. 6-Thioguanine is metabolized initially by deamination and its serum concentration is not increased by allopurinol. Cytarabine and 5-fluorouracil are pyrimidines, which are not metabolized by xanthine oxidase.

44. The answer is B. *(Pathology)*

Inflammation is initiated by recognition that tissues have been damaged. Specific mediators are produced at the site of injury that trigger a cascade of additional mediators, which serve to amplify the inflammatory response. Some mediators are formed from proteins normally circulating in the plasma (e.g., Hageman factor XII), and others are derived from cells involved in the inflammatory response (e.g., histamine, prostaglandins). These are summarized in the table below.

The only two chemical mediators that have the same function in inflammation are complement components C3a and C5a (C4a to a lesser extent). These complement components directly induce mast cell/basophil degranulation in the inflammatory reaction, with subsequent release of preformed elements such as vasoactive amines (histamine and serotonin), proteases, and chemotactic factors for neutrophils and eosinophils. After mast cells degranulate, prostaglandins and leukotrienes are synthesized over the next 2 to 3 hours and are then released into the inflamed tissue as the late phase reaction (secondary release reaction).

Histamine is a vasoactive amine that is derived from mast cells, basophils, and platelets. It is a vasodilator and increases vessel permeability by stimulating endothelial cell contraction in the postcapillary venules. Activated Hageman factor XII interacts with the coagulation, fibrinolytic, and kinin systems, all of which represent cascade systems involving a series of reactions. Histamine activates the intrinsic clotting system to produce a fibrin clot, activates the kinin system to produce bradykinin, and activates the fibrinolytic system to produce plasmin.

C3b is primarily an opsonin. Platelet-activating factor is derived from neutrophils, macrophages, mast cells/basophils, and platelets. It is a vasodilator and platelet aggregator; it increases vessel permeability; and it is an adhering and chemotactic agent.

Activation of cellular phospholipases in the cell membranes of the cellular constituents within the inflammatory process results in the formation of arachidonic acid (synthesized from linoleic acid, an essential

Mediator	Derived	VD/VC	Vessel permeability	Adhesion/ Chemotaxis	Opsonin	Pain
Histamine	Cell	+/–	Increase	–/+ (eosinophils)	No	No
Serotonin	Cell	+/–	Increase	–/–	No	No
LTB4	Cell	–/–	No effect	+/+	No	No
LTC4-D4-E4	Cell	+(E4)/+	Increase	–/–	No	No
Prostaglandins	Cell	+/–	Increase	–/–	No	Yes (PGD2)
PAF	Cell	+/* – or +	Increase	+/+	No	No
C3a	Cell	+/–	Increase	–/–	No	No
C5a	Cell	+/–	Increase	+/+	No	No
C3b	Cell	–/–	No effect	–/–	Yes	No
C567	Cell	–/–	No effect	–/+	No	No
Bradykinin	Plasma	+/–	Increase	–/–	No	Yes

VD = vasodilator
VC = vasoconstrictor
Complement derives from cells but is activated in plasma.
* PAF = a vasodilator in low concentration and a vasoconstrictor in high concentration

fatty acid). Eventually, prostaglandins and leukotrienes are produced. Leukotriene LTB$_4$ is primarily an adhesion and chemotactic agent, whereas leukotrienes LCT$_4$, LTD$_4$, and LTE$_4$ are bronchoconstrictors and vasoconstrictors and increase vessel permeability (operative in the inflammation induced bronchoconstriction of bronchial asthma). Bradykinin derives from the kinin system, which is activated by factor XII. Bradykinin produces pain, is a potent vasodilator, and increases vessel permeability.

Plasmin is an enzyme derived from plasminogen and is important in lysing fibrin; producing some of the complement components (e.g., C3b from C3); and generating fibrin split products, which may increase vessel permeability.

45. The answer is D. *(Microbiology)*
Polyenes (amphotericin B, nystatin) have seven unsaturated double bonds in their macrolide ring structure and a strong affinity for ergosterol, a component of fungal cell membranes not found in bacterial or human cell membranes. This affinity and attachment cause disruption of the fungal membranes, allowing loss of normal function. Polymyxins are cyclic polypeptide antibiotics that are active against gram-negative rods. The positive charged free amino acids act like a cationic detergent to disrupt the phospholipid structure of the cell membrane. Osmotic control is lost, allowing leakage of cytoplasmic contents from the cells.

These compounds and groups of microorganisms do not cross react because of the differences in membrane receptor components for the antimicrobials. Selective toxicity is difficult because of the overall similarities in the cell membranes of humans and microorganisms.

46. The answer is C. *(Pathology)*
The cellular response in acute inflammation consists of the movement of white blood cells out of the blood vessel (i.e., margination, pavementing, and emigration) and into the interstitial tissue followed by chemotaxis to the area of inflammation, and then the phagocytosis and destruction of the offending agent.

Increased vessel permeability due to vasoactive amines, histamine and serotonin, initially slows the flow of blood, which increases the clumping of red blood cells and pushes the leukocytes to the periphery (margination). Leukocyte adhesion by neutrophils and monocytes to the endothelial cells involves interactions between the adhesion molecules on their cell membranes with the corresponding receptors on the endothelial cells. The adhesion molecules on the leukocytes are called integrins (e.g., CD11/CD18 glycoproteins). An intracellular adhesion molecule is intercellular adhesion molecule-1 (ICAM-1). Adhesion molecules on endothelial cells include lectins such as endothelial cell adherence molecule-1 (ELAM-1). Chemical mediators selectively stimulate the synthesis of adhesion molecules on the leukocytes (e.g., C5a and the leukotriene, LTB$_4$), on the vessel endothelium (e.g., interleukin-1 and endotoxin), or on both of the cells (e.g., tumor necrosis factor). Because the neutrophils are lined up along the endothelial surface, the term pavementing is frequently used to describe this event.

Leukocyte emigration of both neutrophils and monocytes into the interstitial space involves their release of collagenase to focally dissolve the basement membrane (type IV collagen) between the endothelial cells, enabling the red blood cells to follow passively (diapedesis) through the defect into the interstitial space. Lymphocytes, basophils, and eosinophils also egress through the defect.

Leukocyte chemotaxis to the area of infection is either a random or a directed response (receptor mediated). Directed chemotaxis represents a purposeful movement of leukocytes along a chemical gradient of chemotactic agents (e.g., bacterial products, C5a, C567, LTB4, and interleukin-1) toward the area of infection. Leukocytes possess microtubules and contractile microfilaments (actin and myosin) that enable them to move through the tissue.

Phagocytosis is the engulfment of microorganisms, foreign particles, and cellular debris by leukocytes. It is an important defense mechanism, particularly in bacterial infections. Phagocytosis consists of four stages: 1) attachment of opsonins such as IgG and C3b to the microorganism or foreign material, 2) attachment of the microorganism or foreign material to the leukocyte, 3) ingestion by the leukocyte, and 4) degradation of the microorganism or foreign material within the phagocytic cell. The phagocytosis of bacteria or foreign materials by neutrophils and/or monocytes is enhanced when the organisms are covered by

IgG immunoglobulins and/or the complement component C3b, a process called opsonization. Fibrinogen, fibronectin, and C-reactive protein aid in localizing bacteria and foreign particles, thus serving as nonspecific opsonizing agents. Neutrophils and monocytes possess membrane receptors for the opsonizing agents, IgG and C3b, thus causing the bacteria or foreign particles to attach to the cell membranes. Bacteria or foreign particles are then engulfed by pseudopodia and drawn into the phagocytic cell. Once internalized the particles are trapped within phagocytic vacuoles (phagosomes) in the cytoplasm. These phagosomes fuse with lysosomes containing proteases, hydrolases, and myeloperoxidase to form phagolysosomes.

Phagolysosomes are visible within neutrophils and monocytes on Wright-Giemsa–stained peripheral smears and provide direct evidence that phagocytosis has occurred. Foreign particles are frequently not capable of being degraded and persist in the injury site, thus serving as a stimulus for chronic inflammation. Regarding the destruction of bacteria, neutrophils and monocytes are armed with both oxygen-dependent and independent mechanisms for killing bacteria. The oxygen-dependent mechanisms include the myeloperoxidase (MPO) system and a system that involves the generation of oxygen-derived free radicals. Oxygen-independent systems use free radicals, pH changes in the phagolysosomes, and lysosomal enzymes to destroy pathogens.

Overall, the MPO system is the most potent of all the bactericidal mechanisms. After phagocytosis has occurred, NADPH oxidase, located in the leukocyte cell membrane, converts molecular oxygen from the surrounding tissue into singlet oxygen, which is a free radical that generates the energy referred to as the respiratory burst. Singlet oxygen is converted into hydrogen peroxide by superoxide dismutase. In the presence of MPO, a lysosomal enzyme present within the phagolysosome, peroxide plus chloride ions are converted into HOCl (bleach), which ultimately destroys the bacteria. The excess peroxide is either neutralized by catalase derived from peroxisomes (microbodies) in the cell or by glutathione in the hexose monophosphate shunt.

47. The answer is A.   *(Behavioral science)*
In a normal distribution, 0.15% of the population will always fall above 3 standard deviations of the mean.

48. The answer is A.   *(Pathology)*
Ultraviolet light is beneficial to wound healing. Factors that interfere with proper wound healing are:

- Infection (most common)
- Vitamin C deficiency (abnormal collagen, because the hydroxylation of proline and lysine residues is deficient)
- Foreign body (infection)
- Malnutrition (insufficient nutrients)
- Tissue hypoxia
- Decreased monocytes (no macrophage-derived growth factor or removal of debris)
- Absolute neutropenia (removes debris, protects against infection)
- Corticosteroids (impairs collagen synthesis)
- Marfan syndrome (fibrillin defect in elastin)
- Ehler-Danlos syndrome (abnormal collagen due to enzyme deficiencies)
- Severe anemia (< 5 g/dl produces significant tissue hypoxia)
- Copper deficiency (cofactor for lysyl oxidase)
- Zinc deficiency (cofactor enzymes in collagen degradation)
- Diabetes mellitus (infection, ischemia, decreased chemotaxis)
- Fibrinogen deficiency (decreased fibrin)
- Radiation injury (decreases healing by decreasing both blood vessels and cell proliferation)

49. The answer is C.   *(Microbiology)*
The appearance of a unilateral, painful vesicular rash after accidental trauma strongly suggests a diagnosis of zoster (shingles) due to reactivation of the varicella-zoster virus (VZV). The maculopapular skin lesions are virtually indistinguishable from those of chickenpox after primary VZV infection. VZV is a single virus, but the manifestations of disease are different after a primary infection versus reactivation.

All of the herpesviruses are thought to become latent after initial infection. Viral persistence is believed to last for the lifetime of the individual.

Herpesvirus	Site of Latency
Herpes simplex virus type 1	Trigeminal ganglion
Herpes simplex virus type 2	Dorsal root ganglion
Varicella-zoster virus (VZV)	Dorsal root ganglion
Cytomegalovirus	Salivary glands and kidney
Epstein-Barr virus	B lymphocytes
Human herpes 6	T lymphocytes
Human herpes 7	T lymphocytes

During latency the virus does not replicate, there are no symptoms, and the individual is noninfectious. However, virus shedding can occur in asymptomatic persons.

Reactivation of herpesviruses is associated with trauma (accidental or surgical), ultraviolet radiation (sunburn), hypothermia, immunosuppressive drugs, and emotional stress. Recurrent disease can occur in spite of preexisting antibodies and cell-mediated immunity. Immunosuppression and advancing age increase the risk for reactivation.

Zoster means belt. Approximately 50% of cases occur in the "belt" region.

The most common complication of zoster is postherpetic neuralgia (persistence of pain for months or years in the area of the rash), especially in persons over the age of 65.

50. The answer is E. *(Pathology)*

Proteins in body fluids are easily separated by electrophoresis. Protein separation is facilitated by the effect of an alkaline pH on altering charges of the different protein fractions. Those protein fractions with the most negative charges (albumin) migrate to the positive pole (anode; A+ is a good grade), whereas those with positive charges (γ globulins) remain at the negatively charged pole (cathode; C- is a bad grade). Beginning from the anode, the proteins separate into 5 major peaks: albumin, α_1 globulins, α_2 globulins, β globulins, and γ globulins. The order of decreasing concentration of the major γ globulins is IgG > IgA > IgM.

Immunoglobulins in the γ globulin region are normally increased as part of the humoral response in the inflammatory process or as a primary disorder of plasma cells (e.g., multiple myeloma). In acute inflammation, IgM is the initial antibody response, which eventually switches over to an IgG antibody response.

When many different clones of plasma cells are synthesizing IgG, the entire γ globulin peak on a serum protein electrophoresis is diffusely elevated, thus producing a polyclonal gammopathy. A polyclonal gammopathy is seen only in chronic inflammation, because IgG antibody synthesis from persistent antigen stimulation produces markedly increased concentrations of IgG (choices D and E). In choice D, there would also be an absence of the α_1 peak, representing α_1 antitrypsin deficiency.

In acute inflammation, the IgM antibodies are not present in high enough concentration to greatly influence the size of the γ globulin peak (choice B). The absence of a polyclonal peak is the key distinguishing factor that separates acute from chronic inflammation on a serum protein electrophoresis. The absence of γ globulins (choice C) results in a flat line in the γ globulin region.

Monoclonal gammopathies are caused by a single clone of plasma cells that produce abnormally high levels in the blood/urine of a homogeneous, intact immunoglobulin, and/or its corresponding light chain (Bence Jones protein) or heavy chain constituent. Instead of a large, diffuse peak, there is a sharp spike (A), or M protein. Most monoclonal gammopathies are of indeterminate significance.

51. The answer is A. *(Biochemistry)*

Precursors of proteins that are to be secreted from the cell or become incorporated into the plasma membrane frequently contain a stretch of hydrophobic amino acids near their amino terminus. Ribosomes synthesizing such proteins are brought to the endoplasmic reticulum (ER), where protein synthesis is completed. The proteins are translocated across the ER as they are synthesized. The signal sequence is cleaved from the protein in the lumen of the ER by the signal peptidase, and therefore is not usually found in the mature final product. The earliest precursors of collagen, a protein that functions outside the cell, have such a signal sequence.

52. The answer is B. *(Microbiology)*

Acyclovir (acycloguanosine) is the most effective drug for herpes encephalitis. It is remarkably nontoxic and can be given intravenously. Treatment is most effective when given early in the disease (before coma).

Acyclovir is also beneficial in oral and genital herpes simplex infections in adults. The severity of symptoms, the length of time that the symptoms are present, and virus shedding are reduced. However, treatment does not prevent latency. The drug is also used for treatment of severe infections with varicella-zoster virus (chickenpox/shingles). It has little or no effect on most other DNA viruses. Oral, topical, and intravenous preparations are available.

Acyclovir is an acyclic analog of guanosine. It is partly phosphorylated by the herpes simplex thymidine kinase enzyme. Phosphorylation is then completed by cell enzymes, and a viral DNA polymerase adds the triphosphorylated analog to the growing viral DNA chain. This action stops the further addition of other nucleosides (i.e., acyclovir is a DNA chain terminator).

Mutations in the thymidine kinase enzyme are often seen in herpesviruses that are resistant to acyclovir. Resistance can also emerge as the result of mutations in the viral DNA polymerase.

Ganciclovir, a methyl guanine derivative related to acyclovir, is approved for cytomegalovirus (CMV) infections. It is frequently used in immunocompromised individuals and organ transplant (especially bone marrow) recipients, either prophylactically or in life-threatening cases of CMV disease.

Foscarnet (phosphonoformic acid) inhibits herpes simplex virus replication; however, resistant mutants emerge easily. Foscarnet also is of some benefit in CMV retinitis in AIDS and in hepatitis B viral infections. Foscarnet accumulates in bone when given systemically.

Idoxuridine (5-iodo-2′ deoxyuridine) is used mostly for topical application in the treatment of corneal lesions due to herpes simplex virus. It is incorporated into newly synthesized viral, as well as host cell, DNA. It is relatively toxic, and drug-resistant mutants can emerge readily. Trifluridine (5-trifluoro-methyl-2′-deoxyuridine) is available for topical treatment of herpes keratitis due to strains of herpes simplex that are resistant to idoxuridine.

Vidarabine (adenine arabinoside, ara-A) is approved for herpes simplex infections, but is more toxic and more difficult to administer than acyclovir. It has been largely replaced by acyclovir, especially for systemic therapy.

53. The answer is B.   *(Behavioral science)*
In the United States, suicide rates are greater in urban than in rural areas. Suicides rates are also highest in the northeastern states and lower in the western mountain and southern states. When compared to European Americans, suicides rates are lower in African Americans and higher in native Americans. Suicide rates are higher in people over age 45 than in people under age 45.

54. The answer is E.   *(Microbiology)*
Rabies is one of the few infectious diseases for which the administration of a vaccine after infection is an effective means of preventing the disease. The postinfection prophylaxis is effective because the incubation period is long enough that an antibody response can be induced. Although the "street" (wild type) virus has a highly variable incubation period, it is generally 2 to 16 weeks. However, the incubation period depends on the strain of the virus, size of the inoculum, and the length of the neural path from the wound to the brain. Cleansing the wound with soap and water disrupts the lipid envelope of the virus and prolongs the incubation time.

All rabies vaccines that are used today in humans are inactivated.

Postexposure immunization with human diploid cell vaccine [HDCV; or adsorbed rabies vaccine (RVA)] is performed as early as possible in persons suspected of having been infected with the rabies virus. Early immunization increases the likelihood that neutralizing anti-rabies antibody will be induced before symptoms appear. The recommended regimen is five total injections over the course of 28 days.

HDCV and the newer RVA are the vaccines of choice. They are now used almost exclusively in the United States and other developed countries. In the preparation of these vaccines, the virus is adapted for growth either in a normal (diploid chromosome number) human fibroblast cell line (HDCV) or in normal fetal rhesus monkey lung cells (RVA). No serious encephalitic or neuroparalytic reactions have been reported with these vaccines (as there are when the virus is harvested from nervous tissues).

Local reactions are common, and a substantial proportion of immunized individuals develop mild systemic symptoms (e.g., headache, nausea, myalgia, dizziness) after HDCV or RVA.

55. The answer is B. *(Biochemistry)*
The ribosome has two binding sites called the "P" (peptidyl) site and the "A" (aminoacyl) site. The P site is the binding site for the transfer RNA (tRNA) molecule covalently linked to the growing polypeptide chain. The A site is the binding site for the tRNA molecule carrying the amino acid specified by the next codon in the messenger RNA. The polypeptide chain grows as the new amino acid is attached to the carboxyl end of the growing polypeptide chain.

56. The answer is A. *(Microbiology)*
The hallmark of subacute sclerosing panencephalitis (SSPE) is an intense infiltration of lymphocytes and plasmacytes into the brain. Some of the cells are cytotoxic T lymphocytes, whereas the activated B cells (plasmacytes) are secreting antibodies against a variant form of the classic measles virus (rubeola). Diagnosis is often based on the presence of a high titer of anti-measles antibody in cerebrospinal fluid.

Rubeola is an enveloped single-stranded RNA virus that belongs to the family Paramyxoviridae. The variant virus of SSPE often exhibits mutations in the M protein, which is critical in viral assembly before budding. It also has increased genetic material of unknown origin; however, it is suspected that it may come from an as yet unidentified animal virus.

SSPE is an encephalitis that occurs primarily in children (peak incidence is at 7 years of age) and young adults. It involves the whole brain (white matter, gray matter, and brain stem), hence the term panencephalitis. It is characterized by insidious onset of intellectual decline, followed by sudden onset of seizures, muscle jerks, visual impairment, and severe intellectual deterioration. Death often results from infection months or years after onset of symptoms. The incidence of SSPE in the United States has declined dramatically since the advent of the measles vaccine.

Creutzfeldt-Jakob disease and kuru are spongiform encephalopathies associated with prions. There is no infiltration of cells of the immune system into the brain in either of these diseases.

Progressive multifocal leukoencephalopathy is a subacute demyelinating disease of the central nervous system. The classic lesions are discrete areas of demyelination due to destruction of oligodendroglia. The Creutzfeldt-Jakob virus (a polyoma virus in the family Papovaviridae) is the etiologic agent.

The agents associated with SSPE, Creutzfeldt-Jakob disease, kuru, and progressive multifocal leukoencephalopathy are persistent and have a very long incubation time (usually measured in years); therefore, they are referred to as "slow viruses" or "prions."

Whitlow's is a primary infection of the digits with herpes simpex virus type 1 or type 2. It occurs in seronegative individuals who come into direct contact with the virus.

57. The answer is C. *(Behavioral science)*
Because both marriage and female sex are associated with a decreased risk for suicide, a divorced 52-year-old man is more likely to commit suicide than a married man or a divorced or single woman of the same age.

58. The answer is D. *(Microbiology)*
The term "prion" is derived from proteinaceous infectious particles. Prions consist of amyloidlike protein that appears to multiply. They are considered to be infectious in that disease can be transmitted from sick to healthy individuals by these particles.

Creutzfeldt-Jakob disease (found worldwide) and kuru (found only among the Fore tribe of New Guinea) are invariably fatal spongiform encephalopathies associated with prions. The disease can be experimentally transmitted to animals (monkeys, rodents) with extracts of brain tissue from patients. Spongiform encephalopathies are characterized by a diffuse loss of neurons, intense astrocyte proliferation, amyloid plaques, and intracytoplasmic vacuolation (brain looks like a sponge).

The prototype disease is scrapie of sheep. Scrapie is a slow degenerative disease of the central nervous system. It also causes intense itching of the skin (sheep scrape against trees and fences). The PrP (prion protein, 27–30,000 MW) from a diseased animal induces disease in healthy animals.

No DNA or RNA has been detected in association with prions. They are not defective viruses, pseudovirions, viroids, or mutated forms of conventional viruses.

Atypical Viruslike Agents

Agent	Composition	Comments
Prions	Protein	Infectious protein, indistinguishable from amyloid, no nucleic acid; resistant to inactivation with common antiviral agents; rod-shaped. Found in humans.
Defective virus	Mutation or deletion in nucleic acid	Viral nucleic acid + proteins, but cannot replicate without a "helper" virus. Formed during growth of most viruses. Found in humans.
Pseudovirions	Viral capsid + cell DNA	Formed during infection with certain types of viruses; fragments of host cell DNA are incorporated into viral capsid protein; can infect cells, but cannot replicate. Found in humans.
Viroids	Single-stranded RNA	One molecule of circular RNA; no protein or envelope; RNA does not code for any protein; replicate by unknown mechanism. Cause of severe diseases in plants. Never found in animals or humans.

Prions are unusually resistant to agents that often inactivate conventional viruses (e.g., formaldehyde, β-propiolactone, proteases, nucleases, heat, ionizing radiation), but are susceptible to phenol, household bleach, ether, acetone, strong detergents, iodine, disinfectants, and autoclaving.

59. The answer is E. (Biochemistry)
The insertion of a single base causes the ribosome to become misaligned on the messenger RNA molecule. Its reading frame then is shifted, so it is not reading the proper codons. The amino acid sequence of a protein is completely garbled after the position of the frameshift mutation.

The substitution of adenine for guanine is a transition, because one purine is substituted for the other purine. The substitution of thymine for adenine is a transversion, because a pyrimidine is substituted for a purine. Transitions and transversions are point mutations that can cause silent, missense, and nonsense mutations, but not frameshift mutations.

60. The answer is B. (Microbiology)
Creutzfeldt-Jakob disease (previously known as subacute presenile dementia) has been transmitted on invasive nonautoclaved medical instruments (e.g., electroencephalogram electrodes). Accidental transmission has also occurred with contaminated growth hormone prepared from human pituitary glands, interferon extracted from leukocytes, corneal transplants, and cadaveric dura mater grafts used for head injury repair. Prions very similar to scrapie PrP (prion protein) have been isolated from the brains of patients with Creutzfeldt-Jakob disease.

Lymphocytic choriomeningitis, which is caused by an arenavirus, is transmitted to humans via urine and feces of infected mice, especially the gray house mouse. The disease is manifested as an acute aseptic meningitis or as a mild influenza-like illness. Transmission of the Creutzfeldt-Jakob virus (a polyoma virus in the Papovaviridae family) probably occurs via inhalation of aerosols. The virus is very small and contains double-stranded cyclic DNA in a supercoiled configuration. The virus is an extremely common one that is found worldwide in humans. Approximately 70% to 80% of people in the United States are seropositive by the age of 15 years. The great majority of infections are asymptomatic; however, after entry and viremia, the virus stays latent in the kidney. Patients with severely depressed cell-mediated immunity (e.g., chronic leukemia, Hodgkin disease, and lymphosarcoma) may develop progressive multifocal leukoencephalopathy (demyelination of the central nervous system due to infection of oligodendroglial cells). It is estimated that 2% to 4% of AIDS patients have progressive multifocal leukoencephalopathy.

Cannibalism, as well as direct contact with contaminated tissues, are believed to be the routes of transmission of kuru, a prion-associated disease. Kuru was prevalent among the Fore tribe of New Guinea before ritualistic cannibalism was outlawed by the government of that country. Kuru is characterized by cerebellar ataxia, tremors, dysarthria, and emotional instability. Kuru means "shivering" in the language of the Fore tribe.

Many viruses can be transmitted by arthropods such as mosquitos, ticks, and sandflies. Viruses transmitted by arthropods are collectively known as arboviruses.

61. The answer is C.   (Pharmacology)
6-Mercaptopurine is the thiol analog of hypoxanthine. It must be converted to the nucleotide form (6-mercaptopurine ribose phosphate) through a process catalyzed by HGPRTase before it can inhibit purine biosynthesis in cancer cells. Neoplastic cells become resistant to mercaptopurine by deleting this enzyme. HGPRTase is not involved in the activation of pyrimidine analogs (cytarabine, fluorouracil) or other anticancer drugs.

62. The answer is D.   (Microbiology)
The expression of at least one viral gene is necessary for a virus to transform a cell. The gene may encode a protein that promotes cell division, inactivates a tumor suppressor protein, or acts as a growth factor or growth factor receptor. A protein product of a transforming virus gene may also act indirectly by activating certain cellular genes whose products, in turn, enhance proliferation.

Viral transformation does not always result in malignant cell growth. For example, epithelial cells immortalized by a human papillomavirus will not produce a tumor when injected into a nude mouse. This indicates that the virus alone is not carcinogenic and that additional factors are needed. The development of cancerous cells is a multistep process that often occurs over a period of years and includes a number of genetic changes.

RNA tumor viruses can both replicate in (with the continuous production of progeny) and transform their natural host cells. In contrast, DNA tumor viruses often replicate well in their natural host cells, but almost never (see question 64) transform the cell.

Heterologous cells transformed by a DNA tumor virus never produce progeny.

Virally transformed cells exhibit a wide spectrum of aberrant characteristics, including 1) morphologic changes (some appear to have reverted to a more immature developmental stage); 2) failure to grow in an organized manner (they do not align themselves like normal cells do); 3) loss of contact inhibition (they fail to stop dividing when they come into contact with other cells; they pile up on each other and form thick foci of growth); 4) decrease in nutritional and growth factor requirements; 5) loss of anchorage dependence (they acquire the ability to divide in suspension); 6) ability to divide indefinitely. Similar changes also can be seen in spontaneously transformed cells in which there is no virus involved.

Cells transformed by viruses tend to be more immunogenic than those that are not associated with a virus. Viral antigens can often be identified on virally transformed cells with monoclonal or polyclonal antisera made in a heterologous species.

Cell transformation is defined as a stable, inheritable change in the growth control properties of the cell. The permanently acquired characteristics are not exhibited by the normal parental cell type.

63. The answer is A.   (Behavioral science)
The Babinski reflex, like the rooting, grasp, and Moro or startle reflexes, is normally seen in the newborn infant.

64. The answer is A.   (Microbiology)
The expression of one or more early genes is essential for a DNA tumor virus to induce cell transformation. The early genes are those that are expressed before replication of the viral DNA. In some oncogenic DNA viruses (e.g., SV40), the protein products of the early genes are referred to as T antigens (tumor antigens).

The specific mechanisms by which DNA tumor viruses contribute to tumorigenesis are largely unknown. However, several significant observations have been made. An early gene product of the virus can bind to 1) chromosomes and initiate cellular DNA synthesis (e.g., large T antigen of SV40); 2) protooncogene proteins and stimulate their activity (e.g., middle T antigen of polyoma binds to pp60 and pp62, which are *c-src* and *c-yes* gene products, respectively); 3) tumor suppressor proteins and inactive them (e.g., E6 of papillomavirus and E1B of adenovirus bind to p53).

Most cells that are transformed by DNA tumor viruses have only one or few viral genes incorporated into their DNA (the entire viral genome cannot be recovered). However, transforming genes can also be found as extrachromosomal plasmids (e.g., some papillomaviruses and some herpesviruses). DNA tumor viruses (unlike retroviruses) do not code for an enzyme (e.g., reverse transcriptase) needed for integration into cell chromosomes. Portions of the viral DNA integrate by nonhomologous genetic recombination using cellular enzymes. The integration event is nonspecific with respect to the site of integration.

The oncogenes of DNA tumor viruses are viral genes and bear little or no homology with the protooncogenes that are found within cells. This is in direct contrast to the oncogenes of RNA tumor viruses (retroviruses), whose oncogenes are thought to be derived from cellular protooncogenes. Thus, the oncogenes of DNA and RNA tumor viruses are very different from each other.

Oncogenic DNA viruses are associated with many animal tumors and several human cancers, including African Burkitt lymphoma (Epstein-Barr virus), nasopharyngeal carcinoma (Epstein-Barr virus), cervical carcinoma (human papillomavirus), and primary hepatocellular carcinoma (hepatitis B virus).

p53 is a tumor suppressor gene ("anti-oncogene") that is present in cells. The p53 protein blocks cell cycle progression. Mutation or inactivation of both alleles can result in tumor formation. More than 50% of all human tumors are functionally defective in p53. The prototype tumor suppressor gene is Rb. It is defective in retinoblastoma (a rare ocular tumor of children), as well as in several other tumor types.

65. The answer is D.   *(Behavioral science)*
Although 20% to 50% of diabetic men eventually have erectile dysfunction, ejaculation often is normal. Although psychological problems may be present, the major cause of sexual problems in diabetic men involves vascular and neurologic changes caused by the disease. The erectile dysfunction associated with poor metabolic control of diabetes can be treated surgically by using penile implants.

66. The answer is A.   *(Behavioral science)*
Children younger than 5 to 6 years of age do not fully understand the meaning of death and may expect the return of a dead relative or pet.

67-69. The answers are: 67-C, 68-E, 69-B.   *(Behavioral science)*
The incidence rate is determined by dividing the number of people who develop an illness in a time period by the total number of people at risk for the illness during that time period. If 300 new cases of lung cancer were identified during the year within a 1,000,000 population base, the incidence rate is 300/1,000,000 or 30/100,000.

The crude mortality rate is determined by dividing the total number of deaths from all causes during the year by the population at midyear and multiplying that number by 1000. If 1200 deaths occurred in a population base of 1,000,000, the crude mortality rate is 1200/1,000,000 or 120/100,000.

The cause-specific mortality rate is determined by dividing the number of deaths related to a given illness by the population at risk for that illness. If 60 people died of lung cancer in a population base of 1,000,000, the cause-specific mortality rate for lung cancer is 60/1,000,000 or 6/100,000.

70. The answer is C.   *(Behavioral science)*
Competitive, driving (type A) individuals are at increased risk for developing coronary artery disease. Pruritus has been associated with repressed anger and anxiety, whereas bronchial asthma has been associated with excessive dependency. Obesity has been associated with oral fixation as well as regression. Psychological factors have not been linked to the development of prostate cancer.

71. The answer is C.   *(Biochemistry)*
An example of a paracrine cell is the mast cell, the product of which affects nearby endothelial cells, resulting in increased vascular permeability and smooth muscle constriction. Mast cells also secrete an eosinophil chemotactic factor, attracting eosinophils to the site of release.

Exocrine cells secrete into a duct system. Endocrine cells secrete into the blood and the product then travels to target organs. Neurocrine cells release a chemical messenger at the terminus of a cytoplasmic extension that affects a target cell. The second messenger is the intracellular messenger that initiates a series of changes through the stimulation of protein kinases.

72. The answer is C. *(Pharmacology)*

Inhibition of cell wall synthesis is one of five mechanisms of action of antimicrobials. These cell wall–acting agents are bactericidal, but they work best against an actively growing organism. Penicillins and cephalosporins interfere with the transpeptidation step at the end of the peptidoglycan layer production. Bacitracin interferes with normal function of the phospholipid carrier molecule in the cytoplasmic membrane; vancomycin prevents the nascent building block unit (N-acetylmuramic acid-N-acetylglucosamine-pentapeptide) from being incorporated into the growing peptidoglycan backbone. Other antibiotics also inhibit protein synthesis, nucleic acid synthesis, membrane function, and metabolic analogs. Erythromycin, chloramphenicol, and clindamycin block protein synthesis in bacteria by affecting the 50S component of the ribosome. Nalidixic acid (and quinolone derivatives) inhibits the bacterial DNA gyrase enzyme. Although penicillin and vancomycin inhibit cell wall synthesis, their pairing with nalidixic acid and polymyxins, respectively, renders combinations that are incorrect answers for the question.

73. The answer is A. *(Biochemistry)*

Cholesterol is an important constituent of cell membranes and a precursor of steroid hormones and the bile acids and salts. Although a sufficient amount is essential for each cell, too much cholesterol contributes to atherosclerotic plaque formation and the problems associated with their development. A feedback mechanism helps to regulate cholesterol production. Preformed cholesterol inhibits the rate-limiting, committed step in cholesterol synthesis, 3-hydroxy-3 methylglutaryl CoA (HMG-CoA) reductase. Unfortunately, too much cholesterol in the diet, or too many calories, particularly as fat, still leads to excess plasma cholesterol. One reason for this excess is simply that intake is more than is required. Another reason is the feedback mechanism itself is inadequate. Important factors contributing to the elevating effect that high-fat diets have on serum levels include a change in the distribution of cholesterol in the body, less cholesterol in membranes and consequently more in the serum, and the fact that high-fat diets are almost invariably diets rich in cholesterol.

Normally, the absorption of ingested cholesterol is efficient. The body does not distinguish between ingested cholesterol and cholesterol synthesized de novo; both are esterified equally well. The bile acid cholic acid is not to be confused with choline.

74. The answer is A. *(Pharmacology)*

High levels of serotonin are believed to delay orgasm and ejaculation. Fluoxetine increases the availability of serotonin at the synapse. Opioid antagonists, α-adrenergic antagonists, nitroglycerine ointment applied to the penis, and intracorporeal administration of vasoactive drugs enhance erectile function and are used to treat erectile dysfunction.

75–77. The answers are: 75-B, 76-A, 77-E. *(Behavioral science)*

In a case-control (retrospective) study, cases (patients with bronchitis) and control subjects (individuals who do not have bronchitis) are identified, and information regarding prior exposure to the risk factor (a history of bronchitis in parents) is obtained and compared using odds ratios. In a cohort study, specific populations (cohorts) that are free of illness are identified and their status is assessed prospectively. In a clinical trial, a cohort receiving one treatment is compared to a cohort receiving a different treatment or placebo. In a cross-sectional study, the health status of a group of individuals is examined at one specific point in time.

The odds ratio is an estimate of relative risk when incidence data are not available, such as in a case-control study.

	Parents had bronchitis	Parents did not have bronchitis
Child with bronchitis	30 (A)	20 (B)
Child without bronchitis	20 (C)	30 (D)

In this study, the odds ratio is calculated by using the formula $A \times D \div B \times C$, in which A represents children with bronchitis exposed to the risk factor (parents had bronchitis in childhood) (n=30), D represents the children without bronchitis whose parents did not have bronchitis in childhood (n=30), B represents the children with bronchitis whose parents did not have bronchitis in childhood (n=20), and C represents the children without bronchitis whose parents had bronchitis in childhood (n=20), yielding 30 × 30÷20 × 20.

Relative risk can only be calculated for cohort studies.

78. The answer is B. *(Anatomy)*
Centrioles are cylindric structures composed of a "pinwheel" of nine triplets of microtubules that are so close together that they share a wall. Centrioles usually are found in pairs, oriented at right angles to one another. These structures and the immediate cytoplasmic area are organizing centers for the microtubules of the mitotic spindle.

To the right of the centriole are the dense granules of glycogen. Basal bodies are at the base of cilia. Whereas centrioles are usually a deeper cytoplasmic structure and rarely approach the cell surface, basal bodies are concentrated at the apical cell border, one per cilium.

A mitochondrion is seen at left. The shelves of cristae are evident, in addition to Ca^{+2} granules, which are storage sites for calcium. The ciliary axoneme is the microtubule core of the cilium. It has nine microtubule doublets surrounding two central microtubules.

79. The answer is B. *(Biochemistry)*
Although fatty acid biosynthesis and degradation are different processes, both are initiated by forming an acyl CoA intermediate. The synthetic process is said to start in the cytosol when acetyl CoA is formed from citrate, which is cleaved by citrate lyase. The degrading process starts when the free fatty acid is transported into a cell and is converted into the CoA derivative by fatty acid CoA synthetase (thiokinase).

In degradation, the fatty acid is transported into the mitochondrion using the carnitine shuttle, where the CoA derivative is reconstituted and subjected to β-oxidation, in which the various acyl moieties are always maintained as the CoA derivative. The reducing equivalents obtained by oxidation of the acyl chain are transferred onto NAD^+ or FAD to form NADH

or $FADH_2$. These cofactors then pass their electrons to the electron transport chain via NADH and succinate dehydrogenase, respectively. Thus, most β-oxidation takes place in the mitochondrial matrix in juxtaposition to the electron transport system. In synthesis, which takes place entirely in the cytosol and uses NADPH as the source of reducing equivalents, the acetyl CoA is transformed to malonyl CoA by a biotin-requiring carboxylation reaction, the rate-limiting and regulated reaction in the synthetic sequence. The malonyl moiety of malonyl CoA is transferred to another – SH group on an acyl carrier protein that is part of the fatty acid synthase complex. The acyl chain then grows in two-carbon increments by the addition of an acetate moiety from acetyl CoA.

The CoA acyl derivative is a molecule that is active or "high energy," a property shared by all thioesters. By activating the acyl group via formation of the thioester, the acyl group can be transferred and transformed in the various reactions just discussed. The high-energy characteristics of the thioester bond are demonstrated by the fact that two ATP equivalents are needed to form a CoA derivative:

$$ATP + CoA + R\text{-}CO \rightarrow AMP + PPi + R\text{-}CSCoA.$$
$$\qquad\qquad \| \qquad\qquad\qquad\qquad\qquad \|$$
$$\qquad\qquad O \qquad\qquad\qquad\qquad\qquad O$$

80. The answer is B. *(Microbiology)*
Antimicrobials that affect bacterial protein metabolism do so because of structural and size differences between human and microbial ribosomes (80S and 70S, respectively). Size differences do not, in themselves, provide selective toxicity; differences in proteins and RNA molecules are the critical factors. Interference occurs at transcriptional or translational levels. At the translation level, either the 30S or 50S subunits are affected. Erythromycin, a bacteriostatic drug with a wide spectrum of activity, binds to the 50S ribosomal subunit and blocks the translocation step by preventing the release of the uncharged tRNA from the donor site once the peptide bond is formed. Resistance occurs primarily because of a plasmid-coded (extrachromosomal genetic element that may be transferred between unrelated bacteria) enzyme that methylates the 23S transfer RNA, thereby blocking the drug attachment. The other choices are incorrect because none of these antimicrobials affects the 50S subunit, although

aminoglycosides and tetracyclines do affect the 30S component, which results in misreading of the messenger RNA.

81. The answer is B. *(Behavioral science)*

The presence of REM erections suggests normal sexual physiology, and such erections indicate that the nature of an erectile disorder is psychological rather than physiologic. In the "postage stamp test," postage stamps connected by perforations are pasted around the penis at the beginning of the night. If erections occur during REM sleep, the perforations are found to be broken on awakening.

82. The answer is D. *(Microbiology)*

The Epstein-Barr virus (EBV) is a herpesvirus that is classified in the gammaherpesvirinae subfamily. These viruses infect lymphoid tissues, induce cell proliferation, and take a variable length of time to complete a single growth cycle.

Other herpesviruses that have been tentatively put into the gammaherpesvirinae subfamily are human herpes 6 and 7.

The alphaherpesvirinae subfamily consists of herpes simplex virus type 1 (HSV-1), HSV-2, and varicella-zoster virus. These are highly cytolytic viruses that infect neurons. They multiply rapidly and take only about 8 to 18 hours to complete one growth cycle.

The cytomegalovirus belongs in the betaherpesvirinae subfamily. These viruses infect cells of the kidney and salivary glands and cause cell gigantism or massive cell enlargement (i.e., they are cytomegalic). One complete growth cycle takes approximately 70 hours.

The herpesviruses have been difficult to classify because of their virtually identical morphology and genetic or antigenic similarity. The current classification is based primarily on their biologic characteristics.

Lentivirinae is the subfamily of the retroviruses to which HIV type 1 (HIV-1) belongs.

Oncovirinae is a retrovirus subfamily consisting of viruses with oncogenic potential. One important member is the human T-cell leukemia virus type I (HTLV-I).

83. The answer is C. *(Microbiology)*

Because normal cells contain genes (protooncogenes) that are similar to the oncogenes found in RNA tumor viruses, it is believed that the viruses acquire oncogenes from a host cell during their multiplication cycle. More than 25 oncogenes, such as *src*, *ras*, *erb*, *myc*, and *myb*, have been identified in RNA tumor viruses. In the viral genome, the genes lack cellular control sequences and most have one or more point mutations, insertions, and/or deletions. These small alterations in the genes presumably result in abnormal proteins that interfere with normal signaling processes. When expressed in the cell, the end result is uncontrolled cell proliferation. This mechanism of tumor induction is common among certain RNA viruses found in animals, but it has not yet been demonstrated for any human cancers.

The Retroviridae family is the only RNA virus family that has oncogenes. In contrast, all but one of the DNA virus families (Parvoviridae) has one or more members that are capable of inducing abnormal cell proliferation under certain conditions.

RNA viruses that contain an oncogene are highly oncogenic. Cell transformation is efficient and rapid. Tumors appear in vivo within a very short period of time and, hence, they are called "acute transforming" agents. As a group, they can induce leukemias, carcinomas, and sarcomas. However, each oncogenic retrovirus exhibits striking specificity for a particular cell type.

The oncogenes found in retroviruses are not required for viral replication. Retroviruses need only three genes to produce progeny: *gag*, *pol*, and *env*. The *gag* gene codes for group-specific, antigens, *pol* codes for the reverse transcriptase enzyme (polymerase), and *env* encodes the proteins that protrude from the envelope of the virus. In many transforming retroviruses, an oncogene replaces one of the three genes needed for replication and therefore are replication defective. A notable exception is the Rous sarcoma virus (found in birds; it is also known as the avian sarcoma virus), which contains *gag*, *pol*, *env*, and *src*. The *src* gene (and a number of other oncogenes) codes for a protein kinase that phosphorylates tyrosine.

In normal cells of the adult, protooncogenes are either silent or are expressed at very low levels. However, during embryogenesis their protein products are often present in large amounts and are thought to play important roles in cell growth, division, and differentiation. Protooncogenes are highly conserved (i.e., they have considerable sequence homology among different species). Within one species, they are found at constant positions of every cell of every individual. Protooncogenes are inherited according to the rules of classical mendelian genetics.

84. The answer is C.   (Biochemistry)

There is a direct correlation between sucrose consumption and dental caries, but no correlation to other diseases, including obesity, diabetes, and hypoglycemia.

There is no essential or minimal requirement for carbohydrates, since all carbohydrates in the body can be synthesized from amino acids. However, if insufficient calories are supplied as carbohydrate, they must come from fat and protein.

Complex polysaccharides, such as starch, are broken down to sugars and are absorbed in the small intestine. They cannot enhance motility of the bowel. The advantage of consuming complex carbohydrates rather than simple sugars is that the monosaccharide component is presented to the liver at a slower rate than is the case for free sugars. Therefore, the blood sugar levels do not increase as much. Moreover, the foods in which complex sugars are found have additional nutritional value, whereas those in which free sugars are found generally supply "empty" calories. A component often found in conjunction with complex carbohydrate is fiber, which does enhance bowel motility. Fiber is a mixture of nondigestible components that provide bulk to the stool.

The dietary recommendation is to increase the caloric percentage of carbohydrate in the diet from 46% to 58% of total calories. This amount makes it possible to reduce the caloric contribution of fat to 30% or less.

85. The answer is D.   (Biochemistry)

Bone is constantly being remodeled. Throughout life it is broken down to maintain serum calcium levels through the action of parathyroid hormone and vitamin D. In this process, both the mineral and the organic matrix is lost. The matrix is replaced under the anabolic influence of hormones: normally estrogen in females and testosterone in males. As individuals age, the level of these sex hormones declines, precipitously in women and gradually in men. The net result is that less bone is built up than is dissolved, resulting in osteoporosis. Anything that either slows the process of dissolution or increases the rate of remodeling slows

and perhaps even reverses the osteoporotic process. Calcitonin release is normally stimulated by an increase in serum calcium and acts to decrease the bone reabsorption and the loss of calcium and phosphate in the urine. Clinical trials have shown that this drug improves bone architecture, relieves pain, and improves function in postmenopausal women. Recently, nasal aerosol preparations have become available.

Addition of calcium to the diet, particularly in conjunction with vitamin D to enhance its absorption, also decreases the rate of bone resorption. The calcium absorbed from the gut keeps blood levels high and thereby inhibits parathyroid function and stimulates endogenous calcitonin release. In supplying calcium, it is important that the daily dose is taken at intervals during the day or else there will be periods in which serum levels decrease and parathyroid function is stimulated and calcitonin release is inhibited.

Estrogen replacement therapy coupled with calcium and vitamin D supplementation also has proved beneficial in the treatment of clinical osteoporosis. The estrogen stimulates bone matrix production and provides a place to deposit calcium. With insufficient matrix the calcium is excreted in the urine. There is very little literature concerning the potential benefits of testosterone supplementation in men to prevent osteoporosis, although it is clear that it does not accelerate the rate of development of osteoporosis.

Oral sodium alendronate (fosamax) inhibits osteoclastic activity and may stimulate osteoblastic activity and is a viable drug for treatment of osteoporosis.

Individuals with a chronic deficiency of calcium approach old age with a greater propensity to develop clinical osteoporosis, since a greater period of each day is spent in resorption of bone, allowing less time for rebuilding. Unfortunately, it is young women who tend to ingest too little calcium. The popularity of vegetarian diets makes this situation worse because it is difficult to obtain sufficient calcium in the typical Western diet without supplementation with dairy products. The addition of dairy products or mineral supplements is important in the prevention of osteoporosis.

During the 1960s and 1970s, massive doses of fluoride were used to treat osteoporosis. Although it was somewhat effective, this therapy was discontinued in favor of estrogen and calcium therapy. Fluoride in large quantities is a poison, but in small amounts it is safe and, when consumed over a period of many years, very likely does afford some protection against osteoporosis. Its major function is to replace some of the critical hydroxyl groups of hydroxyapatite (bone salt). The fluoride atom fits into the crystal matrix better than the hydroxyl group and improves the stability of the crystal. In this way, it reduces the solubility of hydroxyapatite in bone and teeth and increases the resistance of enamel to caries. Fluoride does not enhance the rate of resorption of bone.

Stress also increases the formation of bone. Disuse osteoporosis develops rapidly. As much as half the bone mass may be lost in a limb immobilized for as little as 6 weeks. However, exercise only helps develop the bones that are being stressed. Running decreases the risk of osteoporosis in the legs and to a lesser extent in the whole axial skeleton, which shares part of the weight thrust. It does little, however, for bones that are not stressed, such as those in the arms.

86. The answer is B.   *(Biochemistry)*

The minimal amount of protein required is that which supplies the least prevalent essential amino acid in adequate amounts. The biologic value is a measure of the availability of essential amino acids. The higher the value, the more similar the essential amino acid content of the protein is to the human one, since it will provide these amino acids in quantities that are proportional to that needed. Therefore, the total requirement of a protein with a high biologic value is less than that of one with a low biologic value.

An excess of protein has several adverse effects. The excretion of the end-products taxes the excretory function of the kidneys, and deaths have been reported due to apparent overconsumption of protein among people on fad high-protein diets. Part of the work performed by the kidneys is to regulate the acidosis induced by protein catabolism. This acidosis also contributes to bone dissolution and, if chronic, to development of osteoporosis.

Foods that complement each other with respect to their amino acid content have reciprocal contents of essential amino acids. For example, the addition of a food low in methionine and high in lysine to one high in methionine and low in lysine makes the combination a more complete protein and lesser amounts are required in the diet. However, the two foods should be ingested simultaneously or at least within several hours of each other. Otherwise, the protein first ingested has already undergone catabolic degradation, and the complementary amino acid will no longer be available.

An individual suffering from marasmus has a dietary intake of too few calories but sufficient protein. The amount of protein needed is greater than that required if sufficient calories were consumed, because some protein is used to form glucose. Conversely, if sufficient carbohydrate is consumed, less protein is required. This is called the protein sparing effect of carbohydrates.

Kwashiorkor refers to protein deficiency with sufficient calories. It is most commonly observed in recently weaned infants that have discontinued a relatively high-protein mother's milk diet and have been placed on a low-protein diet. The practice of some underdeveloped societies of maintaining children on mother's milk for 4 or more years helps prevent kwashiorkor.

87. The answer is C.   *(Pathology)*

Aflatoxins predispose to hepatocellular carcinoma, whereas vinyl chloride predisposes to angiosarcoma of the liver. Other important carcinogen associations commonly asked on the USMLE are summarized in the table.

Carcinogen	Tumor Association(s)
Aniline dyes	Bladder cancer (transitional)
Benzidine	Bladder cancer (transitional)
Cyclophosphamide	Bladder cancer (transitional)
Phenacetin	Bladder cancer (transitional)
Vinyl chloride	Angiosarcoma of the liver
Thorotrast	Angiosarcoma of the liver, hepatocellular carcinoma
Arsenic	Angiosarcoma of the liver, squamous carcinoma of the skin, lung cancer
Asbestos	Lung cancer (smoker), mesothelioma (nonsmoker)
Polycyclic hydrocarbons	Lung cancer (squamous and small cell); squamous (smoking) cancers of the oral pharynx, esophagus, larynx; adenocarcinoma of pancreas; bladder (transitional); squamous cervical carcinoma
Chromium	Lung, nasal cavity
Nickel	Lung, nasal cavity
Chewing tobacco	Verrucous carcinoma of the mouth
Alkylating agents	Acute leukemia/lymphoma
Benzene	Acute leukemia (also aplastic anemia)
Oral contraceptives	Liver adenomas, hepatocellular carcinoma
Aflatoxins	Hepatocellular carcinoma
Diethylstilbestrol	Clear cell adenocarcinoma of the vagina
Nitrosamines	Esophageal and gastric cancers
Cadmium	Prostate and lung cancers
Tars, soots, oils	Squamous carcinoma of the skin

88. The answer is D.   *(Biochemistry)*

Ammonia is very toxic to the body. The body best protects itself from ammonia by converting it into the amino acid glutamine, which is the nontoxic storage form of ammonia that circulates in the blood.

$$\text{Glutamate} + NH_4^+ \xrightarrow{\text{Glutamate synthetase}} \text{Glutamine}$$

Glutamine has the distinction of being the amino acid with the highest concentration in the blood. Muscle, liver, and the central nervous system release glutamine rather than ammonia. In the gut, glutamine is removed from the blood to form alanine, citrulline, and ammonium (NH_4^+). In the kidney, glutamine is converted by glutaminase into glutamate and NH_3, the latter diffusing into the tubule lumen and combining with hydrogen ions (H^+) and chloride to form NH_4Cl as an effective method of excreting excess acid.

Converting NH_4^+ into ammonia (NH_3) would be detrimental because it is the diffusible form that is reabsorbed out of the gut into the portal vein. NH_4^+ is nondiffusible, which is the basis for the mechanism of action of orally administered lactulose in decreasing NH_3 concentration in the blood. Bacteria acting on lactulose release hydrogen ions (H^+), which combine with NH_3 to form NH_4^+, which is excreted in the stool rather than reabsorbed into the portal vein.

Combining NH_4^+ with alpha ketoglutarate to form glutamate would be detrimental as well, because alpha ketoglutarate would be used up, depriving the tricarboxylic acid cycle of an intermediate necessary for producing adenosine triphosphate. Some clinicians theorize that this may be one of many detrimental results of excess NH_3 in patients with liver failure or with inborn errors of metabolism resulting in hyperammonemia.

$$\uparrow\uparrow\uparrow \textbf{NH}_3 + \text{alpha ketoglutarate} \xrightarrow{\text{Glutamate dehydrogenase}} \text{Glutamate}$$

Anti-oxidants in the body, such as glutathione, have no effect on NH_3, because it is not a free radical with an unpaired electron in its outer orbit.

Increasing the elimination of NH_4^+ in the stool is not a primary mechanism for excretion, since colon bacteria generate NH_3, the diffusible form, which is reabsorbed into the blood and transported to the liver urea cycle by the portal vein.

89. The answer is C. *(Microbiology)*
Lactose fermentation is a basic laboratory test that will readily distinguish *Esherichia coli* (lactose-positive) from *Salmonella paratyphi* (lactose-negative). Both organisms are gram-negative rods of similar appearance and are capable of fermenting glucose. Because both have fermenting capability, glucose oxidation is not a test usually used to differentiate between them. Hemolysis on blood agar is extremely variable and is not a reliable test for differentiation of these two organisms.

90. The answer is D. *(Microbiology)*
Natural killer (NK) cells account for 5% to 10% of lymphocytes. They participate in antibody-dependent cellular cytotoxicity reactions (type II hypersensitivity reactions). NK cells are not T cells and are sometimes referred to as null cells. They can lyse virally infected cells and tumor cells without prior sensitization. NK cells are frequently referred to as large granular lymphocytes, and would not be confused with small B cells. When activated by interleukin-2, NK cells become lymphocyte-activated killer cells (LAK cells), which can be used to treat certain cancers. NK cells are a source of gamma interferon, which induces class II expression and activates macrophages.

91. The answer is C. *(Behavioral science)*
Pregnancy is more likely to cause death in a 35-year-old woman than methods used to eliminate or prevent it, namely, an abortion, an intrauterine device, an oral contraceptive, or a barrier contraceptive.

92. The answer is A. *(Behavioral science)*
The "sick role" includes the lack, not the acceptance, of responsibility for becoming ill.

93. The answer is A. *(Biochemistry)*
A high-protein diet is contraindicated in a patient with cirrhosis of the liver, because the urea cycle is damaged and is not able to metabolize the ammonia coming from the metabolism of the amino acids. A low-protein diet is the most cost-effective way of lowering ammonia levels in these patients.

Because there is no storage form for amino acids in the body, unlike fatty acids (triacylglycerol) and glucose (glycogen), an excess amount of protein intake increases the number of carbon skeletons. Carbon skeletons form pyruvate, oxaloacetate (OAA), acetyl CoA, acetoacetyl CoA, alpha ketoglutarate, succinyl CoA, and fumarate intermediates. These in turn can enter intermediary pathways to produce

- glucose by gluconeogenesis (OAA, pyruvate, and so forth)
- lipids by increasing fatty acid synthesis (acetyl CoA) and triacylglycerol synthesis (increase formation of dihydroxyacetone phosphate).
- energy by being oxidized to CO_2 and water in the tricarboxylic acid cycle.

The metabolism of amino acids involves the transamination of amino acids into glutamate, followed by oxidative deamination of glutamate into ammonia. The ammonia enters the urea cycle forming urea, which is primarily excreted in the kidneys. Therefore, a person on a high-protein diet (weight lifters) would be expected to have an increase in serum blood urea nitrogen level as well as increased excretion of urea in the urine. This increased excretion imposes a heavy load on the kidneys and creates the potential for renal disease. As expected, those patients who have chronic renal disease should be on a low-protein diet to reduce the urea load imposed on the kidneys.

94. The answer is A. *(Behavioral science)*
Children with attention deficit hyperactivity disorder (ADHD) usually have normal IQs, but commonly exhibit distractibility, impulsiveness, restlessness, and frustration.

95. The answer is E. *(Pathology)*

Acute viral hepatitis is not associated with fatty change but involves either direct cytolysis of the hepatocyte by the infecting virus or alteration of the hepatocyte class I antigens with destruction by CD8 T-cytotoxic cells. The inflammation is primarily lymphocytic.

The accumulation of triglyceride (TG) in the liver (other tissues as well), or fatty change, is a reversible reaction to injury reduced by a number of etiologies, the most common of which is alcohol. Mechanisms for fatty change in the liver include

- an increase in free fatty acids (e.g., starvation, diabetic ketoacidosis, alcohol)
- increased production of acetate (simplest fatty acid) substrate (degradation of alcohol)
- increased release of glycerol to form glycerol 3-phosphate, the carbohydrate backbone for TG synthesis (starvation, diabetic ketoacidosis). Glycerol is only processed in the liver, since glycerol kinase is found only in the liver.

$$\text{glycerol} \xrightarrow[\text{ATP ADP}]{\text{kinase}} \text{glycerol-3 PO}_4 \xrightarrow{\text{fatty acids}} \text{TG}$$

- decreased beta oxidation of fatty acids (alcohol), which leaves more fatty acid for TG synthesis
- decreased synthesis of apolipoproteins (kwashiorkor, CCl_4, other hypoproteinemic states), since there is no carrier protein for TG in the very low-density lipoprotein fraction

In the metabolism of alcohol, there are a number of substrates generated that enhance TG synthesis.
Alcohol$\rightarrow$ acetaldehyde + **NADH$_2$**$\rightarrow$ **acetate** + **NADH$_2$**$\rightarrow$ acetyl CoA

- acetate (fatty acyl CoA) is fed into the production of TG.

$$\text{Glycerol 3 PO}_4 \xrightarrow{\text{fatty acyl CoA (acetate)}} \text{phosphatidic acid} \rightarrow \text{diglyceride} \rightarrow \text{TG}$$

- excess NADH$_2$ favors the formation of dihydroxyacetone phosphate (DHAP) in the glycolytic cycle (reverses the reaction due to excess of NADH$_2$) with production of glycerol 3 phosphate.

$$\text{1,3 diphosphoglycerate} \xrightarrow{\text{NADH}_2 \text{ NAD}} \text{DHAP} \rightarrow \text{glycerol-3 PO}_4 \rightarrow \text{TG}$$

- alcohol decreases the beta oxidation of free fatty acids because NAD is required in the beta oxidation cycle and is tied up as NADH$_2$.

Kwashiorkor produces massive fatty livers because of the decrease in protein intake and reduction in apoprotein synthesis. Apoproteins must coat VLDL before secretion into the blood stream.

Carbon tetrachloride poisoning produces fatty livers from free radical injury, since the CCl_4 is converted by the liver cytochrome system into CCl_3.

Patients taking methotrexate need to have frequent liver enzyme determinations because of tendency for methotrexate to produce fatty livers and hepatic fibrosis.

96. The answer is A. *(Biochemistry)*

In prolonged fasting (starvation), further breakdown of proteins to supply amino acids for gluconeogenesis is counterproductive to the welfare of the body. Therefore, the catabolism of muscle tissue is reduced, resulting in a decrease in the production of urea by the liver and a concomitant reduction of urea excretion in the kidneys.

The urea cycle is located in the hepatocytes. The cycle is as follows:

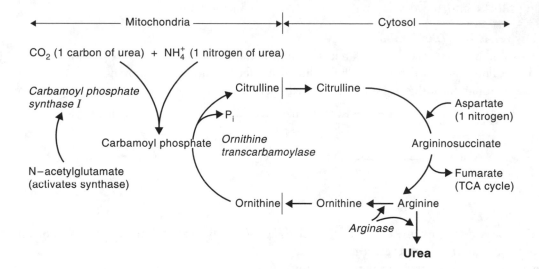

The ammonium ion (NH_4^+) comes from oxidative deamination of glutamate by glutamate dehydrogenase (see figure) and other sources (bacterial degradation of urea in the bowel, amines from the diet, amino acids, amino groups of nucleic acids). It supplies one of the nitrogens of urea. Carbon dioxide (CO_2) provides the carbon atom of urea.

$$\text{Glutamate} \xrightarrow{\text{Glutamate dehydrogenase}} NH_4^+ + \text{alpha ketoglutarate}$$

N-Acetylglutamate, derived from a protein-rich meal and the combination of acetyl CoA + glutamate, is required to activate carbamoyl phosphate synthase I, the rate-limiting enzyme of the cycle that produces carbamoyl phosphate. Ornithine transcarbamoylase removes the high-energy phosphate from carbamoyl phosphate and converts ornithine (a basic amino acid) into citrulline (a basic amino acid). All of this occurs within the mitochondria. The citrulline is transported out of the mitochondria to the cytosol, where it is converted by argininosuccinate synthase into argininosuccinate. Aspartate provides another nitrogen in this reaction. Argininosuccinate is converted into L-arginine by arigininosuccinate lyase and gives off fumarate, which is an intermediate in the tricarboxylic acid cycle.

Arginine is converted into ornithine by arginase, giving off urea, the end-product of amino acid metabolism. Ornithine is transported back into the mitochondria, and the cycle repeats itself. It is understandable why in cirrhosis of the liver the urea cycle would be affected, resulting in a low serum blood urea nitrogen level and an increased serum ammonia level because it cannot be metabolized. Inborn errors of metabolism associated with hyperammonemia due to enzyme deficiencies in the urea cycle are more severe if the enzyme occurs earlier in the cycle (e.g., ornithine transcarbamoylase) rather than later in the cycle (e.g., arginase). The urea cycle enzymes are also disrupted in Reye syndrome, which is responsible for the increase in serum ammonia in these patients.

97. The answer is E. *(Microbiology)*
Five groups of antimicrobials can interfere with cell wall formation. Penicillins and cephalosporins inhibit transpeptidases. Cyclosporine interferes with formation of the polypeptide chain in the cytoplasm of the organism. Vancomycin prevents the incorporation of the building blocks into the developing peptidogly-can backbone. Bacitracin interferes with the function of the phospholipid carrier molecule in the cytoplasmic membrane. Polymyxin molecules incorporate into the cytoplasmic membrane of gram-negative bacteria, distorting the structure sufficiently so that contents of the cytoplasm leak out, and osmotic control is lost.

98. The answer is B. *(Biochemistry)*
In the renal tubules, ammonia (NH_3) is released from glutamine by the action of glutaminase, not glutamate dehydrogenase. This reaction is responsible for the most effective means of removing excess hydrogen ions (H^+) from the body through the kidneys. Glutamate dehydrogenase converts glutamate into NH_4 + alpha ketoglutarate.

$$\leftarrow \text{Blood} \rightarrow \ \leftarrow \text{Renal tubule} \xrightarrow{\hspace{3cm}} \text{Lumen of tubule}$$

$$\underset{\text{Glutaminase}}{}$$

$$\text{Glutamine} \xrightarrow{\hspace{2cm}} \text{Glutamate} + NH_3 \rightarrow \qquad NH_3 + H^+ \rightarrow NH_4^+$$
$$+$$
$$Cl^-$$
$$\downarrow$$
$$NH_4Cl$$

Bacterial ureases acting on urea in the stomach (*Helicobacter pylori*), colon (anaerobes), and urine (*Proteus* species) contribute ammonia to the urea cycle.

Glutamate derived from transamination reactions (see alanine as an example) involving amino acids and ketoacids is converted by oxidative deamination (glutamate dehydrogenase) into NH_4^+ and alpha ketoglutarate. Note that the first step in transamination of alanine is the transfer of the alpha amino group of alanine to the amino acceptor alpha ketoglutarate. This results in the conversion of alanine into the alpha ketoacid pyruvate and alpha ketoglutarate into glutamate. The transaminase in this reaction is alanine aminotransferase (ALT) using pyridoxal phosphate derived from pyridoxine (B_6) as a cofactor. Glutamate undergoes oxidative deamination with the aid of glutamate dehydrogenase into ammonium (NH_4^+) and alpha ketoglutarate, the former entering the urea cycle and the latter returning to combine with another amino group. The transamination reaction is reversible and can be used to synthesize as well as metabolize amino acids.

Amino acids such as histidine, asparagine, serine, and threonine as well as the amino groups in nucleic acids are additional sources of ammonia.

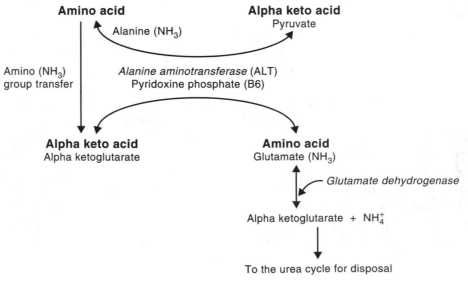

99. The answer is A. *(Pathology)*
Corticosteroids decrease leukocyte adhesion to endothelial cells by decreasing the synthesis of adhesion molecules that cause neutrophils and monocytes to adhere to the endothelial surface. By decreasing leukocyte adhesion, corticosteroids decrease the emigration of leukocytes to the area of inflammation, which reduces the inflammatory reaction. This decrease also results in a neutrophilic leukocytosis, because what was once the marginating pool of neutrophils is now part of the circulating pool. Corticosteroids inhibit phospholipase A2, which reduces the synthesis of prostaglandins and leukotrienes, both of which are involved in the inflammatory process. Corticosteroids are toxic to certain subsets of T lymphocytes and precursor lymphoid cells, the former resulting in a decrease in the total lymphocyte count and the latter leading to suppression of antibody synthesis.

100. The answer is C. *(Biochemistry)*
Primase synthesizes RNA primers during DNA replication. Because it synthesizes RNA, only ribonucleotides can be used as substrates. Thymidine triphosphate (TTP) is a deoxyribonucleotide that is used as a substrate for DNA synthesis. The other choices are appropriate substrates for RNA synthesis.

101. The answer is D. *(Pathology)*
Repair of damaged tissue is dependent on the regenerative capacity of the parenchymal tissue involved (i.e., labile, stable, or permanent cells) as well as the replacement of injured tissue by collagen. Regeneration of epithelium is facilitated when the connective tissue framework remains intact. Removal of both the parenchyma and supportive tissue (e.g., infarction of the lung) leads to replacement of the necrotic material by scar tissue. Labile cells (e.g., squamous epithelium, gastrointestinal epithelium, hematopoietic cells) are replaced by stem cells. Stable cells (e.g., liver, kidney, smooth muscle) must be replaced by prodding G_0 resting cells to move into the cell cycle as a result of tissue loss or by hormone or growth factor stimulation. Permanent cells (striated muscle, skeletal muscle) are replaced by scar tissue (with the exception of the brain). Connective tissue repair occurs via the formation of granulation tissue, consisting of richly vascularized stroma with endothelial cells, and reactive fibroblasts intermixed with chronic inflammatory cells. Factors enhancing granulation tissue formation include fibronectin and various growth factors secreted by cells in the inflammatory response. Fibronectin is derived from fibroblasts and endothelial cells. Its functions include chemotaxis, opsonization, angiogenesis, and cross-linking of collagen to increase the tensile strength of the healing tissue. Growth factors, such as epidermal-derived growth factor and platelet-derived growth factor, have mitogenic properties. Mitogenesis is accomplished by growth factors first binding to receptors, which causes receptor activation and the generation of second messengers, which, in turn, transmit signals to the nucleus resulting in cell division. Integrins are cell-surface adhesion proteins that provide anchorage, cues for migration, and signals for growth and differentiation. They are involved in cellular–extracellular matrix adhesion (integrins binding with fibronectin) and cell–cell adhesion. A control factor that modulates the healing process and prevents the piling up of epithelium is contact inhibition (lost in neoplasia). Cells stop proliferating once they contact another cell surface (lost in malignant cells.) Collagen derived from fibroblasts is first type III collagen, which is later replaced by type I collagen, which has the greatest tensile strength. Type IV collagen is used for basement membranes and does not have a major role in the healing process.

102. The answer is E. *(Pathology)*
Obesity, which is defined as a body weight that is 20% or more over the normal, is least likely to have hypothyroidism as a complication. However, hypothyroidism is commonly associated with obesity.

Obesity beginning in childhood is associated with hyperplasia of fat cells, whereas obesity beginning in adulthood is related to hypertrophy of fat cells. Complications related to obesity include:

- stroke, both atherosclerotic and hypertensive types
- essential hypertension
- coronary artery disease (minor risk factor; increased low-density lipoproteins)
- left ventricular hypertrophy

• an increased risk for endometrial and breast cancer because of the increased aromatization of the 17-ketosteroids (dehydroepiandrosterone and androstenedione) as well as testosterone into estrogens

• the Pickwickian syndrome, which refers to respiratory acidosis from poor movement of the diaphragm when the patient is sitting down. There is retention of carbon dioxide, which results in respiratory acidosis, hypoxemia, and the patient falling asleep.

• cholelithiasis, due to increased cholesterol solubilized in the bile

• type II diabetes mellitus, due to down-regulation of insulin receptor synthesis associated with excess adipose

• osteoarthritis in weight-bearing joints (hips, knees, feet).

103. The answer is C. *(Microbiology)*
Chlamydia organisms are obligate intracellular parasites and as such are not capable of growing in a cell-free environment. The life cycle is unusual; small elementary bodies enter the cell and reorganize into a larger, metabolically active reticulate body, which undergoes repeated binary fission into daughter elementary bodies that are released by cell lysis. *Chlamydia trachomatis* induces the formation of glycogen-containing inclusions within the host cells. *C. trachomatis* is responsible for ocular, genital, and respiratory infections that occur only in humans and are usually transmitted by close personal contact. A clinical diagnosis can be confirmed by observation of elementary bodies by immunofluorescence microscopy or antibody measurement by ELISA. The treatment regimen includes the administration of tetracyclines or erythromycin.

104. The answer is D. *(Biochemistry)*
Tyrosine can be used for the synthesis of catecholamines, thyroid hormone, fumarate, and melanin, but it is not an essential amino acid. The mnemonic for the essential amino acids is AH TV TILL PM (see table below.

Arginine and histidine are required for growth.

Leucine and lysine are the only exclusive ketogenic amino acids, which means that they can be converted into ketone bodies (acetone, acetoacetate, and beta hydroxybutyrate).

Isoleucine, leucine, and valine are branched-chain amino acids that can be used by skeletal muscle for fuel in the fasting state.

Tryptophan is an essential amino acid that can be used for the synthesis of serotonin, melatonin, and the nicotinamide moiety of NAD and NADP.

105. The answer is A. *(Pathology)*
Cytokines are protein products emitted by T cells, macrophages, and other cell types that provide regulatory function for these cells. Interleukin-1 (IL-1) and

A	H	T	V	T	I	L	L	P	M
R	I	R	A	H	S	E	Y	H	E
G	S	Y	L	R	O	U	S	E	T
I	T	P	I	E	L	C	I	N	H
N	I	T	N	O	E	I	N	Y	I
I	D	O	E	N	U	N	E	L	O
N	I	P		I	C	E		A	N
E	N	H		N	I			L	I
	E	A		E	N			A	N
		N			E			N	E
								I	
								N	
								E	

tumor necrosis factor (TNF) are secreted primarily by macrophages and assume an important role in both acute and chronic inflammation. They stimulate acute phase-reactant (APR) synthesis by the liver. APRs include proteins such as complement fibrinogen, coagulation factors, C-reactive protein, and serum-associated amyloid protein. In order to have enough amino acids to generate these APRs, the synthesis of binding proteins such as transferrin and albumin is decreased, and there is a concomitant increase in catabolism of muscle tissue. IL-1 and TNF have many diverse functions, which include:

- Stimulation of the bone marrow to release the postmitotic neutrophil pool, consisting of metamyelocytes, bands, and neutrophils. This influx of neutrophils into the peripheral circulation produces an absolute neutrophilic leukocytosis and "left shift," the latter referring to increased numbers of band neutrophils and fewer mature cells. These white blood cell findings are indicators of infection or, in some cases, a noninfectious acute inflammatory reaction.
- Reduction of the serum concentration of zinc and iron, which normally enhance bacterial reproduction
- Stimulation of production of serum copper, which is involved in hemoglobin synthesis and serves as a cofactor for many of the enzymes that inactivate free radicals
- Stimulation of prostaglandin synthesis in the hypothalamus, which, in turn, stimulates the vasomotor center to increase sympathetic nerve stimulation of peripheral vessels in the skin, reducing heat loss and producing fever
- Stimulation of fibroblasts to synthesize collagen (important for repair)
- Stimulation of B lymphocytes to become plasma cells, which are important in the production of antibodies (immune response)
- Enhancement of the synthesis of adhesion molecules on leukocytes and endothelial cells
- Stimulation of adrenocorticotrophic hormone release with the subsequent release of glucocorticoids (anti-inflammatory agents)

106. The answer is E. *(Physiology)*
Lysine is neither a neurotransmitter nor is it involved in the synthesis of neurotransmitters. Lysine is a key component of collagen and, along with leucine, is a purely ketogenic amino acid.

Glycine is an inhibitory neurotransmitter primarily found in the spinal cord and brain stem. It increases chloride ion conductance. Glycine is blocked by tetanospasmin, the toxin produced by *Clostridium tetani*, thus allowing the afferents to stimulate muscle contraction.

Tryptophan is used in the synthesis of serotonin, a neurotransmitter that is present in high concentration in the brain stem. It is decreased in patients with depression.

Histidine can be converted into histamine, which is a neurotransmitter present in neurons in the hypothalamus.

Glutamine can be converted into glutamate, which is the most prevalent excitatory neurotransmitter in the brain. Glutamate can also be converted into gamma aminobutyrate (GABA), which is an inhibitory neurotransmitter. GABA receptors increase chloride conductance and are the site of action of benzodiazepines and barbiturates.

107. The answer is C. *(Behavioral science)*
Patients rarely know the lethal consequences of their planned suicide method. The majority of suicides can be prevented with psychological intervention and/or the use of antidepressant medication. Many individuals visit their family physicians in the week before a suicide attempt with a variety of medical complaints. The risk of suicide is reduced among married persons. Professional women, particularly female physicians, are at increased risk when compared with nonprofessional women.

108. The answer is A. *(Microbiology)*
The F factor, or sex factor, is a bacterial plasmid that occurs as a small, circular, double-stranded DNA molecule. F^+ cells contain the F factor and act as donors (males) during conjugation. The F pilus, which forms a bridge between the mating cells, is encoded on the F plasmid. During conjugation, a break occurs at a specific site on one strand of the plasmid DNA, and the 5′ end of that single strand moves through the pilus to the recipient F cell in the 5′ to 3′ direction. Following transfer, the single strand is copied, converting the recipient cell to F^+.

109. The answer is C. *(Pathology)*
The cardinal signs of acute inflammation include:

- Localized redness (rubor), which is primarily caused by vasodilatation from the vasoactive amines, histamine and serotonin
- Heat (calor), which is primarily caused by vasodilation from histamine and serotonin
- Swelling (tumor), which is the result of increased vessel permeability with emigration of leukocytes into the interstitial tissue and production of an exudate. It is not a neurogenic response.
- Pain (dolor) is the result of pain fiber stimulation by prostaglandin D and bradykinin.
- Loss of function (functio laesa) is the result of swelling and pain.

Some of the vascular events just described are characteristic of the classic Lewis triple response. If a blunt object is forcibly drawn across the skin:

- A dull red line (stroke line) develops at the site of mild trauma due to capillary dilatation (histamine response).
- A red halo (flare) subsequently develops at the periphery due to arteriolar vasodilatation (neurogenic response).
- Swelling (wheal) occurs due to increased vessel permeability (histamine response).

110. The answer is B. *(Biochemistry)*
Transposons, or jumping genes, are pieces of DNA that can move from one place to another in the genome. They are found in all organisms. The target sites for movement of transposons appear to be randomly selected. Insertion of a transposon causes the duplication of a few nucleotides at the target site, forming a noninverted, or direct, repeat sequence. Insertion of a transposon into the coding region of a gene disrupts that coding region and destroys the function of the gene. Insertion of a transposon into the regulatory region of a gene may turn on or turn off transcription from that gene, depending on the individual circumstance. The antibiotic resistance genes on R factors are often located within transposons.

111. The answer is B. *(Microbiology)*
Rocky mountain spotted fever is caused by *Rickettsia rickettsii*, transmitted by a tick (Ixodid) vector. Although first reported in Rocky Mountain states, this disease is especially important on the east coast of the United States, as well as in Oklahoma and North Carolina.

The typical lesion is a vasculitis, particularly in the endothelial lining of the vessel wall where the organism is found. Damage to the vessels of the skin results in a characteristic rash as well as edema and hemorrhage related to increased capillary permeability. Patients report an acute onset of fever, headache, myalgias, and prostration. The rash proceeds from macules to petechiae and spreads from the extremities to the trunk (centripetal). Diagnosis and treatment decisions are made on clinical grounds because laboratory diagnosis depends on an observed rise in antibody titer. The Weil-Felix test is used to detect antirickettsial antibodies in a serum sample by cross-reacting with antigens of the OX strain of *Proteus vulgaris*, thereby agglutinating the *Proteus* organisms. The treatment of choice for all rickettsial infections is a regimen of tetracycline and chloramphenicol given orally and daily. Recovery depends, in part, on the immune mechanisms of the host.

112. The answer is E. *(Pathology)*
Neutrophils are the key cells for acute rather than chronic inflammation. Chronic inflammation is the host's reaction to persistence of an injurious agent. It consists of both an immune response and a proliferative (cellular) response involving monocytes, macrophages, lymphocytes, plasma cells, fibroblasts, platelets, and endothelial cells. Although the immune response is triggered at injury, it takes several days for immunoreactive molecules to appear, the first representing IgM. Chronic inflammation is characterized by less swelling and hyperemia. Fever either subsides or is episodic. The tissue becomes firm due to the presence of scarring. Types of chronic inflammation include:

- Inflammation resulting from previous acute inflammation (e.g., acute viral hepatitis progressing into chronic hepatitis or acute pyelonephritis progressing into chronic pyelonephritis). This inflammation is frequently the result of inability of an antibiotic to kill an organism or a lack of host immune response to the infection (e.g., AIDS) contributing to an infection becoming chronic.

- Inflammation that occurs in tissue without antecedent acute inflammation. Variants of this type of inflammation include 1) infections by organisms such as tuberculosis, cryptococcosis, and syphilis, which produce granulomatous inflammation; 2) persistence of nondegradable material in the inflammatory site, such as glass, silica, silicone from an implant, and metal; 3) autoimmune diseases where autoantibodies attack host tissue (e.g., systemic lupus erythematosus, rheumatoid arthritis).

The cells of chronic inflammation are different from those of acute inflammation. Normally, monocytes live in the peripheral blood for 24 hours and then emigrate into tissue to become wandering or fixed macrophages in the mononuclear phagocyte system. As a primary effector cell in chronic inflammation, they are important in:

- Phagocytosing and killing microbial agents
- Removing debris (scavenger function)
- Processing antigens for B- and T-lymphocyte responses
- Enhancing host responses via their secretory products (e.g., interleukin-1, tumor necrosis factor, and B- and T-cell growth factors).

Monocytes are activated to kill phagocytized microbial agents by lysosomal enzymes, free radicals, chemotactic factors, and cytokines secreted by CD4 T-helper cells (γ interferon).

B cells are important in antibody production once they become plasma cells. Immunoglobulins act as opsonins (IgG), neutralizing antibodies against toxins and viruses, and are involved in various immune reactions (e.g., allergic reactions). Plasma cells are the key cell seen in the vasculitis associated with syphilis.

T-cell functions related to inflammation include cell-mediated immunity (type IV hypersensitivity); the secretion of cytokines (lymphokines) that help regulate the immune response; and the regulation of B-cell activity by T cells.

Natural killer cells destroy virus-infected cells and tumor cells.

Fibroblasts are important in collagen synthesis for the repair of damaged tissue. Endothelial cells and fibroblasts form granulation tissue, which is the key substrate for wound repair.

Platelets supply platelet-derived growth factor, which is an important mitogen in wound repair.

113. The answer is D. *(Biochemistry)*
Nucleic acid sequences can be exactly related to each other because of the specific base pairs formed in two complementary nucleic acid strands. For this reason, if one knows either the DNA or the RNA sequence, one can predict the other exactly.

Nucleic acid sequences can be related to protein sequences by the genetic code. One can exactly predict the amino acid sequence of a protein from either the DNA or the RNA sequence. The genetic code, however, is degenerate. Several different codons are used to specify the same amino acid. Therefore, knowing the amino acid sequence of a protein only allows one to approximate the original nucleic acid sequence, leaving many of the bases in question.

114. The answer is C. *(Pathology)*
T lymphocytes (CD4 T-helper cells and CD8 T-suppressor/cytotoxic cells) are primarily involved in cellular immunity. Natural killer cells, which have different markers than T cells (null cells), are involved with antibody-dependent cytotoxicity reactions (type II hypersensitivity).

Although neutrophils are the key cells involved in most acute inflammatory reactions, there are some exceptions to the rule in other types of inflammation. Eosinophils are the dominant cells in allergic reactions (e.g., hay fever) and those reactions against invasive helminthic infections (e.g., strongyloides, ascaris, hookworms, but not protozoal infections or noninvasive helminths such as pinworms). Eosinophils are attracted to the area of inflammation by both eosinophil chemotactic factor and histamine released by mast cells/basophils after degranulation by the anaphylatoxins, C3a and C5a. Eosinophils contain arylsulfatase and histaminase, which neutralize leukotrienes and histamine, respectively. Eosinophils also contain major basic protein and crystalline material seen on electron microscope examination (e.g., Charcot-Leyden crystals seen in sputum samples in people with asthma derive from these crystals).

Mast cells/basophils contain primary mediators in their basophilic granules, such as histamine, heparin, chemotactic factors for neutrophils and eosinophils, proteases, and platelet activating factor. Mast cells/basophils have a secondary release reaction of chemical mediators including prostaglandins and leukotrienes.

Mast cells/basophils are the key cell of type I hypersensitivity reactions.

Normally, monocytes live in the peripheral blood for 24 hours and then emigrate into tissue to become wandering or fixed macrophages in the mononuclear phagocyte system. As a primary effector cell in chronic inflammation, they are important in:

- Phagocytosing and killing microbial agents
- Removing debris (scavenger function)
- Processing antigens for B- and T-lymphocyte responses
- Enhancing host responses via their secretory products (i.e., interleukin-1, tumor necrosis factor, B- and T-cell growth factors)

Monocytes are activated to kill phagocytized microbial agents by lysosomal enzymes, free radicals, chemotactic factors, and cytokines secreted by CD4 T-helper cells (γ interferon).

B cells are important in antibody production once they become plasma cells. Immunoglobulins act as opsonins (IgG), neutralizing antibodies against toxins and viruses, and are involved in various immune reactions (e.g., allergic reactions and antibody-dependent cytotoxicity reactions). Plasma cells are the key cell seen in the vasculitis associated with syphilis.

T-cell functions related to inflammation include cell-mediated immunity (type IV hypersensitivity); the secretion of cytokines (lymphokines) that help regulate the immune response; and the regulation of B-cell activity by T cells.

115. The answer is D.   *(Microbiology)*

Cytokines are a large and diverse group of proteins released by lymphoctyes and other lymphoreticular cells. They help to regulate immune function and inflammation and include the interferons, interleukins, colony-stimulating factors, and tumor necrosis factors. Platelet-activating factor (PAF), a lysophosphatidylcholine derivative formed as a by-product of the arachidonic acid reacylation cycle, is a powerful mediator of asthma and shock and increases interleukin-1 expression.

116. The answer is D.   *(Biochemistry)*

Messenger RNA (mRNA) molecules carry information coding for the amino acid sequence of a protein molecule. In eukaryotes, mRNA undergoes a series of processing events as it is being produced. A modified guanosine residue (the cap) is attached to the 5′ end. A poly A tail is attached to the 3′ end. Introns are moved by splicing, leaving only the exons in the final mature mRNA molecule.

117. The answer is E.   *(Behavioral science)*

Homicide rates are increasing as confirmed by the fact that homicide is the second-to-third most common cause of death in people from ages 15 to 24 years.

118. The answer is D.   *(Pharmacology)*

The treatment of steroid-sensitive tumors includes the removal or antagonism of hormones promoting tumor growth and the administration of hormones inhibiting tumor growth. Prostate cancer is treated with estrogens, such as diethylstilbestrol; antiandrogens, such as flutamide; and gonadotropin-releasing hormone agonists (leuprolide and goserelin). When administered continuously in the form of long-acting injectables or implants, the releasing hormone agonists inhibit the release of gonadotropins, resulting in decreased testosterone production. Tamoxifen is an antiestrogen with partial agonist activity that is used in treating estrogen-sensitive breast cancer.

119. The answer is C.   *(Behavioral science)*

This man is likely to be homosexual. According to the DSM-IV, homosexuality is not a sexual dysfunction; rather, it is a normal variant of sexual expression. Homosexual individuals have normal gender identity and normal testosterone levels. Evidence of a genetic influence in homosexuality has been reported, and many homosexual individuals have a homosexual relative. Homosexual individuals often exhibit cross-gender behavior during childhood.

120. The answer is B.   *(Microbiology)*

Spores of *Clostridium botulinum* contaminate vegetables and meat. When foods are canned without adequate sterilization, spores survive and germinate in an anaerobic environment. As vegetative cells grow, toxin (eight types) is produced and released. Botulism is the poisoning that occurs after ingestion of the preformed toxin, which blocks the release of acetylcholine and results in muscle paralysis. Most of the *Clostridium botulinum* organisms are dead and likely do not contribute to the disease. Therefore, antibiotic therapy is not necessary. Appropriate management involves the use of antitoxin and assisted ventilation.

The other organisms listed grow in tissue and produce toxins and enzymes that relate to specific disease presentations. Antibiotics are beneficial in this setting.

121. The answer is E.   *(Biochemistry)*
N-acetylneuramic acid (NANA) is found frequently in glycoproteins and glycolipids and less frequently in glycosaminoglycans. It also is found in gangliosides, which are a subset of the glycolipids. NANA is never found in the phospholipids, which contain no carbohydrate.

122. The answer is E.   *(Microbiology)*
Ramsay-Hunt syndrome is caused by zoster (shingles) involving the VIIIth nerve. Vesicular lesions are noted in the ear canal. Zoster results from reactivation of latent varicella-zoster virus, a member of the herpesvirus family. Primary infection with the virus causes chickenpox.

The herpes simplex viruses (HSV) are responsible for a wide spectrum of disease states. Transmission of HSV type 1 (HSV-1) is primarily through saliva, whereas HSV type 2 (HSV-2) is transmitted primarily by direct sexual contact or from mother to newborn during birth.

Most primary infections are asymptomatic. Symptomatic infection with HSV-1 is seen most often in young children in the oral and perioral areas. Vesicular and ulcerative lesions, fever, sore throat, and edema occur approximately 3 to 5 days after infection. Swelling and tenderness of the gums (gingivostomatitis) are the most common features.

In adults, primary HSV-1 infection usually is seen as a pharyngitis or pharyngotonsillitis, with or without local lymphadenopathy.

A primary eye infection with HSV-1 can result in keratoconjunctivitis. Dendritic ulcers and vesicles on the eyelids are frequently seen. Recurrences are common in the eye and can lead to decreased visual activity.

HSV-1 is the most common cause of sporadic, fatal encephalitis in the United States. Involvement of the temporal lobe and presence of lymphocytes in the cerebrospinal fluid are characteristic of the disease.

Definitive diagnosis, however, usually requires isolation of the virus from a brain biopsy during the illness or at autopsy.

Neonatal herpes is acquired primarily at the time of birth from a mother with active genital disease due to HSV. However, infection of the newborn may also occur in utero or sometime shortly after birth. Approximately 75% of cases are caused by HSV-2. In newborns, lesions may be confined to the skin; encephalitis may be present without skin involvement; or the infection may be disseminated and involve many organs including the central nervous system.

123. The answer is E.   *(Pathology)*
The lesion in the lung represents a loosely formed granuloma with a prominent Langhan's multinucleated giant cell along the periphery of the lesion. The formation of granulomas involves cellular immunity, or type IV hypersensitivity. Some antigenic agents evoke a granulomatous type of chronic inflammation with the formation of discrete granulomas containing eosinophilic-staining epithelioid cells (activated macrophages), multinucleated giant cells (fused epithelial cells), and a rim of chronic inflammatory cells. Granulomas are formed as a reaction against an inert foreign body (e.g., glass) or as an immune response to a poorly degradable antigenic material (e.g., tuberculosis, systemic fungi).

Using tuberculosis (TB) as an example, the pathogenesis of a granuloma is as follows. Nonactivated alveolar macrophages phagocytize the TB organisms inhaled into the alveoli by droplet infection. The alveolar macrophages disseminate throughout the body. In these various locations, the macrophages process the TB antigens without killing the organisms. The macrophages eventually present the processed TB antigens to CD4 T-helper cells in 30 to 50 days. These cells interact with each others' class II antigen sites. Both cells are activated, resulting in the release of interleukin 1 (IL-1)/tumor necrosis factor (TNF) from the macrophages and lymphokines from CD4 T-helper cells, which include γ interferon (formerly called macrophage activating factor) and macrophage inhibitory factor. IL-1 and TNF recruit more CD4 helper T cells and stimulate B cell proliferation. γ interferon activates the macrophages, which results in the destruction of the TB organisms. The granular debris remaining from both dead macrophages and bacteria resembles cheese on macroscopic examination of the tissue, thus the term caseous necrosis. Macrophage inhibitory factor restrains the macrophages from leaving the inflammatory site, which contributes to the formation of well-circumscribed granulomas. Activated macrophages resemble epithelial cells on hematoxylin/eosin-stained slides, thus the term epithelioid cells. Fusion of the epithelioid cells results in the formation of multinucleated giant cells. Healing of a granuloma is by fibrosis often complicated by dystrophic calcification that is visible on a chest radiograph as a circumscribed nodule ("coin lesion") with flecks of calcification. These granulomas are the most common cause of a solitary coin lesion in the lung. Not all diseases that produce granulomas are associated with caseous necrosis. In tuberculosis and certain of the systemic fungi (e.g., histoplasmosis, coccidioidomycosis), granulomas start out without caseation (hard granulomas) and often progress into caseation at a later stage. Granulomas associated with sarcoidosis, Crohn disease, berylliosis, syphilitic gummas, tularemia, and other causes of granulomatous inflammation do not have caseation.

Antibodies and complement are the least important components in the pathogenesis of granulomas. CD4 T-helper cells, macrophages, γ interferon, and macrophage inhibitory factor all play a critical role.

124. The answer is B.   *(Biochemistry)*

The liver microsomal cytochrome P-450 mono-oxygenase system is the major pathway for the hydroxylation of aromatic and aliphatic compounds including drugs, steroids, and various alcohols. These oxidations serve to detoxify drugs and foreign compounds and convert them into water-soluble forms that are more readily excreted through the kidneys. The general reaction is as follows:

$$NADPH + O_2 + RH \text{----------> } NADP^+ + H_2O + ROH$$

Substrate RH can be a drug, steroid, fatty acid, or other chemical. This formation of ROH is called mono-oxygenation.

Cytochromes are heme proteins with a single iron protoporphyrin group (heme of hemoglobin has 4 irons attached to protoporphyrin) for binding with oxygen and substrate. They are present in all tissues except mature red blood cells. The supply of NADPH is critical for the functioning of the system. The cytochrome P-450 system can be induced ("revved up") by various compounds such as alcohol, phenobarbital, and rifampin (antibiotic). Cytochrome oxidase in the oxidative system can be inhibited by carbon monoxide.

Functions of cytochrome P-450 include:

- the synthesis of steroids in the adrenal cortex (e.g., aldosterone, cortisol)
- aromatization reactions (introduce an aromatic ring into the structure) in adipose tissue and the ovaries where androgens (e.g., testosterone, androstenedione) are converted into estrogens (e.g., estradiol, estrone).
- the oxidization of xenobiotics, which are lipophilic substrates that are foreign to the body (e.g., drugs, industrial chemicals, food additives, environmental contaminants). Addition of an –OH group makes compounds more polar and water soluble so they can be excreted in the urine.
- the generation of toxic metabolites called free radicals (unstable compounds with an unpaired electron in the outer orbit) that can damage tissue. For example, carbon tetrachloride (CCl_4) is used in the cleaning industry. When ingested, it is metabolized to a free radical (CCl_3) that severely damages the liver. Acetaminophen toxicity is another example of formation of a free radical with subsequent damage to the liver. Free radicals can be neutralized by glutathione (GSH), vitamin E, and vitamin C.

125-126. The answers are: 125-E, 126-C.   *(Behavioral science)*

Severe weight loss would occur as part of a pathological grief reaction involving depression, rather than a normal grief reaction. In a normal grief reaction, this 62-year-old woman might be expected to show mild anxiety, mild insomnia, and intermittent crying spells. Illusions, such as believing one sees a dead loved one, are not uncommon in a normal grief reaction.

Antidepressants are not indicated in a normal grief reaction. Providing reassurance and advice, increasing the frequency of medical appointments, and prescribing benzodiazepines if needed for insomnia are indicated in a normal grief reaction.

127-131. The answers are: 127-B, 128-F, 129-C, 130-E, 131-B. *(Biochemistry)*

Hepatocytes are one of the few types of cells in the body that can liberate free glucose; most cell types lack glucose 6-phosphatase. Therefore, in most nonhepatic cells, glucose, once phosphorylated, is fated to be metabolized. In contrast, the liver stores glucose as glycogen; it can then manufacture glucose, via glycogenolysis and then gluconeogenesis, and supply the rest of the body with glucose as the need arises. The last step of both gluconeogenesis and glycogenolysis is liberation of free glucose due to the action of glucose 6-phosphatase, which converts glucose 6-phosphate into glucose plus inorganic phosphate. Gluconeogenesis also takes place in the kidney cortex, in which gluconeogenic cells also express glucose 6-phosphatase. Individuals with Von Gierke disease, an autosomal recessive glycogen storage disease, have a deficiency of this enzyme in all cells.

Phosphocreatine is an alternative emergency-energy storage form in skeletal muscle, heart muscle, and brain tissue. The phosphate group is transferred from the creatine moiety to ADP by the action of phosphocreatine kinase to create ATP. Two different allelic sets express peptides that are active as a dimer, M and B. Therefore, the three isozymic forms of the enzyme are M_2(CK-3), B_2(CK-1), and MB(CK-2). [Recall that isozymes (isoenzymes) are enzymes that have the same catalytic function, but a different molecular structure.] Muscle uses exclusively the M_2-phosphocreatine kinase isozyme; brain, the B_2 isozyme; and, heart, a mixture of the M_2 and MB-isozymes. An increased serum level of MB-phosphocreatine kinase is the definitive sign of damage to the heart muscle. Serum enzyme levels begin to rise within 6 to 8 hours of an acute myocardial infarction, peak in 24 hours, and return to normal after 3 days.

The brain uses only glucose and ketone bodies as fuel. Under normal conditions, glucose is the primary source. In starvation, ketone bodies as well as glucose are used by the brain for fuel, only glucose by the erythrocytes, and fatty acids by muscle and some other tissues. Hypoglycemia, in the early fasting state, is characterized by symptoms relating to neuroglycopenia, or a brain without fuel, resulting in fatigue, mental state aberrations, and other behavioral disorders.

The metabolic activity of erythrocytes, which lack a nucleus and mitochondria, primarily consists of glycolysis and, when under oxidative stress, the hexose monophosphate shunt. The end product of glycolysis is lactate, which is used by the hepatocyte to synthesize glucose via gluconeogenesis. The production of lactate via anaerobic glycolysis in red blood cells, or by muscle cells during periods of oxygen debt, and its return to the liver and kidney for reconversion to glucose via gluconeogenesis is called the Cori cycle.

In humans, only hepatocytes have glycerol kinase activity, which converts glycerol into glycerol 3-phosphate. Therefore during triacylglyceride synthesis, the adipocyte cell must generate its glycerol de novo from glucose via glycolysis. Recall that insulin is required for fatty acid uptake in the adipocyte. Fatty acids derived from the action of capillary lipoprotein lipase are added to this newly synthesized glycerol to form triacylglycerides.

132-134. The answers are: 132-C, 133-A, 134-D. *(Behavioral science)*

The use of biofeedback training to raise peripheral temperature is effective in the treatment of Raynaud disease. If a teacher consistently fails to call on a child who is raising his hand, the hand-raising behavior will eventually disappear, or become extinct. Treating pedophilia by using electric shock paired with photographs of undressed children is based on the concept of classical conditioning and is known as aversive conditioning.

135-136. The answers are: 135-B, 136-C. *(Biochemistry)*

A Lineweaver-Burke plot (double-reciprocal plot) is useful because it gives a straight line when $1/V_0$ is plotted versus $1/[S]$. The intercept on the x axis is $-1/K_m$. The intercept on the y axis is $1/V_{max}$. Inhibitor #2 gives a line characteristic of a competitive inhibitor. Point B is equal to $-1/K_m$ in the presence of competitive inhibitor #2. Competitive inhibitors increase the apparent K_m of an enzyme for its substrate, but do not affect V_{max}.

Inhibitor #1 gives a line characteristic of a noncompetitive inhibitor. Point C is equal to $1/V_{max}$ in the presence of noncompetitive inhibitor #1. Noncompetitive inhibitors decrease the V_{max} of an enzyme without affecting the K_m.

137-141. The answers are: 137-B, 138-D, 139-E, 140-C, 141-A. *(Pharmacology)*
Erythropoietin is produced by the kidney in response to hypoxia. This agent is now available as a recombinant DNA product to treat or prevent anemia in patients with renal failure as well as bone marrow disorders, including aplastic anemia and various malignancies. Cyclosporine is a peptide antibiotic that not only is effective in the treatment of "graft-versus-host" syndrome in organ transplant patients, but also appears to block antigen activation of T cells. Cytokines approved for clinical use include two colony-stimulating factors (CSF), granulocyte CSF and granulocyte-macrophage CSF, used in reversing chemotherapy-induced leukopenia; interleukin-2 for treating metastatic renal cell carcinoma; and interferon-α for the treatment of such neoplastic disorders as Kaposi sarcoma and hairy cell leukemia.

142-143. The answers are: 142-D, 143-E. *(Biochemistry)*
The Michaelis constant, K_m, is a measure of the affinity of an enzyme for its substrate. It is defined as the substrate concentration that gives one half of the maximal velocity (V_{max}). A small K_m indicates high affinity, whereas a large K_m indicates low affinity.

When the sustrate concentration is much higher than the K_m (for example, point E), the velocity approaches V_{max}. The velocity is then independent of substrate concentration (zero order). At substrate concentrations much less than K_m (for example, point C), the velocity is directly proportional to the substrate concentration (first order).

144-148. The answers are: 144-D, 145-B, 146-A, 147-C, 148-E. *(Behavioral science)*
In this example of a concurrent cohort (prospective) study, a specific population (ninth-grade girls) that is free of the condition (pregnancy) at the start of the study is identified. Following assessment of exposure to the risk factor (not receiving sex education lectures), exposed and nonexposed subjects are compared to see who develops the condition (pregnancy).

In this example of a case-control (retrospective) study, subjects who have the disorder (fibrocystic breast disease) and subjects who do not have the disorder (disorders not involving the breast) are identified.

Information regarding prior exposure to the risk factor (birth control pill use) is obtained and compared using odds ratios.

The telephone sample is an example of a cross-sectional study, which provides information on possible risk factors (smoking) and health status (presence of upper respiratory infections) of people at one point in time.

In this example of a nonconcurrent cohort study, some activities may have taken place in the past (chemical exposure 30 years ago).

In this example of a clinical treatment trial, which is essentially a prospective study, the incidence of a condition (hemorrhoids) is determined in a cohort receiving one treatment (surgery) versus a cohort receiving a different treatment (diet).

149-153. The answers are: 149-F, 150-D, 151-B, 152-E, 153-C. *(Pharmacology)*
All of these substances are believed to act as cotransmitters and neuromodulators in the enteric nervous system and elsewhere. Neuropeptide Y causes long-lasting vasoconstriction, whereas dopamine is a vasodilator in renal blood vessels and nitric oxide dilates many vascular beds and mediates penile erection. Vasoactive intestinal peptide is widely distributed in the central and peripheral nervous systems. It also relaxes gastrointestinal smooth muscle and stimulates the release of several hormones. The enkephalins and substance P are found in secretomotor neurons in the enteric nervous system.

154-157. The answers are: 154-D, 155-B, 156-E, 157-C. *(Physiology)*
Dihydrotestosterone is responsible for masculinization of the external genitalia during prenatal development. Testosterone is the female libido hormone, whereas progesterone has a negative influence on sex drive in women. Deficient cortisone production during fetal life is a factor in the etiology of the adrenogenital syndrome.

158-162. The answers are: 158-D, 159-E, 160-C, 161-B, 162-A. *(Pharmacology)*
These enzyme inhibitors are used to treat neoplastic disease or tissue hypertrophy. Finasteride inhibits 5α-

testosterone reductase, which converts testosterone to dihydrotestosterone. Finasteride is used to treat benign prostatic hypertrophy and may be a future treatment for prostate cancer. Aminoglutethimide inhibits adrenal steroid synthesis and the enzyme aromatase, which converts adrenal androgens to estrone in adipose tissue. Aminoglutethimide is used to treat breast cancer and adrenal hyperplasia. Etoposide, which is used to treat small-cell lung cancer and testicular cancer, is a podophyllotoxin that inhibits topoisomerase II, causing DNA strand breaks. Methotrexate inhibits mammalian dihydrofolate reductase and the formation of active folic acid, which is required for purine and thymidine synthesis. Hydroxyurea inhibits ribonucleotide reductase, which converts ribonucleotides to deoxyribonucleotides in DNA synthesis. Hydroxyurea is a secondary agent for a variety of tumors, including those of the head, neck, and melanoma.

163-165. The answers are: 163-C, 164-E, 165-D. *(Microbiology)*
The child most likely has chickenpox, which is caused by the varicella-zoster virus (VZV), a member of the herpesvirus family. Both "chickenpox" and "varicella" refer to the disease that follows primary VZV infection. A unique feature of the varicella is the appearance of successive crops or waves of lesions, so that at any one given time the lesions may be in various stages of development (i.e., nonsynchronous pock development). Appearance of the rash correlates with viremia.

The distribution of the skin rash (as described in the case history), especially its presence in the scalp area, is typical of varicella. Vesicles are also frequently found on mucous membranes of the mouth, the conjunctivae, and the vaginal area. The thin-walled vesicles of varicella have the hallmark appearance of a "dew-drop on a rose petal." The rash is not painful, but it is very itchy. Excessive scratching may lead to scarring and superinfection with bacteria.

Varicella is a relatively mild, but highly contagious, disease of childhood. Peak incidence is from 3 to 5 years of age. Complications are rare, and the mortality rate is very low. Varicella has an incubation period of 14 to 21 days.

Cytomegalovirus (CMV), which is the etiologic agent of cytomegalic inclusion disease in newborns, is a common herpesvirus. About 90% of infants with the disease exhibit signs of central nervous system damage within the first 2 years of life. Severe hearing loss, ocular abnormalities, and mental retardation are common. Congenital or perinatal infection can result in fetal death. CMV is a leading cause of mental retardation in the United States.

Diagnosis of cytomegalic inclusion disease is often based on identification of large cells with "owl eye" intranuclear inclusion bodies (eccentric inclusions surrounded by a clear halo) in desquamated cells in the urine (best fluid for diagnosis) or in tissues. Inclusion bodies with this type of morphology are a hallmark of CMV disease.

Many pregnant women who have been previously infected with CMV will shed the virus in cervical secretions during the last trimester of gestation. The virus can also be shed in saliva, breast milk, semen, and urine. Most congenital infections are thought to be caused by transmission of reactivated virus in utero. However, clinical disease in infants is most often associated with primary CMV infection of the mother during pregnancy (transplacental, or vertical, transmission).

The student most likely has infectious mononucleosis caused by infection with the Epstein-Barr virus (EBV), a herpesvirus, which is primarily transmitted in the saliva by kissing. Approximately 35% to 75% of young adults will develop at least some signs of the disease after primary EBV infection. In addition to the symptoms experienced by this student, individuals with the disease may have hepatosplenomegaly and a petechial rash at the junction of the soft and hard palate. The hepatitis is usually anicteric (normal bilirubin) and rarely becomes chronic.

166-170. The answers are: 166-B, 167-E, 168-D, 169-A, 170-C. *(Pharmacology)*
Most antineoplastic agents cause reversible bone marrow suppression, and several drugs produce dose-limiting toxicities affecting vital organs. Although some toxicities may be prevented or treated (e.g., hydration and diuretics minimize cisplatin renal toxicity), most target organ effects are irreversible. Hydration can avert the cystitis that results from cyclophosphamide. Pulmonary fibrosis is a less common toxicity associated with bleomycin, but this condition is potentially fatal and should be monitored.

171-174. The answers are: 171-I, 172-G, 173-D, 174-O. *(Biochemistry)*
During posttranscriptional modification of mRNA in eukaryotes, a "cap" containing 7-methylguanosine is attached at the 5′ end of the molecule.

Intervening sequences, or "introns," are spliced out during posttranscriptional processing of eukaryotic mRNA. Such introns begin at their 5′ end with the sequence GU and end at their 3′ end with the sequence AG. The remainder of the intron can be of essentially any length or sequence.

During posttranscriptional processing of tRNA, the base sequence CCA is added to the 3′ end of the molecule. Amino acids become covalently attached to this portion of tRNA.

The process of translation, or protein synthesis, ends when the ribosome encounters a termination (nonsense) codon. The three nonsense codons are UGA, UAG, and UAA. CAAT, TATA, the Hogness box, and the Pribnow box are all associated with promoter regions for the initiation of transcription. The attenuator is a special termination signal for transcription that is sometimes used for prokaryotic genetic regulation. The polyadenylation sequence indicates where the poly A tail is to be attached during processing of eukaryotic mRNAs. The Shine-Delgarno sequence is a binding site for ribosomes on prokaryotic mRNA. AUG (adenosine-uracil-guanine) is the codon for methionine and is used as the initiation codon during protein synthesis. Formylmethionine, or fmet, is the amino acid used for initiation of protein synthesis in prokaryotes. GAATTC is a palindrome that is recognized by the restriction endonuclease *Eco* RI.

175-176. The answers are: 175-C, 176-D. *(Pathology)*
Although the early stages of acute inflammation are stereotyped regardless of the type of injurious agent, there is considerable variation in the tissue's response on a macroscopic level depending on the magnitude of this response and the nature and texture of the tissues involved.

A 45-year-old man with chronic renal failure and a pericardial friction rub would most likely have fibrinous inflammation, which consists of an exudate rich in fibrinogen that forms excess fibrin, producing a shaggy, "bread and butter" appearance to the surface of the pericardium. Increased vessel permeability and the deposition of fibrin are the key elements in this type of inflammation. Fibrinous pericarditis is also seen in rheumatic fever or in an acute transmural myocardial infarction.

An 8-year-old child with dysphonia, a gray-white exudate in the oropharynx and cervical lymphadenopathy most likely has pseudomembranous inflammation due to diphtheria. Pseudomembranous inflammation refers to toxin-induced superficial mucosal damage, with the formation of a necrotic membrane along the surface of the mucosa. Another example is the pseudomembrane of antibiotic-induced colitis from toxins elaborated by an overgrowth of *Clostridium difficile*.

Serous inflammation refers to the elaboration of a thin, watery exudate with insufficient amounts of fibrinogen to form fibrin material. This type of inflammation frequently occurs in body cavities (e.g., a viral-induced inflammation of the pleura) or in blister fluid in a second-degree burn.

Catarrhal (phlegmonous, coryza) inflammation connotes the excessive production of mucous secretions (e.g., a runny nose due to a rhinovirus infection, coryza in rubeola, the catarrhal stage of whooping cough).

Suppurative (purulent) inflammation refers to the collection of pus with localized liquefactive necrosis of the tissue to form an abscess (e.g., lung abscess). One organism that classically produces abscesses is coagulase positive *Staphylococcus aureus*. Coagulase helps generate fibrinous material to localize the infection. Pus consists of an exudate containing viable and nonviable neutrophils and microorganisms, along with debris from the digestion of parenchymal cells and their supporting stroma.

Some antigenic agents evoke a granulomatous type of chronic inflammation with the formation of discrete granulomas containing eosinophilic staining epithelioid cells (activated macrophages), multinucleated giant cells (fused epithelioid cells), and a rim of chronic inflammatory cells. Granulomas are formed as a reaction against an inert foreign body (e.g., glass) or as an immune response to poorly degradable antigenic material (e.g., tuberculosis, systemic fungi). Granulomatous inflammation involves interactions between T cells and macrophages and is a type of cellular immunity, or type IV hypersensitivity.

177-180. The answers are: 177-B, 178-C, 179-A, 180-E. *(Microbiology)*

Cephalosporins and penicillins are β-lactam antibiotics that interfere with development by blocking the final step of cross-linking. They block the transpeptidization step, resulting in incomplete cell walls that allow lysis to occur in an unfavorable osmotic situation.

Quinolones are synthetic analogues of nalidixic acid. They are active against many gram-positive and gram-negative bacteria. The mechanism of action of all quinolones involves the inhibition of bacterial DNA synthesis by blocking the DNA gyrase enzyme.

Rifampin is a derivative of rifamycin, an antibiotic produced by *Streptomyces* organisms. In vitro, it is active against some gram-positive cocci and gram-negative cocci, some enteric bacteria, mycobacteria, and chlamydiae. The prolonged use of rifampin as a single drug permits the selection and emergence of resistant mutants. There is no cross-resistance to other antimicrobial drugs. Rifampin binds strongly to DNA-dependent RNA polymerase and inhibits RNA synthesis in bacteria. It can penetrate phagocytic cells and kill intracellular microorganisms. Rifampin-resistant mutants exhibit an altered RNA polymerase.

Polymyxins are basic, cationic polypeptides that are nephrotoxic and neurotoxic. Polymyxins can be bactericidal for many gram-negative rods, including *Pseudomonas* and *Serratia*, by binding to cell membranes rich in phosphatidylethanolamine, interfering with the membrane's ability to function in active transport and as a permeability barrier. Because of toxicity, polymyxins are used primarily as topical agents.

Erythromycin inhibits protein synthesis by interfering with translocation reactions and with the formation of initiation complexes. Sulfonamides are bacteriostatic. Once removed, bacterial growth can resume. Sulfonamides affect a wide range of microorganisms.

Test 4

QUESTIONS

DIRECTIONS:

Each of the numbered items or incomplete statements in this section is followed by answers or by completions of the statement. Select the ONE lettered answer or completion that is BEST in each case.

1. IQ is normally distributed with a mean of 100 and a standard deviation of 15. Among 2000 people, how many will have IQs at or above 145?

(A) 3
(B) 15
(C) 25
(D) 135
(E) 270

2. A woman whose husband died 3 months ago complains that she has slept poorly since his death. Although she cries at dinnertime each evening, she goes out with a neighbor to play bingo every Tuesday night and sees her children on weekends. After you have talked to her for a few minutes, she reveals that she thinks she saw her husband walking down the street yesterday. As her primary care physician, what should you do?

(A) Prescribe a barbiturate for sleep
(B) Prescribe antidepressant medication
(C) Prescribe antipsychotic medication
(D) Refer her to a psychiatrist
(E) Provide support and reassurance

3. Which of the following characteristics classifies rubella or German measles as a Togavirus?

(A) Protein capsid
(B) Nucleic acid genome
(C) Lipid envelope
(D) Hemagglutinin
(E) Method of transmission

4. A 72-year-old woman who lives alone presents with numerous ecchymotic areas on her skin, glossitis, perifollicular hemorrhages, and swollen gums that bleed easily when touched. She also complains of pain in her legs. Her diet primarily consists of tea, crackers, and bologna. She is mildly anemic, and has a normal platelet count and a prolonged bleeding time. The patient most likely has

(A) scurvy
(B) pellagra
(C) von Willebrand disease
(D) a qualitative platelet disorder
(E) marasmus

5. A patient with diabetic ketoacidosis is likely to have

(A) oliguria secondary to dehydration
(B) an increased effective arterial blood volume
(C) a hyperchloremic normal anion gap metabolic acidosis before treatment
(D) an initial dilutional hyponatremia
(E) expansion of the intracellular fluid compartment

6. If $\Delta G^{0'}$ = -10.3 kcal/mol for the reaction

$$\text{phosphocreatine} \rightarrow \text{creatine} + \text{phosphate}$$

and $\Delta G^{0'}$ = +7.3 kcal/mol for the reaction

$$\text{adenosine diphosphate (ADP)} + \text{phosphate} \rightarrow \text{adenosine triphosphate (ATP)}$$

then what is the value of $\Delta G^{0'}$ for the following reaction?

$$\text{phosphocreatine} + \text{ADP} \rightarrow \text{ATP} + \text{creatine}$$

(A) -17.6 kcal/mol
(B) -10.3 kcal/mol
(C) -3.0 kcal/mol
(D) +3.0 kcal/mol
(E) +17.6 kcal/mol

7. The following are the arterial blood gases of two patients who are breathing room air.

	pH (7.35–7.45)	PaCO$_2$ (33–44 mm Hg)	PaO$_2$ (75–105 mm Hg)	Bicarbonate (22–28 mEq/L)
Patient A	7.20	70	50	27
Patient B	7.34	59	50	31

Which of the following statements concerning these patients is correct?

(A) Patients A and B have different primary acid–base disorders

(B) Patient A is less compensated than patient B

(C) Patients A and B most likely have normal oxygen saturations

(D) Patients A and B most likely have normal oxygenation of tissue

(E) Patient A has respiratory acidosis as compensation, whereas patient B has metabolic alkalosis as compensation

8. Which of the following viruses is most likely to be the cause of retinitis in a patient with AIDS?

(A) Epstein-Barr virus

(B) Varicella-zoster virus

(C) Herpes simplex virus type 1

(D) Herpes simplex virus type 2

(E) Cytomegalovirus (CMV)

9. A patient with diabetic ketoacidosis is vomiting. Both the ketoacidosis and vomiting are of equal severity. The arterial blood gases are most likely to exhibit which of the following changes in arterial pH, arterial carbon dioxide tension (PaCO$_2$), and bicarbonate (HCO$_3^-$)?

	pH	PaCO$_2$	HCO$_3^-$
(A)	Normal	Normal	Normal
(B)	Decreased	Increased	Decreased
(C)	Increased	Decreased	Increased
(D)	Normal	Increased	Increased
(E)	Normal	Decreased	Decreased

10. An increase in the serum level of creatine kinase isozyme 2 (CK$_2$) indicates that damage has occurred in the

(A) liver

(B) heart

(C) skeletal muscle

(D) lungs

(E) kidneys

11. A patient with chronic obstructive pulmonary disease, blue bloater type, is vomiting. Both the pulmonary disease and vomiting are of equal severity. Which of the following changes in arterial pH, arterial carbon dioxide tension (PaCO$_2$), and bicarbonate (HCO$_3^-$) would occur?

	pH	PaCO$_2$	HCO$_3^-$
(A)	Normal	Normal	Normal
(B)	Decreased	Increased	Decreased
(C)	Increased	Decreased	Increased
(D)	Normal	Increased	Increased
(E)	Normal	Decreased	Decreased

12. During a medical check-up for a new insurance policy, a 55-year-old grandmother tests positive in the screening assay for antibodies against HIV type 1. She has no known risk factors for exposure to the virus. Which of the following is the most appropriate next step?

(A) Perform the screening test a second time
(B) Attempt to grow the virus in cell culture
(C) Request that a polymerase chain reaction be performed
(D) Tell the patient that she is likely to develop AIDS
(E) Immediately begin therapy with azidothymidine

13. A patient with the following electrocardiogram would most likely

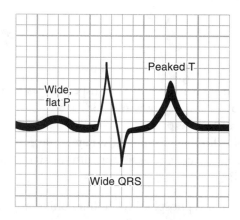

(A) be taking a loop diuretic
(B) have chronic renal failure
(C) have chronic diarrhea
(D) have been vomiting
(E) have been hyperventilating

14. Which of the following factors is most useful for predicating the direction of a chemical reaction?

(A) The change in entropy
(B) The change in free energy
(C) The change in enthalpy
(D) The temperature
(E) The heat of combustion of the substrate

15. Respiratory acidosis is most likely compensation for a patient who

(A) has overdosed on barbiturates
(B) is on nasogastric suction
(C) has chronic renal failure
(D) has Addison disease
(E) has salicylate intoxication

16. A diploid genome within a cylindric nucleoid is present in

(A) Influenza A
(B) Hantavirus
(C) Lassa virus
(D) HIV type 1 (HIV-1)
(E) Rotavirus

17. A normal anion gap metabolic acidosis most likely occurs in a patient who has

(A) diarrhea
(B) renal failure
(C) lactate acidosis
(D) diabetic ketoacidosis
(E) methyl alcohol poisoning

18. In biosynthesis, monosaccharides are most often added to growing oligosaccharide chains as the

(A) adenosine diphosphate (ADP) derivative
(B) coenzyme A (CoA) derivative
(C) adenosine monophosphate (AMP) derivative
(D) uridine diphosphate (UDP) derivative
(E) inosine monophosphate (IMP) derivative

19. A 55-year-old woman with Sjögren syndrome complains of muscle weakness. She has the following laboratory results:

Serum sodium	139 mEq/L	(135 to 147 mEq/L)
Serum potassium	2.0 mEq/L	(3.5 to 5.0 mEq/L)
Serum chloride	112 mEq/L	(95 to 105 mEq/L)
Serum bicarbonate (HCO_3^-)	15 mEq/L	(22 to 28 mEq/L)
Serum blood urea nitrogen	20 mg/dl	(7 to 18 mg/dl)
Serum creatinine	1.6 mg/dl	(0.6 to 1.2 mg/dl)
Urine pH	6.0	Varies with diet

Which of the following conditions does this patient most likely have?

(A) Acute tubular necrosis

(B) Uremia

(C) A renal defect in reabsorbing bicarbonate

(D) An increased anion gap metabolic acidosis

(E) Normal renal function

20. Antiviral proteins are induced in a host cell as a result of

(A) viral genome replication

(B) interferon attachment to a cytoplasmic membrane receptor

(C) interferon attachment to a nuclear receptor

(D) virion attachment to a receptor

(E) repression of an interferon gene that is normally consistently expressed

21. A patient with right-sided heart failure has dependent pitting edema. Which of the following is the most appropriate management of the patient's sodium and water intake?

	Sodium intake	Water intake
(A)	No change	Decrease
(B)	Increase	Increase
(C)	Decrease	No change
(D)	Decrease	Decrease
(E)	No change	No change

22. A newborn girl, with a suspected gestation age of 7 to 8 months, presents with labored breathing, hypoxia, and respiratory acidosis. A sample of the amniotic fluid is obtained. What is the most likely biochemical finding consistent with the symptoms described?

(A) A dioleicphosphatidylcholine:sphingomyelin ratio of more than 2:1

(B) A dipalmitoylphosphatidylcholine:sphingomyelin ratio of more than 2:1

(C) A dipalmitoylphosphatidylethanolamine:sphingomyelin ratio of less than 2:1

(D) A dipalmitoylphosphatidylethalanolamine:sphingomyelin ratio of more than 2:1

(E) A dipalmitoylphosphatidylcholine:sphingomyelin ratio of less than 2:1

23. Destruction of the juxtaglomerular apparatus results in

(A) a loss of hydrogen ions in the urine
(B) hyperaldosteronism
(C) an increase in angiotensin II
(D) metabolic alkalosis
(E) hyperkalemia

24. Which of the following is a lentivirus?

(A) Human papilloma virus (HPV) type 18
(B) HIV type 1
(C) HPV type 3
(D) Human T-cell leukemia virus type I
(E) Human herpesvirus 6

25. Hyponatremia and clinical evidence of dehydration are most likely to occur in a patient with

(A) an isotonic loss of fluid
(B) a hypotonic loss of pure water
(C) a hypertonic loss of fluid
(D) an isotonic gain of fluid
(E) a hypertonic gain of fluid

26. A gerontologist has several patients who complain that they have difficulty driving at night. Their specific complaint is that they can see only a few yards ahead after an approaching car has passed, even if the car did not have on its high beams. Some of these patients have gall bladder trouble, and others have been watching the fat content of their diets. The patients watching their fat content are on diets that are almost vegetarian. Most of their calories come from fat-free commercial cereals, which they eat with fat-free milk. They also eat fresh green salads with few red and orange vegetables, and they use little or no dressing. Some patients are taking a multivitamin supplement with their morning fat-free meal. The group with normal bile function is prescribed a geriatric multivitamin supplement to be taken with a tablespoon of canola oil. When they return in 6 months, most of the patients who complied with their prescription say that their ability to drive at night has markedly improved. Which of the following most likely explains what has occurred?

(A) The patients were developing cataracts due to essential fatty acid deficiency
(B) They were suffering from the first symptoms of vitamin E deficiency
(C) The patients were experiencing an age-related problem involving the absorption of fat-soluble vitamins
(D) Their diets were deficient in fat, and the fat-soluble vitamins were not being absorbed
(E) The patients were deficient in essential fatty acids, which were then supplied in the oil supplement prescribed

27. If an increased amount of sodium is presented to the distal tubule in the presence of aldosterone, an individual would most likely

(A) develop hypokalemia
(B) develop metabolic acidosis
(C) retain hydrogen ions
(D) have reduced exchange of sodium for potassium
(E) have decreased reabsorption of bicarbonate

28. Of the following risk factors for suicide, the one that is associated with the highest risk is

(A) male gender
(B) prior psychiatric illness
(C) age over 45 years
(D) recent divorce
(E) serious medical illness

29. The *arrows* represent the degree of magnitude of the gain (↑) or loss (↓) of sodium and water. Which of the following represents a patient who has a decrease in serum osmolality?

Total body sodium (TBNa)	Total body water (TBW)
(A) ↓	↓
(B) ↔	↓↓
(C) ↑↑	↑
(D) ↑	↑↑
(E) ↑	↑

30. Which of the following statements concerning vitamin A and its related compounds is most accurate?

(A) Mild cases of acne are treated by oral administration of all-*trans* retinoic acid (tretinoin)
(B) All-*trans* retinoic acid binds to opsin to form the visual pigment rhodopsin
(C) Retinol produces its effect via the generation of second messengers
(D) Spermatogenesis is dependent on the presence of all-*trans* retinoic acid
(E) Children on a vitamin A–deficient diet develop neural problems associated with bone resorption in the area of foramina

31. Respiratory alkalosis is expected to occur as compensation in a patient who

(A) has a pulmonary embolus
(B) has chronic bronchitis
(C) has a history of drinking antifreeze
(D) has hyperemesis gravidarum
(E) is taking a loop diuretic

32. Which of the following statements about HIV type 1 infection is correct?

(A) Only CD4+ T lymphocytes are infected with the virus
(B) Studies strongly suggest that the virus is a mutated simian virus
(C) Viral replication proceeds continually during the asymptomatic period
(D) Neurologic abnormalities are present only in a few patients with AIDS
(E) Infected individuals who develop AIDS do not produce neutralizing antibody

33. In the pathophysiology of right heart failure, which of the following is most likely to occur?

(A) An increase in venous return to the heart
(B) Inhibition of antidiuretic hormone release
(C) Secondary aldosteronism
(D) Decreased sodium reabsorption in the proximal tubules
(E) An increase in the effective arterial blood volume (EABV)

34. Which of the following disaccharides is the major repeating unit of dermatan sulfate?

(A) Galactosyl-β-1,4-glucose
(B) Galactosyl-β-1,4-acetylglucosamine
(C) Iduronate-β-1,3-acetylgalactosamine-4-sulfate
(D) Glucuronate-β-1,3-acetylglucosamine
(E) Glucuronate-β-1,3-acetylgalactosamine-6-sulfate

35. Which of the following sites is most susceptible to damage during hypovolemic shock?

(A) Purkinje cells in the cerebellum
(B) Renal tubules in the renal medulla
(C) Subendocardial tissue
(D) Hepatocytes around the central vein
(E) Tips of the villi in the small intestine

36. Children often have repeated pharyngeal infections with *Streptococcus pyogenes* because

(A) host immunity to *Streptococcus* is of short duration
(B) group A streptococci have multiple antigenic types of M protein
(C) antigenic drift or shift occurs frequently
(D) penicillin resistance is common with this bacterium
(E) children do not develop high titers of antibodies to streptolysins

37. Which of the following glycogen storage diseases is caused by a deficiency of a lysosomal enzyme?

(A) Pompe's disease
(B) McArdle's disease
(C) Von Gierke's disease
(D) Cori's disease
(E) Andersen's disease

38. Transmission of HIV type 1 (HIV-1) is most likely to occur through

(A) a mosquito bite
(B) a contaminated swimming pool
(C) kissing with exchange of saliva
(D) transfusion of factor VIII concentrate
(E) anal intercourse between men

39. A pediatrician examines a patient who has all the classic symptoms of rickets. A vitamin D supplement and exposure to sunlight are prescribed. However, the patient's condition does not improve. This patient most likely suffers from an inability to

(A) absorb vitamin D from the gut
(B) convert 7-dehydrocholesterol to cholecalciferol
(C) form 25-hydroxycholecalciferol in the liver
(D) form 25-hydroxycholecalciferol in the kidney
(E) form 1,25-dihydroxycholecalciferol in the kidney

40. Which one of the following statements is true about both doxorubicin and dactinomycin?

(A) Both agents are used to treat hypercalcemia
(B) Both agents are cell cycle–specific agents
(C) Both agents are plant alkaloids
(D) Both agents produce cardiac toxicity
(E) Both agents act by intercalating between DNA base pairs

41. Which of the following statements concerning vitamin K is most accurate?

(A) Vitamin K deficiency is the most common cause of prolonged clotting times
(B) It acts by influencing transcription in a manner similar to vitamins D and A
(C) It is a lipid-soluble antioxidant
(D) It enhances the calcium-binding properties of specific proteins
(E) It inhibits blood clotting by inactivating clotting factors synthesized in the liver

42. Which one of the following is an endogenous infection that occurs following oral trauma?

(A) Nocardiosis
(B) Chromoblastomycosis
(C) Histoplasmosis
(D) Dermatomycosis
(E) Actinomycosis

43. A boy whose mother has died suddenly can appreciate death's finality and feels guilty and responsible for her death. What is the most likely age of this child?

(A) 4 years
(B) 8 years
(C) 12 years
(D) 14 years
(E) 16 years

44. A febrile 28-year-old heroin addict who is HIV positive presents with tachypnea and severe hypoxemia. The patient most likely has pulmonary disease caused by

(A) *Streptococcus pneumoniae*
(B) *Haemophilus influenzae*
(C) *Mycoplasma pneumoniae*
(D) *Pneumocystis carinii*
(E) *Legionella pneumophila*

45. Sal I is a type-2 restriction endonuclease commonly used in recombinant DNA work. Of the following DNA sequences, the one most likely to be the recognition sequence for Sal I is

(A) GTAGTA
(B) GTCCTG
(C) GTCGAC
(D) GTACAT
(E) GCTCTG

46. A retrovirus most likely activates a cellular oncogene by

(A) insertional mutagenesis
(B) synthesizing a nuclease
(C) producing a cytolytic enzyme
(D) expressing no genes
(E) binding to cell ribosomes

47. Compliance with medical advice is most closely associated with which one of the following?

(A) Marital status
(B) Race
(C) Religion
(D) Educational level
(E) Quality of patient instruction (e.g., written directions)

48. Which of the following viruses is associated with the development of cancer in humans?

(A) JC virus
(B) Feline leukemia virus
(C) Hepatitis B virus
(D) Adenovirus
(E) Simian sarcoma virus

49. If a DNA molecule contains 22% adenine (molar percentage), then what is its cytosine content?

(A) 22%
(B) 28%
(C) 44%
(D) 56%
(E) 78%

50. The enzyme carried in the mature HIV type 1 virion is

(A) DNA-dependent RNA polymerase
(B) RNA-dependent RNA polymerase
(C) RNA-dependent DNA polymerase
(D) DNA-dependent DNA polymerase
(E) Integrase

Questions 51-52

The age of onset of disease X is normally distributed with a mean of 50 years and a standard deviation of 12 years.

51. The median age for contracting disease X is

(A) 38 years
(B) 50 years
(C) 55 years
(D) 62 years
(E) 74 years

52. The percentage of people that would be expected to develop disease X between the ages of 38 and 62 years is

(A) 34%
(B) 68%
(C) 95%
(D) 98%
(E) 99.3%

53. A cancer researcher conducted a medical experiment and failed to reject the null hypothesis although the experiment was successful. What type of error did this researcher make?

(A) A type I error
(B) A type II error
(C) A type III error
(D) An experimental error
(E) An inferential error

54. Which of the following is the most severe life stressor?

(A) Divorce
(B) Marriage
(C) Serious medical illness
(D) School graduation
(E) Birth of a child

55. A researcher is asked to develop a study to examine the relationship between the use of aspirin and gastric bleeding. What is the independent variable in this study?

(A) The presence of gastric bleeding
(B) The age of the patient
(C) The patient's history of tobacco use
(D) The patient's history of alcohol consumption
(E) The patient's use of aspirin

56. Each time an arthritis patient exercises, her joint pain is reduced. As a result, the patient increases the number of times she exercises per week. What is this an example of?

(A) Sensitization
(B) Habituation
(C) Positive reinforcement
(D) Negative reinforcement
(E) Extinction

57. Investigators identified 255 women with breast cancer and 790 women without breast cancer seen at two hospitals in Newark, New Jersey in 1985. On the basis of interviews and data analyses, it was determined that women with breast cancer are more likely to have a first-degree relative with breast cancer than women with disorders not involving the breast. This study is a

(A) cross-sectional study
(B) case-control study
(C) prospective cohort study
(D) historical cohort study
(E) randomized clinical treatment trial

58. Which one of the following statements is true regarding the prevalence of schizophrenia in the United States?

(A) Schizophrenia is more prevalent among men than women

(B) Schizophrenia is more prevalent among Catholics than Protestants

(C) Schizophrenia is more prevalent among blacks than whites

(D) The prevalence of schizophrenia is approximately 1%

(E) The prevalence is the same in all socioeconomic groups

59. Six patients were hospitalized for different lengths of time: 6, 5, 4, 2, 5, and 20 days. What is the most appropriate measure of central tendency for these data?

(A) Range

(B) Median

(C) Mean

(D) Standard deviation

(E) Standard error

60. A medical student who was uncomfortable in the gross anatomy lab at the beginning of the semester becomes more comfortable as the semester progresses. What is this an example of?

(A) Sensitization

(B) Habituation

(C) Positive reinforcement

(D) Negative reinforcement

(E) Extinction

61. A researcher wants to assess the strength of association between height and body weight. Which of the following is the most appropriate statistical test?

(A) Correlation

(B) Independent t-test

(C) Analysis of variance

(D) Dependent t-test

(E) Chi-squared test

62. Even after consulting with a consultation-liaison psychiatrist, a 37-year-old woman who is 7 months pregnant refuses treatment that is required to save the life of her fetus. Both her physician and the consulting psychiatrist determine that the woman is mentally competent. What should the physician do next?

(A) Get a court order to do the procedure

(B) Tell the patient that she will be prosecuted if she does not consent to the procedure

(C) Force the patient to have the procedure

(D) Tell the patient that she is killing her child if she does not consent to the procedure

(E) Accept that the woman does not want to undergo the procedure

63. If a strand of DNA with the base sequence AGTACTGC is used as a template for transcription, what sequence would the RNA product have? (All distractors are written in the conventional 5′ to 3′ direction.)

(A) AGTACTGC

(B) AGUACUGC

(C) UCAUGACG

(D) GCAGUACU

(E) GCAGTACT

Questions 64-65

Use these scores to answer the following questions: 5, 7, 4, and 8

64. What is the standard deviation?

(A) $\sqrt{10}/3$
(B) $\sqrt{3}/10$
(C) $\sqrt{10}/4$
(D) $\sqrt{4}/10$
(E) $\sqrt{10}/6$

65. What is the standard error?

(A) $1.83/\sqrt{2}$
(B) $2/1.83$
(C) $1.83/4$
(D) $4/1.83$
(E) $1.83/\sqrt{4}$

66. A liver cell is most likely to differ from a kidney cell in its

(A) nuclear DNA
(B) mitochondrial DNA
(C) ribosomal RNA
(D) transfer RNA
(E) messenger RNA

67. Which one of the following statements is true about both cyclophosphamide and cisplatin?

(A) Both agents crosslink DNA strands
(B) Both agents must be activated by cytochrome P-450 enzymes
(C) Both agents are cell cycle–specific agents
(D) Both agents cause relatively little myelosuppression
(E) Both agents are inorganic metal complexes

68. Which of the following is more likely to involve women than men?

(A) Homocide
(B) Suicide
(C) Alcoholism
(D) Major depression
(E) Obsessive-compulsive personality disorder

69. Which antibiotic enhances rickettsial growth?

(A) Erythromycin
(B) Sulfonamides
(C) Tetracycline
(D) Penicillin
(E) Chloramphenicol

70. The minimal inhibitory concentration (MIC) and minimal bactericidal concentration (MBC) are reflective of

(A) selective toxicity
(B) range
(C) sensitivity
(D) resistance
(E) growth rate

71. A researcher wants to assess the strength of association between age and blood pressure. Which of the following is the most appropriate statistical test?

(A) Correlation
(B) Independent t-test
(C) ANOVA
(D) Dependent t-test
(E) Chi-square test

72. Soluble substances found in the matrix of a mitochondrion include all of the

(A) enzymes of the tricarboxylic acid (TCA) cycle
(B) enzymes involved in β-oxidation of fatty acids
(C) DNA responsible for the synthesis of the proteins associated with oxidative phosphorylation
(D) enzymes of the urea cycle
(E) enzymes associated with the electron transport system

73. The Epstein-Barr virus is associated with the development of African Burkitt lymphoma. Which of the following statements regarding this association is correct?

(A) *Plasmodium* species is often recovered from the neoplastic cells
(B) The neoplastic cells do not express virus-specific antigens
(C) The viral DNA cannot be detected in neoplastic cells
(D) Ingestion of aflatoxin increases the risk for tumor development
(E) Overexpression of the *c-myc* gene is a common finding

74. Azidothymidine (AZT) blocks replication of HIV type 1 because it

(A) binds to the *tat* gene and prevents viral transcription
(B) is a nucleoside analog that is incorporated into viral DNA
(C) binds to the long terminal repeats of the viral genome
(D) induces mutations in the *env* gene so that the virus cannot bind to cells
(E) enzymatically degrades viral mRNA

75. A 29-year-old technician in a primate research laboratory develops fever, myalgia, paraesthesia, and diplopia. Acute ascending paralysis and other signs of nervous system involvement appear during the next 2 weeks. The patient dies shortly thereafter of respiratory paralysis. Which of the following viruses is most likely implicated in this case?

(A) Herpes simplex virus type 1
(B) Herpes simplex virus type 2
(C) Herpes B virus
(D) Cytomegalovirus
(E) Rabies virus

76. Measurement of the initial velocity (V_0) of an enzyme-catalyzed reaction as a function of substrate concentration [S] produces the following data.

[S] (mmol/L)	V_0 (μmol/min)
0	0
0.5	5
2	20
5	40
10	60
20	80
100	80

The approximate K_m of the enzyme for the substrate is

(A) 5 mmol-L
(B) 10 mmol-L
(C) 20 mmol-L
(D) 40 mmol-L
(E) 50 mmol-L

77. If the pK_a for acetic acid is 4.8, what is the pH of a solution containing 0.1 mol-L acetate and 0.01 mol-L acetic acid?

(A) 2.8
(B) 3.8
(C) 4.8
(D) 5.8
(E) 6.8

78. The mutant enzyme from a patient with a genetic disease is isolated, and its kinetic properties are studied. The following diagram shows results of a study of initial reaction velocity (V_0) as a function of a substrate concentration [S].

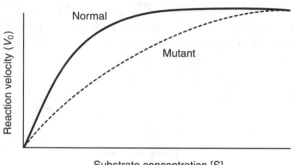

The mutant enzyme differs from the normal enzyme in that

(A) the mutant enzyme has a higher K_m

(B) the mutant enzyme has a lower K_m

(C) the mutant enzyme has a higher maximum velocity (V_{max})

(D) the mutant enzyme has a lower V_{max}

(E) the equilibrium constant for the reaction is lower in the presence of the mutant enzyme

79. A patient with AIDS is likely to have

(A) a normal hemoglobin concentration

(B) intact directed chemotaxis by neutrophils and monocytes

(C) decreased p24 core protein

(D) intact activation of macrophages

(E) hypergammaglobulinemia

80. Exposure of an arterial blood gas specimen to room air would most likely have which of the following effects on the arterial oxygen tension (PaO_2) and arterial carbon dioxide tension ($PaCO_2$)?

	PaO_2	$PaCO_2$
(A)	No change	No change
(B)	Decreased	Increased
(C)	No change	Increased
(D)	Increased	Decreased
(E)	Increased	No change

81. A patient with the following electrocardiogram would most likely have

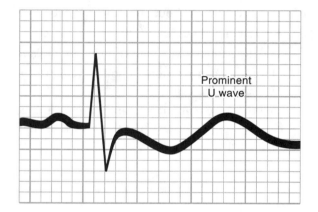

(A) Addison disease

(B) an acute myocardial infarction

(C) primary hyperparathyroidism

(D) primary aldosteronism (Conn syndrome)

(E) acute tubular necrosis

82. Which of the following is more characteristic of vitamin D deficiency in children, rather than adults?

(A) Looser lines (pseudofractures) in the metaphysis of bone

(B) Osteopenia on radiograph

(C) Bowing of the legs

(D) Craniotabes

(E) Decreased mineralization of bone

83. A gram-positive coccus was isolated from a wound. It was β-hemolytic, catalase positive, and coagulase positive. It would be identified as

(A) *Streptococcus pneumoniae*
(B) *Streptococcus pyogenes*
(C) *Enterococcus faecalis*
(D) *Staphylococcus aureus*
(E) *Staphylococcus epidermidis*

84. Your 75-year-old male patient had a stroke 3 weeks ago. During an examination, you discover that he has prostate cancer. His wife asks you not to tell him about the cancer because the shock and fear will kill him. What should you do?

(A) Tell the patient about the cancer immediately
(B) Avoid telling the patient about the cancer
(C) Tell the patient's wife to tell him about the cancer
(D) Have the consultation–liaison psychiatrist tell him about the cancer
(E) Tell the patient about the cancer if in your medical opinion you believe that this information will not harm him

Questions 85-86

The following diagram shows the pedigree of a family in which some members may have the ΔF508 allele for cystic fibrosis. The ΔF508 allele contains a three-base deletion in the coding region of the gene for the cystic fibrosis transmembrane regulator (CFTR) protein. Also shown are DNA fragments produced by framing the site of the mutation with two oligonucleotide primers, performing the polymerase chain reaction (PCR), and separating the products by electrophoresis. M probe = 63 bp, Z probe = 60 bp.

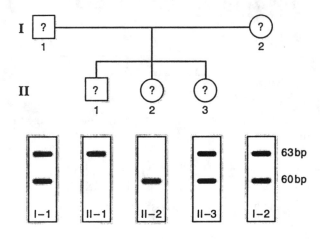

85. In this family, the individual who is affected by cystic fibrosis is

(A) I-1
(B) I-2
(C) II-1
(D) II-2
(E) II-3

86. What is the effect of the ΔF508 mutation on the CFTR protein?

(A) The amino acid sequence is garbled as a result of a frameshift mutation.
(B) The protein is shortened as a result of a nonsense mutation.
(C) One amino acid is missing from the protein.
(D) The protein contains a single amino acid substitution.
(E) The amino acid sequence is unchanged.

Questions 87-88

Severe pulmonary complications arose after surgery on an obese middle-aged male. An arterial PO_2 of 60 mm Hg was obtained after the administration of 40% O_2. Assume that TBP = 760 mm Hg and R = 0.8 and an ideal $PACO_2$ of 40 mm Hg.

87. What is the A-a gradient for O_2?

(A) 4 mm Hg
(B) 65 mm Hg
(C) 40 mm Hg
(D) 109 mm Hg
(E) 175 mm Hg

88. What is the most likely cause of his hypoxemia?

(A) Hypoventilation due to central nervous system depression
(B) Extensive pulmonary edema as a result of lung injury, in this situation, adult respiratory distress syndrome (ARDS)
(C) Anemia, due to overtransfusion of fluids
(D) Inadequate tidal volume resulting from obesity

DIRECTIONS:

Each of the numbered items or incomplete statements in this section is negatively phrased, as indicated by a capitalized word such as NOT, LEAST, or EXCEPT. Select the ONE lettered answer or completion that is BEST in each case.

89. All of the following relate to patient compliance EXCEPT

(A) the patient's understanding of the instructions
(B) the patient's belief that the regimen will work
(C) the provision of written instructions about the regimen
(D) the patient's level of education
(E) the quality of the patient's relationship with the physician

90. Which of the following clinical findings is **LEAST** likely to be associated with mumps infections?

(A) Meningitis
(B) Parotitis
(C) Gastritis
(D) Pancreatitis
(E) Orchitis

91. All of the following are characteristic of scurvy, rather than rickets, EXCEPT

(A) disruption of epiphyseal bone growth
(B) normal mineralization of bone
(C) loss of teeth
(D) hemarthroses
(E) anemia

92. All the following viruses are associated with fetal or neonatal infections EXCEPT

(A) herpes simplex virus type 2
(B) cytomegalovirus
(C) rubella virus
(D) hepatitis A virus
(E) hepatitis B virus

93. Multinucleated cells are LEAST likely associated with which of the following combinations of diseases?

(A) Histoplasmosis and rubeola
(B) Congenital toxoplasmosis and cytomegalovirus infection
(C) Rubeola and dementia in AIDS
(D) Herpes virus infections and Crohn disease
(E) Sarcoidosis and anaplastic cancers

94. *Chlamydia trachomatis* and *Chlamydia pneumoniae* share all of the following properties and characteristics EXCEPT

(A) infective stage as the elementary body
(B) growth in cell culture
(C) susceptibility to doxycycline
(D) reproduction by binary fission within the host cell lysosome
(E) implication in inclusion conjunctivitis and interstitial pneumonia of the newborn

95. Which of the following vitamin relationships is NOT correct?

(A) Riboflavin deficiency—scaly dermatitis in nasolabial folds and scrotum
(B) Niacin deficiency—Cassal necklace
(C) Vitamin A deficiency—Bitot spot
(D) Pyridoxine deficiency—convulsions in newborns
(E) Vitamin E deficiency—keratomalacia

96. All of the following statements about positive-sense RNA viruses are true EXCEPT

(A) viral messenger RNA is synthesized using a virion associated with RNA transcriptase
(B) virus particles lack a virion associated with RNA transcriptase
(C) viral RNA is messenger RNA
(D) replication of viral RNA occurs in the presence of inhibitors of DNA synthesis
(E) replication of viral RNA occurs in the presence of actinomycin D

97. Which of the following relationships is NOT correct?

(A) Pantothenic acid—component of coenzyme A (CoA) and fatty acid synthase
(B) Thiamine—cofactor in transketolase reactions and pyruvate dehydrogenase complex
(C) Niacin—essential component of flavin adenine dinucleotide (FAD) and flavin mononucleotide
(D) Pyridoxine—transaminase reactions
(E) Biotin—carboxylase reaction involved in the synthesis of oxaloacetate

98. Which of the following sets of laboratory data causes an osmotic gradient with the LEAST movement of water into the intracellular fluid compartment? Assume the normal serum osmolality is 275 to 295 mOsm/kg.

	Serum sodium (mEq/L)	Serum glucose (mg/dl)	Serum blood urea nitrogen (mg/dl)
(A)	120	90	12
(B)	130	108	24
(C)	140	90	72
(D)	145	126	90
(E)	145	126	120

99. Which of the following relationships is NOT correct?

(A) Magnesium—cofactor for adenylate cyclase
(B) Chromium—component of glucose tolerance factor, which potentiates insulin
(C) Copper—component of lysyl oxidase, cytochrome c oxidase, ferroxidase, and superoxide dismutase
(D) Selenium—component of glucose-6-phosphate dehydrogenase
(E) Zinc—cofactor for enzymes involved in collagen metabolism

100. Polyvalent crotalid antivenins may be used to neutralize the toxic effects of venoms of all of the following snakes EXCEPT the

(A) eastern coral snake
(B) western diamond rattlesnake
(C) copperhead snake
(D) cottonmouth snake
(E) eastern diamond rattlesnake

101. Which of the following is NOT a dietary recommendation for cancer prevention?

(A) Avoidance of obesity
(B) Decrease in total fat intake to less than 30% of total calories
(C) Decrease in the intake of caffeine products
(D) Increase in the intake of dark green, deep yellow, and orange vegetables
(E) Reduced intake of salt-cured, smoked, and nitrite-cured foods

102. Which of the following is LEAST likely to be involved in the pathophysiology of endotoxic shock?

(A) Decreased production of nitric oxide
(B) Activation of the alternate complement pathway
(C) Increased release of interleukin-1 and tumor necrosis factor
(D) Generation of anaphylatoxins
(E) Production of myocardial depressant factor

103. Nutritional changes associated with aging include all of the following EXCEPT

(A) decreased absorption of vitamin A
(B) decline in the need for calories
(C) decreased absorption and utilization of pyridoxine (B_6)
(D) reduction in the need for iron in women
(E) increased need for calcium

104. All of the following microorganisms are prokaryotes EXCEPT

(A) *Mycoplasma*
(B) *Chlamydia*
(C) *Rickettsia*
(D) *Corynebacterium*
(E) *Aspergillus*

105. Which of the following associations is NOT correct?

(A) Biotin deficiency—increased consumption of raw egg whites
(B) Folate deficiency—alcoholism
(C) Iron deficiency—pure vegetarian diet with no iron supplements
(D) Vitamin B_{12} deficiency—ovolactovegetarian diet
(E) Pyridoxine deficiency—therapy with isoniazid

106. For all of the following clinical disorders, the primary alterations in Starling forces are correct EXCEPT for

	Clinical disorder	Hydrostatic pressure	Oncotic pressure
(A)	Pulmonary edema in heart failure	↑	↔
(B)	Dependent pitting edema in heart failure	↑	↔
(C)	Pitting edema in kwashiorkor	↔	↓
(D)	Ascites in malabsorption	↔	↓
(E)	Ascites in cirrhosis	↑	↔

↑ Increase
↓ Decrease
↔ No effect

107. Which of the following relationships is NOT correct?

(A) Hartnup disease—defect in the intestinal and renal uptake of neutral and essential amino acids resulting in a pellagra-like disorder

(B) Cystinuria—defect in the intestinal and renal uptake of cysteine, lysine, ornithine, and arginine, leading to an increase in hexagonal-shaped cystine crystals in the urine and stone formation

(C) Tyrosinemia—deficiency of tyrosinase resulting in severe liver disease and renal tubular acidosis

(D) Histidinemia—increase in urinary imidazole pyruvic acid and mental retardation in some cases

(E) Maple syrup urine disease—deficiency of branched chain α-ketoacid dehydrogenase resulting in a sweet-smelling urine, neurologic problems, and increased mortality

108. All of the following are true about hospitalized medical patients EXCEPT

(A) depression is commonly experienced by medical inpatients

(B) approximately 20% of medical inpatients have psychiatric disorders

(C) psychotherapy is useful for medical inpatients with psychological problems

(D) behavioral therapy is useful for medical inpatients with psychological problems

(E) patients with a history of psychiatric illness are at particular risk for developing psychological problems if they are hospitalized

109. Which one of the following statements regarding *Streptococcus* is LEAST accurate?

(A) Viridans streptococci, important causes of diarrhea, are identified on the basis of their ability to ferment lactose

(B) Group B β-hemolytic streptococci, an important cause of neonatal sepsis, are identified on the basis of their ability to hydrolyze hippurate

(C) *Streptococcus faecalis*, an important cause of urinary tract infections, can grow in 6.5% sodium chloride (NaCl)

(D) *Streptococcus pneumoniae*, an important cause of pneumonia, is inhibited by optochin

(E) *Streptococcus mutans* is the most significant organism involved in caries production

110. Which type of histone is LEAST likely to be found in the nucleosome core?

(A) H1
(B) H2A
(C) H2B
(D) H3
(E) H4

111. A 30-year-old male homosexual presents with unexplained weight loss, swollen lymph nodes, and raised, red skin lesions on his chest. Which of the following would confirm a diagnosis of AIDS?

(A) Identification of the skin lesions as Kaposi sarcoma
(B) A CD4+ cell count of greater than 200/µl of blood
(C) Generalized lymphadenopathy
(D) Disseminated adenocarcinoma of the colon
(E) Positive antibody test for HIV

112. Which of the following is LEAST likely to be true about sexuality in a 55-year-old postmenopausal woman, as compared with sexuality in a 35-year-old premenopausal woman?

(A) Her libido is decreased
(B) Her sexual activity is decreased
(C) She experiences more vaginal dryness
(D) She experiences more discomfort during intercourse
(E) Her vaginal walls are thinner

113. Virus isolation in cell culture is useful for all of the following conditions EXCEPT

(A) genital herpes
(B) zoster
(C) influenza
(D) genital warts
(E) mumps

114. Unlike bacterial resistance to antibiotics, tumor cell resistance to antineoplastic drugs does NOT usually involve

(A) enzymatic inactivation of antineoplastic drugs
(B) increased drug efflux from tumor cells
(C) increased repair of tumor cell DNA
(D) decreased affinity of the target enzyme for the drug
(E) amplification of the target enzyme of a drug

115. All of the following are true about the correlation between drugs of abuse and sexuality EXCEPT

(A) marijuana enhances the enjoyment of sex primarily by physiological means
(B) marijuana use often results in an immediate increase in libido
(C) cocaine use is associated with priapism
(D) heroin impairs ejaculation
(E) long-term use of alcohol is associated with decreased male potency

116. In which one of the following conditions would blood culture provide the LEAST information?

(A) Osteomyelitis
(B) Brucellosis
(C) Typhoid fever
(D) Tetanus
(E) Bacterial pneumonia

117. All of the following wound repair relationships are correct EXCEPT

(A) third-degree burns—keloid formation
(B) liver injury—regeneration, scar tissue formation, or both
(C) lung injury—repair of alveolar epithelium by type I pneumocytes
(D) central nervous system injury—gliosis secondary to astrocytes
(E) peripheral nervous system injury—axon regeneration

118. A patient with a chronic stenosing lesion of the common bile duct would LEAST likely have a problem with

(A) follicular hyperkeratosis
(B) bleeding
(C) mineralization of bone
(D) tetany
(E) deficiency of B$_{12}$

119. Latex agglutination tests are routinely used to diagnose infections caused by all the following organisms EXCEPT

(A) *Streptococcus pneumoniae*
(B) group A streptococcus
(C) *Neisseria meningitidis*
(D) *Haemophilus influenzae*
(E) *Chlamydia trachomatis*

Questions 120-121

A 54-year-old man has been diagnosed with hypertension. Answer the following questions regarding his likelihood of complying with medical advice.

120. Which of the following variables is LEAST likely to be related to whether he takes his prescribed medication?

(A) Complexity of the treatment regimen
(B) Duration of treatment
(C) Presence of symptoms
(D) Educational level
(E) Waiting-room time

121. According to the Health Belief Model, the likelihood of this patient complying with medical advice increases with all of the following factors EXCEPT

(A) the patient feels ill
(B) the patient's activities have been disrupted by illness
(C) the patient believes that the cost of the treatment outweighs its benefits
(D) the patient feels that it is practical to obtain health care
(E) the patient believes he can overcome impediments to obtain needed care

DIRECTIONS:

Each set of matching questions in this section consists of a list of four to twenty-six lettered options (some of which may be in figures) followed by several numbered items. For each numbered item, select the ONE lettered option that is most closely associated with it. To avoid spending too much time on matching sets with large numbers of options, it is generally advisable to begin each set by reading the list of options. Then for each item in the set, try to generate the correct answer and locate it in the option list, rather than evaluating each option individually. Each lettered option may be selected once, more than once, or not at all.

Questions 122-123

Match each patient with the appropriate personality type.

(A) Schizoid
(B) Obsessive-compulsive
(C) Passive-aggressive
(D) Schizotypal
(E) Paranoid

122. An obese patient who is subconsciously angry with her physician begins arriving late for her weekly appointments with him and continues to gain weight.

123. A faculty member in a medical school wrongly claims that his research productivity is poor because someone took his research ideas.

Questions 124-128

For each drug, select the steroid receptor(s) it binds.

(A) Aldosterone
(B) Estrogen
(C) Androgen, progesterone, and glucocorticoid
(D) Glucocorticoid and progesterone
(E) Androgen
(F) Androgen and aldosterone

124. Danazol

125. Mifepristone

126. Clomiphene

127. Cyproterone and flutamide

128. Spironolactone

Questions 129-133

For each patient described, select the most closely associated personality type.

(A) Passive–aggressive
(B) Antisocial
(C) Paranoid
(D) Schizoid
(E) Obsessive–compulsive
(F) Dependent
(G) Borderline
(H) Histrionic
(I) Depressive
(J) Avoidant

129. A 56-year-old single man who has voluntarily limited his contact with others has been content with his solitary job as a night watchman for the past 25 years.

130. A 35-year-old female patient says that she has fallen in love with you. When you recommend that she see another physician, she attempts suicide.

131. A 56-year-old female patient arrives in your office dressed in a low-cut blouse and describes her flu symptoms in an emotional, colorful fashion.

132. A 45-year-old male patient always arrives 15 minutes late for his appointment.

133. A 60-year-old male patient tells you that he has filed three lawsuits against the town for infringing on his property and has filed complaints against two doctors who formerly treated him.

Questions 134-138

For each description, choose the appropriate complex carbohydrate or lipid.

(A) Chondroitin sulfate
(B) *N*-linked glycoprotein
(C) Dermatan sulfate
(D) Ganglioside
(E) *O*-linked glycoprotein
(F) Sphingomyelin
(G) Glycogen
(H) Hyaluronic acid

134. Dolichol phosphate is required for synthesis.

135. The difference between A and B red blood cell antigens resides in the sugar bound in this type of structure

136. Storage of this substance is associated with Niemann-Pick disease

137. Storage of this substance is associated with Tay-Sachs disease

138. Storage of this substance is associated with Pompe's disease

Questions 139-143

For each disease, select the biologic material the vaccine is made from.

(A) Bacterial toxoid
(B) Killed bacteria
(C) Killed virus
(D) Live attenuated virus
(E) Bacterial polysaccharide

139. Whooping cough

140. Diphtheria

141. Tetanus

142. Hepatitis B, influenza, and rabies

143. Measles, mumps, polio, and rubella

Questions 144-149

Match each description with the type of reinforcement it describes.

(A) Continuous
(B) Fixed ratio
(C) Fixed interval
(D) Variable ratio
(E) Variable interval

144. A patient needs to reach a very busy doctor, but keeps getting a busy signal. The only way she is going to get through is if she manages to call when the doctor is between conversations. She begins dialing the doctor's office very frequently.

145. A medical student who has a failing average in one of his courses studies harder as the final approaches to avoid failing the course.

146. A medical student allows himself a candy bar after each set of 50 pages of a physiology text he reads.

147. An office worker patronizes a vending machine that is in good working order.

148. A gambler continues to play the same slot machine in Atlantic City.

149. A fisherman spends the morning fishing.

Questions 150-152

For each of the following descriptions, select the appropriate disease.

(A) Phenylketonuria
(B) Alcaptonuria
(C) Maple syrup urine disease
(D) Homocystinuria
(E) Histidinemia

150. A patient's urine darkens when voided.

151. It is caused by a deficiency of phenylalanine hydroxylase.

152. It is caused by a deficiency of branched-chain α-keto acid dehydrogenase used in the breakdown of the branched-chain amino acids.

Questions 153-154

For each set of physical findings, select the most likely associated virus.

(A) Epstein-Barr virus
(B) Human papilloma virus (HPV) type 18
(C) Human T-cell leukemia virus type I (HTLV-I)
(D) Hepatitis B virus
(E) Herpes simplex virus type 2

153. A 45-year-old female presents with profuse intermenstrual bleeding and pain in the lumbosacral region. Severe koilocytic dysplasia is noted in a Pap smear.

154. A 60-year-old male presents with moderate lymphadenopathy, skin lesions, and hepatosplenomegaly. Hypercalcemia and a high white blood cell count are noted. The lymphocytes in the peripheral blood appear to be abnormal. Histologic examination of skin biopsy shows prominent dermal and subcutaneous infiltration by lymphocytes.

Questions 155-158

Match each of the following descriptions with the appropriate term.

(A) Anticodon
(B) A site
(C) Attenuator
(D) Chain termination codon
(E) Elongation factor
(F) Enhancer
(G) Operator
(H) Promoter
(I) P site
(J) Release factor
(K) Repressor
(L) Rho factor
(M) Shine-Delgarno sequence
(N) σ Factor

155. A protein subunit of *Escherichia coli* RNA polymerase involved in initiation of transcription

156. A binding site on DNA for RNA polymerase

157. A regulatory sequence in eukaryotic DNA that does not have to be in a fixed location and influences the rate of transcription

158. The part of the ribosome to which fMet-tRNA binds

Questions 159-163

Match each cancer with the drug used to treat it.

(A) Chlorambucil
(B) Mechlorethamine
(C) Prednisone
(D) Cytarabine
(E) Busulfan

159. Chronic myelogenous leukemia

160. Hodgkin disease

161. Acute lymphocytic leukemia

162. Acute myelogenous leukemia

163. Chronic lymphocytic leukemia

Questions 164-169

Match each of the following descriptions with the appropriate vitamin.

(A) Vitamin A
(B) Vitamin D
(C) Vitamin K
(D) Vitamin E
(E) Ascorbic acid
(F) Thiamine
(G) Riboflavin
(H) Niacin
(I) Biotin
(J) Folic acid
(K) Vitamin B_{12}
(L) Vitamin B_6 (pyridoxine)
(M) Pantothenic acid

164. It is a water-soluble vitamin that is stored in the liver.

165. It is primarily involved in amino acid metabolism.

166. It is a precursor of NAD^+ and $NADP^+$.

167. It is synthesized in the body from tryptophan.

168. It is the precursor of coenzyme A.

169. It is required for hydroxylation of proline and lysine.

Questions 170-171

For each of the following descriptions, select the associated disease.

(A) Respiratory acidosis
(B) Respiratory alkalosis
(C) Metabolic acidosis
(D) Metabolic alkalosis

170. The bicarbonate (HCO_3^-) concentration is increased and the arterial pH is decreased.

171. The HCO_3^- concentration is decreased and the arterial pH is decreased.

Questions 172-175

Match each of the following descriptions with the appropriate element.

(A) Chromium
(B) Cobalt
(C) Copper
(D) Iodine
(E) Iron
(F) Manganese
(G) Magnesium
(H) Molybdenum
(I) Selenium
(J) Zinc

172. It is a required cofactor in all kinase reactions.

173. A deficiency of this element in adults causes loss of taste and smell.

174. It helps lower blood glucose levels.

175. A deficiency of this element causes goiter.

Questions 176-180

For each term, choose the word or phrase with which it is most closely associated.

(A) Habituation
(B) Sensitization
(C) Modeling
(D) Shaping
(E) Discriminative stimulus
(F) Extinction
(G) Conditioned response
(H) Unconditioned stimulus
(I) Continuous reinforcement
(J) Variable ratio reinforcement

176. A woman who has received five intravenous chemotherapy treatments becomes nauseated when she sees the needle at the start of the sixth treatment.

177. A child receives candy each time he prints a letter more clearly.

178. A third-year medical student observes a surgeon doing a procedure on a patient before attempting it herself.

179. After 4 weeks of Gross Anatomy lab, a medical student no longer notices the smell of formaldehyde.

180. After 4 weeks of Gross Anatomy lab, a medical student is more bothered by the smell of formaldehyde that she was on the first day of lab.

ANSWER KEY

1. A	31. C	61. A	91. A	121. C	151. A
2. E	32. C	62. E	92. D	122. C	152. C
3. B	33. C	63. D	93. B	123. E	153. B
4. A	34. C	64. A	94. E	124. C	154. C
5. D	35. B	65. E	95. E	125. D	155. N
6. C	36. B	66. E	96. A	126. B	156. H
7. B	37. A	67. A	97. C	127. E	157. F
8. E	38. E	68. D	98. C	128. A	158. I
9. A	39. E	69. B	99. D	129. D	159. E
10. B	40. E	70. C	100. A	130. G	160. B
11. D	41. D	71. A	101. C	131. H	161. C
12. A	42. E	72. B	102. A	132. A	162. D
13. B	43. B	73. E	103. A	133. C	163. A
14. B	44. D	74. B	104. E	134. B	164. K
15. B	45. C	75. C	105. D	135. E	165. L
16. D	46. A	76. A	106. E	136. F	166. H
17. A	47. E	77. D	107. C	137. D	167. H
18. D	48. C	78. A	108. B	138. G	168. M
19. C	49. B	79. E	109. A	139. B	169. E
20. B	50. C	80. D	110. A	140. A	170. A
21. D	51. B	81. D	111. A	141. A	171. C
22. E	52. B	82. D	112. A	142. C	172. G
23. E	53. B	83. D	113. D	143. D	173. J
24. B	54. C	84. E	114. A	144. E	174. A
25. C	55. E	85. D	115. A	145. C	175. D
26. D	56. D	86. C	116. D	146. B	176. G
27. A	57. B	87. E	117. C	147. A	177. D
28. C	58. D	88. B	118. E	148. D	178. C
29. D	59. B	89. D	119. E	149. E	179. A
30. E	60. B	90. C	120. D	150. B	180. B

ANSWERS AND EXPLANATIONS

1. The answer is A. *(Behavioral science)*
Among 2000 people, 3 people (0.15% of the population of 2000) would be expected to have an IQ of 145 or greater.

2. The answer is E. *(Behavioral science)*
You should provide support and reassurance to this woman whose husband died 3 months ago; she is experiencing a normal grief reaction. Although she cries at dinnertime each evening, she is showing an effort to get back to her former lifestyle by going out with her neighbor and seeing her children weekly. The illusion that she thinks she saw her husband walking down the street is not uncommon in a normal grief reaction. You need not prescribe medication or refer this woman to a psychiatrist at this time.

3. The answer is B. *(Microbiology)*
Rubella virus is the only member of the *Rubivirus* genus in the Togaviridae family. It is not transmitted by arthropods.

Rubella is often compared with measles (rubeola), a paramyxovirus, because both involve rashes in infected individuals. Paramyxoviruses have negative-sense RNA (opposite base composition from messenger RNA), a helical capsid, lipid envelope, and a hemagglutinin, as does rubella. The main difference is that rubella contains a positive-sense RNA genome. Positive-sense indicates that the RNA has the same base composition as messenger RNA.

Although rubella is transmitted in aerosol droplets, similar to those of measles, the method of transmission has nothing to do with placement in the togavirus grouping.

4. The answer is A. *(Pathology)*
The patient has scurvy, caused by vitamin C deficiency from a diet lacking citrus fruits, green vegetables, and other fruits and vegetables.
Key clinical findings in scurvy include:

- subperiosteal hemorrhages secondary to vessel instability from defective collagen synthesis; this is one of the reasons for severe bone pain in this patient.

- hemarthroses (bleed into joints), which is another reason for bone pain
- hemorrhagic folliculitis (ring hemorrhages around the hair follicles)
- poor wound healing
- gum hyperplasia, bleeding, periodontal disease, loss of teeth, and glossitis
- ecchymoses from vessel instability
- a scorbutic rosary in children from increased abnormal osteoid in the epiphyses

Laboratory findings include:

- anemia (iron deficiency and/or folate deficiency)
- an increased bleeding time (unstable vessels)
- decreased amount of ascorbic acid in leukocytes or platelets

Pellagra is caused by a niacin deficiency. It is characterized by the 3 Ds—diarrhea, dementia, and dermatitis. The dermatitis involves increased pigmentation in sun-exposed areas, like Cassal necklace, which is a classic finding.

Classic von Willebrand disease is an autosomal dominant disease with absence of von Willebrand factor (defect in platelet adhesion producing a prolonged bleeding time) and decreased factor VIII antigen and VIII coagulant. The disease would not present in the manner described in the question because it is not related to a nutritional problem.

A qualitative platelet disorder refers to a functional platelet abnormality, rather than a quantitative problem (thrombocytopenia or thrombocytosis). An example is aspirin blocking cyclooxygenase and preventing synthesis of thromboxane A_2 (platelet aggregating agent) in the platelet. This prolongs the bleeding time, but does not produce the findings in this patient.

Marasmus is characterized by a low caloric intake. Dietary deficiencies are compensated for by the breakdown of protein and fats. Although this patient could have developed or will develop marasmus, the clinical findings are more specific for scurvy.

5. The answer is D. *(Pathology)*
A patient with diabetic ketoacidosis is likely to have an initial dilutional hyponatremia because of the osmotic effect of glucose in the extracellular fluid drawing water

out of the intracellular fluid compartment, which dilutes the sodium concentration. The following formula corrects for this dilutional effect.

Corrected serum sodium = measured serum sodium + (glucose/100 x 1.5)

For example, if glucose is 1000 mg/dl and serum sodium is 130 mEq/L, then

Corrected serum sodium = 130 mEq/L + (1000/ 100 x 1.6) = 146 mEq/L

Eventually, sodium depletion occurs caused by a loss of water and sodium from the osmotic effect of glucose in the urine (osmotic diuresis). Because the renal loss is hypotonic, hypernatremia usually occurs.

6. The answer is C. *(Biochemistry)*
The final reaction is obtained by adding the first two reactions. The standard free energy change, $\Delta G^{0'}$, for the overall reaction is calculated by adding the two $\Delta G^{0'}$s for the two independent reactions. A negative $\Delta G^{0'}$ predicts that the reaction will proceed spontaneously in the direction written, whereas a positive $\Delta G^{0'}$ predicts that the reaction will proceed in the opposite direction. An energetically unfavorable reaction can be driven forward by coupling it to a reaction that releases a large amount of free energy.

7. The answer is B. *(Pathology)*
To interpret arterial blood gas disorders, define respiratory disorders by comparing the patient's measured arterial carbon dioxide tension ($PaCO_2$) to the reference intervals in the laboratory; in this case, it is 33 to 44 mm Hg. A patient with respiratory alkalosis, or increased clearing of carbon dioxide (hyperventilation), has a $PaCO_2$ less than 33 mm Hg. A patient with respiratory acidosis, or hypoventilation, has a $PaCO_2$ greater than 44 mm Hg. Similarly, metabolic

acidosis and alkalosis are defined by the reference limit for bicarbonate; in this case, it is 22 to 28 mEq/L. Metabolic acidosis is defined as a bicarbonate less than 22 mEq/L, whereas metabolic alkalosis is defined as a bicarbonate greater than 28 mEq/L. The pH (normal range 7.35 to 7.45) defines whether the primary process is an acidemia (pH less than 7.35) or an alkalemia (pH greater than 7.45). As shown in the table below, compensation for an alkalosis is always acidosis, and compensation for acidosis is always alkalosis. With rare exceptions, compensation does not bring the pH back to the normal range. The pH reflects the primary process in the patient.

For example, consider a patient with a $PaCO_2$ less than 33 mm Hg (respiratory alkalosis), a bicarbonate less than 22 mEq/L (metabolic acidosis), and a pH greater than 7.45 (alkalemia). This patient has a primary respiratory alkalosis, because the pH is alkalemic, with a compensatory metabolic acidosis. If the bicarbonate was normal, it would be an uncompensated respiratory alkalosis.

Patient A has findings that are consistent with a primary respiratory acidosis that is uncompensated, because the bicarbonate is not outside the normal range. Because the pH is acidic in patient B, the patient has a primary respiratory acidosis with partial compensation with metabolic alkalosis. It is partial compensation because the pH is not in the normal range. Full compensation (pH in the normal range) does not normally occur.

8. The answer is E. *(Microbiology)*
Cytomegalovirus (CMV) retinitis is a common finding in patients with AIDS, particularly when the patient's CD4+ cell count falls below 50 cells/µl. The condition usually begins as a painless decrease in vision. If untreated, the lesion expands outward and may lead to complete blindness. Although initially only one eye may be involved, the contralateral retina is likely to

Disorder	pH	Bicarbonate	$PaCO_2$	Compensation
Metabolic alkalosis	Alkalemia	Increased	Increased	Respiratory acidosis
Metabolic acidosis	Acidemia	Decreased	Decreased	Respiratory alkalosis
Respiratory alkalosis	Alkalemia	Decreased	Decreased	Metabolic acidosis
Respiratory acidosis	Acidemia	Increased	Increased	Metabolic alkalosis

be affected in untreated cases. ocular *Toxoplasma* infection may occasionally mimic CMV retinitis.

The Epstein-Barr virus is prevalent in AIDS patients and has been associated with the development of lymphoma, particularly lymphoma of the central nervous system (CNS). Nucleic acid sequences specific for the virus are detectable in virtually all AIDS-associated CNS lymphomas. Epstein-Barr virus is also implicated as the cause of oral hairy leukoplakia, white frond-like lesions on the tongue, which is frequently seen in individuals infected with HIV type 1.

Because most individuals with AIDS are adults who have already been infected with the varicella-zoster virus during childhood, zoster (i.e., shingles) may appear as the result of reactivation of latent virus. The zoster is usually self-limiting, even in patients with relatively advanced HIV 1 infection.

Oral and genital lesions, because of reactivation, account for most of the morbidity associated with the herpes simplex viruses in patients with AIDS. The frequency and extent of reactivation episodes are more severe than in the general population. Herpes simplex virus is a relatively common cause of acute retinal necrosis in patients with AIDS and is associated with mild to moderate pain, myositis, and optic neuritis. Ocular structures in addition to the retina are frequently involved and can lead to concurrent conjunctivitis, scleritis, and keratitis.

9. The answer is A.   *(Pathology)*

This question explores the concept of mixed acid–base disorders, in which there are two or more disorders present simultaneously. Conceptually, consider each acid–base disorder as a teaspoon of that disorder being added to a pot. The result is a combination of the individual pHs, arterial carbon dioxide tensions (Pa_{CO_2}), and bicarbonates (HCO_3^-) of the acid–base disorders. The following is an example, with the arrows representing degrees of increase or decrease:

	pH	Pa_{CO_2}	HCO_2^-
Metabolic acidosis	↓	↓	↓↓
Respiratory acidosis	↓	↑↑	↑
Final results	↓↓	Normal to ↑	Normal to ↓

An additive effect on pH occurs in cardiorespiratory arrest: metabolic acidosis + respiratory acidosis.

Note that the pH is markedly decreased, whereas the Pa_{CO_2} and HCO_3^- vary from normal to immediately outside the normal range.

The opposite effect on pH occurs in a patient with uremia who is vomiting: metabolic acidosis + metabolic alkalosis.

	pH	Pa_{CO_2}	HCO_3^-
Metabolic acidosis	↓	↓	↓↓
Metabolic alkalosis	↑	↑	↑↑
Final results	Normal	Normal	Normal

Note that the pH, Pa_{CO_2}, and HCO_3^- neutralize each other because the acid–base disorders are exactly opposite of each other.

Therefore, if a patient with diabetic ketoacidosis is vomiting and both conditions are of equal severity, the arterial blood gases exhibit the same findings as shown for metabolic acidosis (ketoacidosis) and metabolic alkalosis (vomiting); that is, a normal pH, normal P_{CO_2}, and a normal HCO_3^-.

10. The answer is B.   *(Biochemistry)*

There are three isozymes of creatine kinase that are distinguished by their electrophoretic mobilities. Myocardial muscle contains a relatively large fraction of creatine kinase isoenzyme 2 (CK_2). Following a myocardial infarction, CK_2 is released from the damaged heart muscle and begins to appear in the plasma in about 4 to 8 hours. It reaches peak plasma levels at about 24 hours and disappears in 36 to 72 hours.

11. The answer is D.   *(Pathology)*

This question involves the concept of mixed acid–base disorders, in which there are two or more disorders present simultaneously. Consider each acid–base disorder a teaspoon of that disorder being added to a pot. The result is a combination of the individual pHs, arterial carbon dioxide tensions (Pa_{CO_2}), and bicarbonates (HCO_3^-) of the acid–base disorders.

A patient with chronic obstructive pulmonary disease would have respiratory acidosis, and vomiting would produce metabolic alkalosis. The combination of these two conditions should normalize the pH and have an additive effect on both the Pa_{CO_2} and HCO_3^-.

	pH	PaCO$_2$	HCO$_3^-$
Metabolic alkalosis	↑	↑	↑↑
Respiratory acidosis	↓	↑↑	↑
Final results	Normal	↑↑↑	↑↑↑

12. The answer is A. *(Microbiology)*

In populations with a low prevalence of HIV type 1 infection, a positive result in the enzyme-linked immunosorbent assay (ELISA) may be a false positive. A blood sample should be tested a second time. If the repeat ELISA is positive, the results should be confirmed using a test such as the Western blot; radio-immune precipitation and immunofluorescence assays are also available.

The Western Blot test is less likely to give a false positive than the ELISA because the viral antigens are separated electrophoretically before addition of serum. Direct comparisons are made with known positive and negative controls. Also, a small proportion of individuals may have antibodies against cell components that may be present as contaminants in the viral preparations used in the ELISA. Recent immunization with the influenza vaccine has also been reported to give transient false-positive ELISA results in a few individuals.

13. The answer is B. *(Pathology)*

The electrocardiogram exhibits a peaked T wave, which indicates hyperkalemia. Chronic renal failure is a common cause of hyperkalemia, because tubular damage interferes with the excretion of potassium.

Hyperkalemia is less common than hypokalemia. It is potentially more dangerous to cardiac function than hypokalemia, because it decreases the intracellular–extracellular potassium ratio, which hypopolarizes the cell membrane. Hypopolarization of the cell membrane causes a higher resting transmembrane electrical potential that is closer to the membrane threshold. This produces the following electrocardiographic findings:

- Between 5.6 and 6.0 mEq/L, tall, peaked T waves are best observed in the precordial leads. They are the result of enhanced repolarization.
- Between 6.0 and 6.5 mEq/L, there is a reduction in impulse conduction, which often causes prolonged PR and QT intervals.

- Between 6.5 and 7.0 mEq/L, there are diminished P waves and depressed S-T segments, which is also seen in angina and cerebrovascular accidents because of catecholamine release.
- Above 7 mEq/L, an intracardiac block occurs. The block begins in the atria, then involves the atrioventricular node, and finally involves the ventricles, causing the heart to stop during diastole. In the presence of hyponatremia and hypocalcemia, this situation is worsened.

In patients with severe hyperkalemia (less than 7.0 mEq/L), intravenous calcium gluconate reverses the electrocardiographic findings immediately by raising the threshold potential of neuromuscular tissue, thus reestablishing the difference between the resting transmembrane potential and the threshold potential.

14. The answer is B. *(Biochemistry)*

The change in free energy, ΔG, can be used to predict the direction of a chemical reaction. If ΔG is negative, then the reaction proceeds spontaneously as written. If ΔG is positive, then the reaction proceeds in the opposite direction. Neither the change in entropy, ΔS, nor the change in enthalpy, ΔH, can by itself predict the direction of the reaction. Likewise, the temperature and the heat of combustion of the substrate have no predicative value.

15. The answer is B. *(Pathology)*

According to the Henderson-Hasselbalch equation, the arterial pH is proportional to the ratio of HCO$_3^-$/ PCO$_2$, which is normally approximately 20 to 1. Because the relationship is a ratio, an increase or decrease in either the HCO$_3^-$ or PCO$_2$ concentration automatically alters the arterial pH. For example, a primary increase in serum HCO$_3^-$ causes an increase in arterial pH, or metabolic alkalosis. A primary increase in arterial PCO$_2$ decreases arterial pH, causing respiratory acidosis. Compensation for acid–base disorders is an attempt to bring the ratio back to 20 to 1, which should bring the pH back to the normal range (full compensation).

Except for individuals who live in the Andes mountains in Peru, who have a fully compensated chronic respiratory alkalosis, full compensation rarely occurs. Instead, the arterial pH is brought close to, but not into, the normal range (partial compensation). By looking at the ratio of HCO_3^-/P_{CO_2}, it can be noted that for compensation to occur, it must always move in the same direction as the primary process. For example, if metabolic alkalosis (increased bicarbonate) is the primary process, respiratory acidosis (increased P_{CO_2}) must occur as compensation to bring this ratio as close as possible to 20 to 1.

16. The answer is D. *(Microbiology)*

All retroviruses, including HIV type 1 (HIV-1), have a diploid genome (i.e., there are two complete copies of the RNA carried within mature virions). The nucleocapsid of retroviruses has both icosahedral and helical symmetry; HIV-1, which has a cylindrical or bar-shaped nucleoid, is an exception. Presence of a core with this type of morphology is unique and is diagnostic for HIV-1.

Influenza A has single-stranded RNA in 8 segments, which are prone to genetic reassortment. This virus is responsible for major epidemics and pandemics of influenza.

Hantavirus has single-stranded RNA, which is triple-segmented. It is a rodent-borne bunyavirus associated with severe respiratory distress and rapidly progressive pulmonary edema.

Lassa virus is in the arenavirus family and has single-stranded, double-segmented RNA. It is the etiological agent of a severe hemorrhagic fever.

Rotaviruses have double-stranded RNA in 8 to 12 segments. They are a major cause of diarrheal illness in infants.

17. The answer is A. *(Pathology)*

A normal anion gap metabolic acidosis is expected in a patient who has diarrhea, because there is a loss of bicarbonate in the stool that is counterbalanced by an equal gain of chloride to normalize the anion gap.

Metabolic acidosis is classified into two types: increased anion gap and normal anion gap. Because there is an equal number of positive and negative charges, there is no anion gap (which refers to less negative than positive charges). However, to separate the two types of metabolic acidosis, the following formula was devised to differentiate them. Only sodium (Na), chloride (Cl), and bicarbonate (HCO_3^-) are used in the formula:

$$\text{Anion gap} = Na - (Cl + HCO_3^-) = 140 \text{ mEq/L} - (104 \text{ mEq/L} + 24 \text{ mEq/L}) = 12 \text{ mEq/L}$$

According to this relationship involving the most common cation (Na) and the most common anions (Cl and HCO_3^-), there are 12 anions unaccounted for, which are the anions not represented in the formula, mainly albumin, phosphate, and organic acids. Thus, an increase in the anion gap indicates the presence of other anions (e.g., lactate, acetoacetate) that are not normally increased in the plasma.

An increased anion gap metabolic acidosis involves the addition of an acid to the extracellular fluid compartment. Some of the hydrogen ions from the acid are buffered by HCO_3^-, and the loss of HCO_3^- caused by buffering is replaced by the anion of the acid to maintain electroneutrality. Examples of this type of metabolic acidosis include ketoacidosis (diabetes, starvation, alcoholism), lactic acidosis, uremia, salicylate poisoning, methyl alcohol poisoning, and ethylene glycol poisoning.

For example, if a patient has lactic acidosis and the HCO_3^- is lowered to 14 mEq/L (normal is 24 mEq/L), the anion gap is:

$$\uparrow\text{Anion gap} = 140 - (104 + 14) = 22 \text{ mEq/L } (12 \pm 2)$$

The 10 mEq/L unaccounted-for anions greater than the normal of 12 mEq/L represent the lactate anions.

Normal anion gap type involves losing HCO_3^-; the loss of negative charges is counterbalanced by an equal gain in Cl anions (hyperchloremic metabolic acidosis). This occurs when HCO_3^- is lost in the gastrointestinal tract or in the urine. Examples of this include diarrhea, cholestyramine (resin binds HCO_3^-), renal tubular acidosis (proximal and distal types), primary hyperparathyroidism (increased parathormone decreases HCO_3^- reabsorption in the proximal tubule), and carbonic anhydrase inhibitors (which block HCO_3^- reabsorption in the kidneys).

Because the HCO_3^- that is lost is counterbalanced by an equal gain in Cl anions, the anion gap remains the same. For example, assume the serum HCO_3^- decreases to 14 mEq/L. This decrease is counterbalanced by an equal gain in serum Cl from a normal of 104 mEq/L to 114 mEq/L. Assuming the serum Na remains the same, the anion gap equals 140 − (114 + 14) = 12 mEq/L, which is normal.

18. The answer is D.   *(Biochemistry)*
Sugars are most often involved in reactions with uridine triphosphate (UTP) to form the uridine diphosphate (UDP) derivative plus free pyrophosphate (PP$_i$). The monosaccharide is then incorporated into a growing polysaccharide chain as the UDP derivative. This is the procedure used for the synthesis of glycogen, the glycosaminoglycans, and the O-linked glycoproteins. The major exception is in the synthesis of the *N*-linked glycoproteins, during which a polysaccharide containing *N*-acetylglucosamine, mannose, and glucose is coupled to dolichol, an 80- to 100-carbon chain lipid. In this case, the mannose units are added as the guanosine diphosphate (GDP) derivative.

19. The answer is C.   *(Pathology)*
The patient has renal tubular acidosis with a normal anion gap metabolic acidosis, which is commonly associated with tubulointerstitial disease in patients with Sjögren syndrome.

Metabolic acidosis is divided into increased anion gap and normal gap types. Because there is an equal number of positive and negative charges, there is no anion gap. However, to differentiate the two types of metabolic acidosis, the following formula was devised. Only sodium, chloride, and bicarbonate (HCO$_3^-$) are used in the formula:

$$\text{Anion gap} = \text{Na} - (\text{Cl} + \text{HCO}_3^-) = 140 \text{ mEq/L} - (104 \text{ mEq/L} + 24 \text{ mEq/L}) = 12 \text{ mEq/L}$$

Normal anion gap type involves losing HCO$_3^-$; the loss of negative charges is counterbalanced by an equal gain in chloride anions (hyperchloremic metabolic acidosis). This occurs when HCO$_3^-$ is lost in the gastrointestinal tract or in the urine. Examples of this include diarrhea, cholestyramine (resin binds HCO$_3^-$), renal tubular acidosis (proximal and distal types), primary hyperparathyroidism (increased parathormone decreases HCO$_3^-$ reabsorption in the proximal tubule), and carbonic anhydrase inhibitors (block HCO$_3^-$ reabsorption in the kidneys).

In proximal renal tubular acidosis type 2, there is a defect in reabsorbing HCO$_3^-$ in the proximal tubule due to lowering of the renal threshold of bicarbonate reabsorption (e.g., 15 mEq/L instead of the normal 24 mEq/L), causing a loss of HCO$_3^-$ in the urine. It also causes an alkaline urine pH, which becomes more acidic when the serum HCO$_3^-$ drops to 15 mEq/L.

Bicarbonaturia results in a normal anion gap metabolic acidosis. The increased negative charge in the tubule urine from the HCO$_3^-$ draws out positive charges, similar to potassium, thus hypokalemia also occurs. Because the ratio of intracellular to extracellular potassium concentration is the principal determinant of membrane potential in excitable tissue, hypokalemia increases the ratio, which results in hyperpolarization of the cell membranes. Thus, the resting transmembrane electrical potential is lowered and the distance from the threshold potential is increased, causing muscle weakness.

In distal renal tubular acidosis type 1, there is a defect in the aldosterone-dependent hydrogen ion/potassium pump in the collecting tubules. The inability to secrete hydrogen ions hinders HCO$_3^-$ reabsorption. Hydrogen ions are needed to bind with HCO$_3^-$ in the tubular lumen to form carbonic acid, which dissociates into water and carbon dioxide. The carbon dioxide diffuses into the renal tubular cell to form carbonic acid again, and this dissociates into hydrogen ions and HCO$_3^-$, the latter being reabsorbed. Therefore, inability to secrete hydrogen ions results in a loss of HCO$_3^-$ in the urine, which alkalinizes the urine pH. Inability to secrete hydrogen ions also results in potassium loss in the urine, thus producing hypokalemia. The hydrogen ions that diffuse back into the cell combine with chloride that is reabsorbed to offset the HCO$_3^-$ loss, thus producing a normal anion gap metabolic acidosis.

The type of renal tubular acidosis in this patient (type 1) requires special testing (e.g., infusion of acid to document an inability to excrete hydrogen ions). The hypokalemia was responsible for her muscle weakness. Her serum blood urea nitrogen and creatinine concentration are slightly increased, indicating tubular dysfunction that is most likely related to tubulointerstitial disease associated with Sjögren syndrome.

20. The answer is B.   *(Microbiology)*
The role of interferons (IFNs) in limiting viral growth was one of the first functions of these cytokines to be recognized. Interferons are produced by white blood cells (lymphocytes) and fibroblasts. Viral attachment and entry into a permissible host cell (cell #1) allows a virus growth cycle to occur that results in the assembly and release of mature virions. As a result of viral nucleic acid replication, IFN genes in host cell #1 are

activated and IFN is produced and released from the cell. IFN then binds to a receptor on a second permissible host cell (cell #2) and a signal is sent to the nucleus of cell #2, resulting in the production of an antiviral protein that interferes with the growth cycle of any viruses attempting to grow in cell #2. Viral messenger RNA (mRNA) is degraded without significantly affecting cellular mRNA metabolism. This sequence of events takes place within hours of virus infection and lessens the virus load that must be eliminated by the host's immune system. α- and β-IFN are more efficient in controlling viral growth than γ-IFN.

21. The answer is D.   (Pathology)

In right-sided heart failure, there is a hypotonic gain of water and sodium from the kidneys because of a decrease in effective arterial blood volume (EABV). Because both water and sodium are reabsorbed, they should both be restricted.

22. The answer is E.   (Biochemistry)

The most likely biochemical finding would be a dipalmitoylphosphatidylcholine:sphingomyelin ratio of less than 2:1. The type II granular pneumocytes begin synthesizing surfactant at approximately the 33rd week of gestation. The major lipid component of lung surfactant is dipalmitoylphosphatidylcholine. (Lecithin is the common name for the phosphatidylcholine family, individual members of which have different fatty acids esterified on carbons 1 and 2 of the glycerol backbone.) After the 33rd week of gestation (approximately 7.5 months), the dipalmitoylphosphatidylcholine concentration increases and the dipalmitoylphosphatidylcholine:sphingomyelin ratio decreases. This change can be measured in the amniotic fluid and serves as an index of fetal maturity. Lack of sufficient surfactant leads to alveolar collapse and is responsible for approximately 15% of the neonatal deaths in developed countries.

23. The answer is E.   (Physiology)

Destruction of the juxtaglomerular apparatus causes a decrease in renin production, which ultimately causes a decrease in angiotensin II and aldosterone. Hypoaldosteronism leads to an inability to reabsorb sodium in the late distal and early collecting ducts (hyponatremia) and an inability to excrete potassium (hyperkalemia) and hydrogen ions (metabolic acidosis) in exchange for sodium. Destruction of the juxtaglomerular apparatus occurs in diabetics who develop hyaline arteriolosclerosis of the afferent arteriole (i.e., the location of the juxtaglomerular apparatus) and the efferent arteriole. Tubulointerstitial disease can also cause destruction of this apparatus. Hyporeninemic hypoaldosteronism is the same as type IV renal tubular acidosis and is usually suspected when patients develop hyperkalemia with token increases in potassium intake.

24. The answer is B.   (Microbiology)

HIV type 1 is a member of the lentiviriniae (lentivirus) subfamily within the Retroviridae family. There are three subfamilies of retroviruses: oncovirinae, lentivirinae, and spumavirinae.

25. The answer is C.   (Physiology)

To have hyponatremia in the presence of dehydration, the latter indicating a reduction in total body sodium (TBNa), the patient must have a hypertonic loss of fluid, in which there is proportionately more sodium lost than water. Hypertonic loss of fluid occurs in patients who have Addison disease and patients who are on diuretics.

Serum sodium is proportional to the ratio of TBNa to total body water (TBW)

$$\text{Serum sodium} \sim \text{TBNa} / \text{TBW}$$

This ratio is frequently altered by access or lack of access to water. For example, a patient with an isotonic loss of fluid should have a normal serum sodium because equal amounts of sodium and water are lost ($\downarrow$ TBNa / $\downarrow$ TBW). However, if there is an access to water, hyponatremia ($\downarrow$ TBNa / $\uparrow\uparrow$ TBW) is likely to occur, because the excess water alters the ratio in favor of hyponatremia. A physical examination determines TBNa status. Because sodium is limited to the extracellular fluid compartment and the interstitial fluid compartment is larger than the plasma volume, a decrease in TBNa is associated with signs of dehydration, whereas an increase in TBNa is associated with pitting edema. If neither dehydration nor pitting edema is present, the TBNa is normal. The following chart lists the types of fluid losses and their effect on the serum Na and TBNa.

Type of fluid loss/gain	Ratio alteration	Serum sodium	Findings on physical examination	Examples
Isotonic loss	↓TBNa/↓TBW	Normal	Dehydration	Adult diarrhea; third-degree burns
Isotonic gain	↑TBNa/↑TBW	Normal	Pitting edema	Excess isotonic saline (intravenous)
Hypotonic loss	↓TBNa/↓↓TBW	Hypernatremia	Dehydration	Osmotic diuresis (glucose, urea, mannitol); sweating; infant diarrhea
Hypotonic loss	TBNa/↓↓TBW	Hypernatremia	Normal	Diabetes insipidus; water loss caused by fever
Hypotonic gain	↑TBNa/↑↑TBW	Hyponatremia	Pitting edema	Edema in right heart failure, cirrhosis, nephrotic syndrome, and malabsorption
Hypotonic gain	TBNa/↑↑TBW	Hyponatremia	Normal	Inappropriate antidiuretic syndrome
Hypertonic loss	↓↓TBNa/↓TBW	Hyponatremia	Dehydration	Patients taking diuretics; Addison disease
Hypertonic gain	↑↑TBNa/↑TBW	Hypernatremia	Pitting edema	Excess $NaHCO_3^-$

26. The answer is D. *(Biochemistry)*
The patients' symptoms describe night blindness (nyctalopia), an early symptom of vitamin A deficiency. Many elderly people describe these symptoms, which are not necessarily an age-related abnormality in absorption of fat-soluble vitamins. Normally, the fat-soluble vitamins are absorbed with fat and packaged into chylomicrons. However, if these vitamins are not consumed with sufficient lipid to form the chylomicrons, they are not adequately absorbed and a marginal deficiency occurs. The patients were doing what many elderly patients do—that is, trying to maintain a healthy lifestyle by eliminating fatty foods. However, lipids aid in the absorption of fat-soluble vitamins. Moreover, the bulk fat and the vitamin must be ingested simultaneously. It is counterproductive to take vitamins in the morning and consume fat at the evening meal.

Night blindness is not caused by an essential fatty acid or vitamin E deficiency, although these patients are liable to have an essential fatty acid deficiency. An essential fatty acid deficiency is most likely characterized by dry, itchy skin, which is also a common ailment in the elderly. In order to avoid potential toxicity, as well as for its antioxidant effect, the vitamin A supplements should be taken as β-carotene.

27. The answer is A. *(Physiology)*
If an increased amount of sodium is presented to the distal tubule in the presence of aldosterone, an individual would most likely develop hypokalemia because of the augmented exchange of sodium for potassium in the aldosterone-enhanced sodium–potassium pump.

Also, an increased exchange for hydrogen ions once the potassium becomes depleted is likely to occur. Because hydrogen ion excretion in the distal tubule is a mechanism for the reclamation of bicarbonate, the excess in bicarbonate reabsorption causes metabolic alkalosis. Hydrogen ions in the lumen interact with bicarbonate to form carbonic acid, which dissociates into carbon dioxide and water. Carbon dioxide diffuses back into the renal tubular cell, combines with water to form carbonic acid, and again dissociates into bicarbonate and hydrogen ions.

28. The answer is C. *(Behavioral science)*
In order of decreasing risk, the risk factors for suicide are age over 45 years, alcohol and drug abuse, prior suicide attempts, male gender, serious prior psychiatric illness, recent divorce or death of a spouse, serious medical illness, unemployment, and unmarried status.

29. The answer is D. *(Physiology)*
To decrease the serum osmolality with the choices listed, a patient must have a hypotonic gain in fluid; that is, the patient must gain more water than sodium.

Recall that the serum osmolality is primarily a reflection of the serum Na concentration:

Serum osmolality = 2 (serum sodium) + serum glucose/18 + serum blood urea nitrogen/2.8

The serum sodium, in turn, is proportional to the ratio of total body sodium (TBNa) to total body water (TBW):

Serum sodium ~ TBNa/TBW

This ratio is frequently altered by access or lack of access to water. For example, if the patient receives a hypotonic solution ($\uparrow$TBNa/$\uparrow\uparrow$TBW), the serum sodium and the serum osmolality are decreased. A patient with an isotonic loss of fluid ($\downarrow$TBNa/$\downarrow$TBW) should have a normal serum Na (normal osmolality) because an equal amount of sodium and water is lost. A patient with a loss of only pure water ($\leftrightarrow$TBNa/$\downarrow\downarrow$TBW) would have hypernatremia (increased osmolality). An individual who is given a hypertonic fluid ($\uparrow\uparrow$TBNa/$\uparrow$TBW), such as sodium bicarbonate, would most likely have hypernatremia (increased osmolality). A patient with an isotonic gain of fluid ($\uparrow$TBNa/$\uparrow$TBW) would have a normal serum sodium and osmolality.

30. The answer is E. *(Biochemistry)*
Vitamin A has many functions, including regulation of bone development. Children deprived of vitamin A develop nerve damage, because the rate of bone reabsorption is decreased. Because of this decrease, the hole in the foramina through which the nerves pass does not increase in size rapidly enough to keep up with the growth of the nerve. Consequently, nerves passing through the foramina suffer encroachment and compression.

All-*trans* retinoic acid (tretinoin) is formed endogenously from retinol in epithelial cells, after the retinol is taken up by the target cell. In these cells, the retinoic acid binds to an intracellular receptor and receptor–retinoate complex activates enhancer sequences on the DNA, thereby influencing transcription. The mode of action is analogous to that of the steroid hormones, vitamin D and thyroxine. The hormone does not bind to a membrane receptor to generate a second messenger, such as cyclic adenosine monophosphate (cAMP).

All-*trans* retinoic acid is too toxic to be administered orally. It is primarily used as a topical preparation to treat mild cases of acne, psoriasis, and skin changes associated with aging. Severe acne resistant to tretinoin is often managed by the topical administration of 13-*cis* retinoic acid (isotretinoin).

Retinoic acid has no function in the visual cycle or in the support of spermatogenesis. In the visual cycle, it is 11-*cis* retinal that binds to opsin to form rhodopsin. Exposure of rhodopsin to light reconverts the 11-*cis* retinal back to all-*trans* retinal, which is then released from opsin. This process triggers a nerve impulse and light is perceived by the brain.

31. The answer is C. *(Pathology)*
According to the Henderson-Hasselbalch equation, the arterial pH is proportional to the ratio of bicarbonate (HCO_3^-) to carbon dioxide tension (P_{CO_2}), which is typically approximately 20:1. Because the relationship is a ratio, an increase or decrease in either the HCO_3^- or P_{CO_2} concentration automatically alters the arterial pH. For example, a primary increase in serum HCO_3^- causes an increase in arterial pH, or metabolic alkalosis.

Compensation is an attempt to bring the ratio back to 20:1, which should bring the pH back to normal range (full compensation). Full compensation rarely occurs. Instead, the arterial pH is brought close to normal range (partial compensation). It should be clear by looking at the ratio of HCO_3^-:P_{CO_2} that for compensation to occur, it must always move in the same direction as the primary process. For example, if metabolic alkalosis (increased HCO_3^-) is the primary process, respiratory acidosis (increased P_{CO_2}) must occur as compensation to bring the ratio close to 20:1. Antifreeze (ethylene glycol) is converted to oxalic acid (metabolic acidosis), so respiratory alkalosis is the compensation. The following chart summarizes these relationships:

Primary disease	Primary process	Compensation
Metabolic alkalosis	Increase in HCO_3^-	Respiratory acidosis with an increase in P_{CO_2}
Metabolic acidosis	Decrease in HCO_3^-	Respiratory alkalosis with a decrease in P_{CO_2}
Respiratory alkalosis	Decrease in P_{CO_2}	Metabolic acidosis with a decrease in HCO_3^-
Respiratory acidosis	Increase in P_{CO_2}	Metabolic alkalosis with an increase in HCO_3^-

32. The answer is C. *(Microbiology)*
It was originally thought that the HIV type 1 virus lies latent and produces little or no progeny after an initial wave of replication. This belief arose because free virus particles or antigens were difficult to detect in the blood during much of the clinically silent period. It has now been established that viral replication proceeds continually within lymphoid tissues during the majority of the time that the patient is infected with HIV type 1, regardless of whether or not symptoms are present.

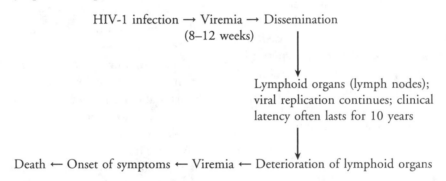

33. The answer is C. *(Pathology)*
In right-sided heart failure, secondary aldosteronism is likely to occur as a compensation for a decrease in effective arterial blood volume (EABV), or that volume of blood that is necessary to stimulate the baroreceptors.

When the cardiac output decreases because of right heart failure, the EABV decreases, which stimulates the vagus nerve, innervating the baroreceptors to release antidiuretic hormone from the hypothalamus to reabsorb free water in the distal and collecting tubules of the kidneys. The reduction in renal blood flow also stimulates the renin-angiotensin-aldosterone system, thus aldosterone is present (secondary aldosteronism) to reabsorb sodium in isotonic proportions in the late distal and early collecting ducts. The low cardiac output decreases the peritubular capillary hydrostatic pressure, which automatically increases the peritubular capillary oncotic pressure, so the proximal tubule reabsorption of sodium is increased (reabsorption is in isotonic proportions). The tonicity of the reabsorbed fluid from the proximal, distal, and collecting tubules is hypotonic. The fate of this hypotonic fluid when it returns to the extracellular compartment depends on the serum sodium concentration and Starling forces. If hyponatremia is present and Starling forces are normal, then most of the fluid moves into the intracellular compartment by osmosis. If hyponatremia is present and there is an alteration in Starling forces (e.g., increased hydrostatic pressure, decreased oncotic pressure), the fluid still moves from the extracellular to the intracellular compartment. However, when the fluid reaches the venous side of the circulation, the altered Starling forces move the fluid out of the plasma and into the interstitial space, resulting in pitting edema.

In summary, serum sodium determines movement of fluid between the extracellular and intracellular compartments by the law of osmosis, whereas Starling forces (hydrostatic and oncotic pressure) determine the movement of fluid in the extracellular compartment between the plasma and interstitial space. When the cardiac output increases, the EABV is increased and the opposite occurs—that is, antidiuretic hormone is not released, renin is not stimulated, and the peritubular capillary hydrostatic pressure is increased, resulting in a loss of sodium and water.

34. The answer is C.   *(Biochemistry)*

The glycosaminoglycans are a group of negatively charged heteropolysaccharides. In general, they exist as complexes in which the amount of carbohydrate greatly exceeds that of the protein in the complex. The negative charges induce these complexes to fan out and form gels with a large amount of associated water. A common feature of the glycosaminoglycans is that they consist of repeating disaccharide units. The structure of the repeating disaccharide units is illustrated in the figure on page 276.

Heparin

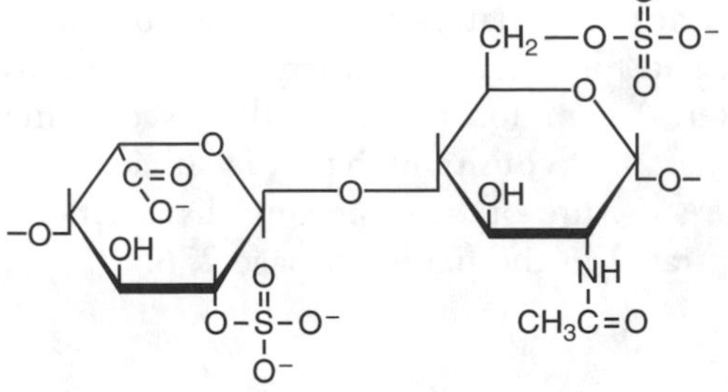

β–Iduronic acid
2–Sulfate

N–Acetyl–α–
Glucosamine
6–Sulfate

Keratin sulfate

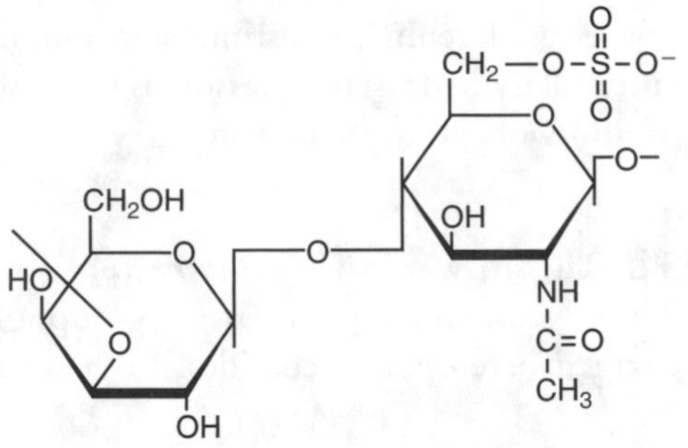

β–Galactose

N–Acetyl–α–
Glucosamine
6–Sulfate

Dermatan sulfate

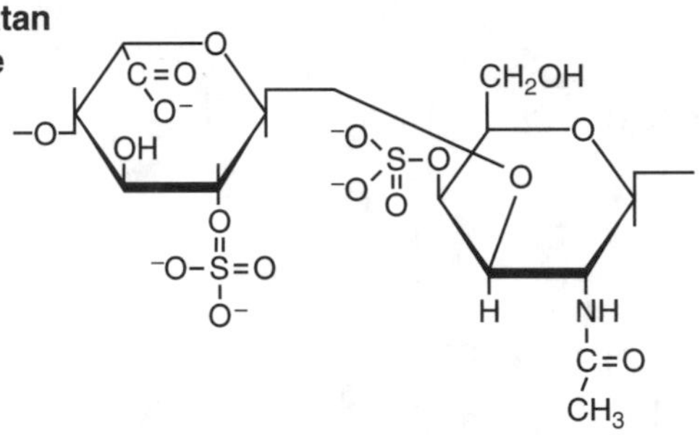

β–Iduronic acid
2–Sulfate

N–Acetyl–β–
Galactosamine
4–Sulfate

Heparan sulfate

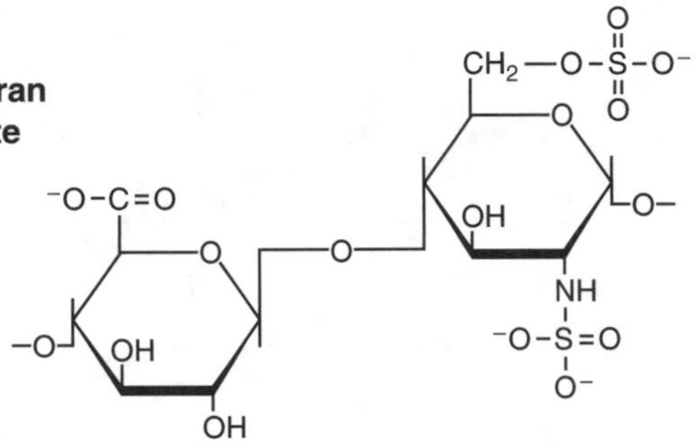

β–Glucuronic acid

β–Glucosamine
N,6–Sulfate

Hyaluronic acid

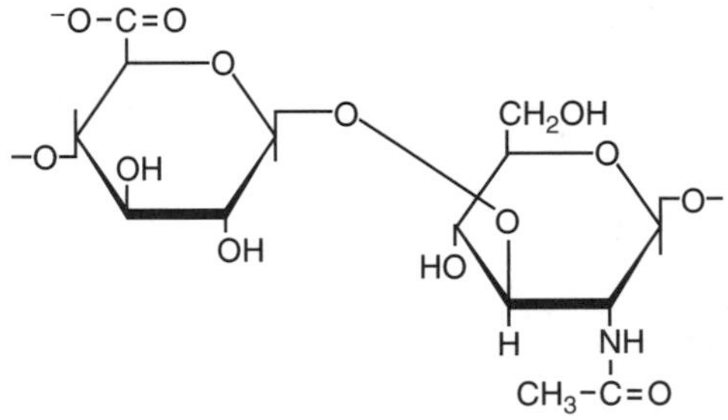

β–Glucuronic
acid

N–Acetyl–β–
Glucosamine

Chondroitin sulfate

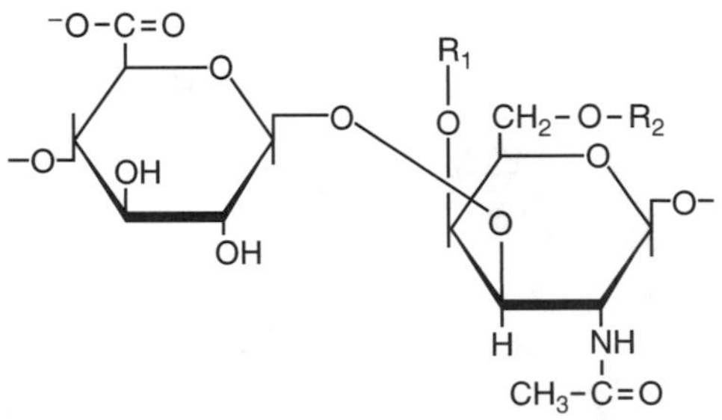

β–Glucuronic
acid

N–Acetyl–β–
Galactosamine

	Chondroitin 4–Sulfate	Chondroitin 6–Sulfate
$R_1 =$	SO_3^-	H
$R_2 =$	H	SO_3^-

In all but one glycosaminoglycan, keratan sulfate, one of the repeating units is a uronic acid, a sugar in which the hydroxyl that is usually located at carbon 6 is oxidized to a carboxyl group. This carboxyl group is negatively charged at physiologic pHs. In all of the glycosaminoglycans except dermatan sulfate and heparin, the uronic acid is glucuronic acid. In dermatan sulfate and heparin, the uronic acid is iduronic acid. In all of the glycosaminoglycans except heparin sulfate, one of the sugars of the repeating disaccharide unit is an acetylated amino sugar. The acetylated amino sugar is either glucosamine or galactosamine. Dermatan sulfate has iduronic acid and *N*-acetylgalactosamine as its repeating disaccharide units.

35. The answer is B.   *(Pathology)*
Many organs are affected during shock. However, the kidneys are affected most significantly because the renal medulla, where the tubules are primarily located, normally receives the least amount of blood. Ischemic acute tubular necrosis with renal failure is the most common cause of death in patients with shock.

36. The answer is B.   *(Microbiology)*
Currently, more than 80 types of M protein have been recognized; therefore, an individual can have repeated infections with group A organisms, such as *Streptococcus pyogenes*, because antibody to M protein provides only type-specific immunity. The M protein is associated with virulence and directly interferes with phagocytosis by white blood cells. Group A streptococci are responsible for approximately 95% of human streptococcal infections. These organisms are β-hemolytic (i.e., they cause complete red blood cell destruction in blood agar) and sensitive to penicillin, erythromycin, and bacitracin. Host immunity to streptococci is long-lasting. Antigenic changes (drift or shift) do not routinely occur in group A streptococci. Streptolysins are antigenic and can induce the production of antibodies.

37. The answer is A.   *(Biochemistry)*
Pompe's disease is a glycogen storage disease caused by a deficiency of lysosomal enzyme. The table below briefly summarizes the eight types of glycogen storage diseases.

Deficient Enzyme	Type	Affected Organ	Glycogen Structure
Glucose 6-phosphatase	I	Liver, kidney	Normal
α-1,4-Glucosidase	II	All	Normal
Amylo-1,6-glucosidase	III	All	Many short branches
Glucosyl α-4,6-transferase	IV	Liver, spleen	Fewer, longer branches
Phosphorylase	V	Muscle	Normal
Phosphorylase	VI	Liver	Normal
Phosphofructokinase	VII	Muscle	Normal
Phosphorylase kinase	VIII	Liver	Normal

All but type II (Pompe's disease) involve enzymes of energy metabolism (e.g., glycogenesis, glycogenolysis, glycolysis, or gluconeogenesis). Pompe's disease affects a lysosomal enzyme, α-1,4-glucosidase, and involves all cells that store glycogen, including liver, heart, and muscle cells.

38. The answer is E.   *(Microbiology)*
HIV type 1 (HIV-1) is transmitted primarily during sexual contact, particularly anal intercourse; through exposure to blood or blood products (e.g., transfusion, sharing needles); from mother to fetus; and from mother to infant. An individual with a sexually transmitted disease, such as syphilis or gonorrhea, is at greater risk for infection because of the lesions that may be present in the genital area and elsewhere. Promiscuous individuals with numerous partners are at greater risk than those in monogamous relationships. Asymptomatic HIV-1 positive individuals can transmit the virus.

Under experimental conditions, it has been demonstrated that HIV-1 can survive in the gut of mosquitos that have been fed or injected with contaminated blood. However, the virus does not persist in the mosquito for more than a few days, and it does not infect or replicate in insect cells. Epidemiologic studies also indicate that transmission by insect vector is highly unlikely.

Infection from swimming in an HIV-1 contaminated pool is highly unlikely. The virus is completely inactivated after a 10-minute treatment with 10% household bleach, 50% ethanol, 0.3% hydrogen peroxide, 0.5% Lysol, and other agents at room temperature. Heating of liquids for 10 minutes at 56°C also results in inactivation. However, survival of HIV-1 outside of the body is prolonged in dried proteinaceous materials.

HIV-1 can be isolated occasionally from saliva but is present in very low titers. Studies of health care workers who have come in contact with saliva of HIV-1 positive patients report no cases of seroconversion. The risk for transmission by one mucous membrane exposure to blood or other body secretions is estimated to be less than 0.1%.

Hemophiliacs no longer receive factor VIII concentrate from a large pool of donors. Instead, a cryoprecipitate is prepared from a single donor and infectivity is destroyed by heating the factor prior to administration. In addition, the blood is screened for HIV antibody.

The risk of infection from the transfusion of blood or blood products has dropped dramatically in the last decade, partly because of testing blood from donors for antibodies against HIV-1 and excluding high-risk individiuals from donating. Unfortunately, antibodies against HIV-1 antigens are usually not detectable until 2 to 8 weeks after infection. Thus, a person could donate contaminated blood during this window period. The risk for HIV-1 infection after blood transfusion is currently estimated to be 1:450,000 to 1:660,000 units transfused.

39. The answer is E. *(Biochemistry)*
Cholecalciferol, or vitamin D_3, is formed from 7-dehydrocholesterol in the skin through ultraviolet light, or it is ingested from animal sources. Ergocalciferol, or vitamin D_2, is found in plants. Either form of vitamin D is carried to the liver where it is first hydroxylated at the 25-position, which is the major vitamin D derivative in the circulation and the liver. The 25-hydroxy form is further activated by a second hydroxylation, 1-α-hydroxylase, at the 1-position in the kidney or inactivated by hydroxylation at the 24-position. The active 1,25-derivative circulates to targeted cells in the kidney, bone, and intestine, where it binds to nuclear receptors and influences transcription.

This person has a form of rickets that does not respond to nutritional supplementation or sunlight. However, it will respond to supplementation with 1,25-dihydroxycholecalciferol (calcitrol). Because in this case the rickets is caused by a deficiency of functional vitamin D, this inherited autosomal recessive disease is termed type I vitamin-D–dependent rickets. Because of nutritional supplementation and the prevalent tendency to expose more of the body to sunlight, this disease is more common in developed countries than is classic rickets, caused by dietary deficiency and lack of sunshine, which is still the prevalent form in some developing countries.

A very rare form of rickets is caused by aberrant 1,25-dihydroxycholecalciferol receptors. This disease is given the somewhat misleading name of type II vitamin-D–dependent rickets. The name vitamin-D–resistant rickets is reserved for an X-linked dominant trait in which excess phosphate is lost in the renal tubules, causing an hypophosphatemia.

40. The answer is E. *(Pharmacology)*
Both doxorubicin and dactinomycin are antitumor antibiotics that act in part by intercalating between adjacent DNA base pairs and disrupting nucleic acid synthesis. Dactinomycin preferentially inhibits RNA polymerase. Doxorubicin blocks both RNA and DNA synthesis and has other actions, including inhibition of topoisomerase II and formation of free radicals, leading to DNA strand breakage. Both drugs are cell cycle–nonspecific. Only doxorubicin causes cardiac toxicity. Neither drug is a plant alkaloid or is used in treating hypercalcemia. (Plicamycin, another antitumor antibiotic, is used to treat hypercalcemia.)

41. The answer is D. *(Biochemistry)*
Vitamin K is the only fat-soluble vitamin that acts as a cofactor. It does not affect transcription nor does it act as an antioxidant. It is a required cofactor in the carboxylation of specific glutamic acid residues to form γ-carboxyglutamic acid. This posttranslational modification allows coagulation factors II, VII, IX, X, and

proteins C and S to bind calcium, because the γ-carboxyglutamic acid residues are good chelators. Once they bind calcium, their proteolytic activity is activated and the coagulation cascade is stimulated to form a clot.

γ-Carboxyglutamic acid proteins have also been reported in bone, kidney, and placenta, suggesting vitamin K–dependent carboxylation reactions may play a role in the metabolism of these tissues as well.

Vitamin K is abundant in the diet and is synthesized by the bacterial flora, thus deficiencies are rare. Vitamin K deficiency is most commonly observed in newborn infants, between days 2 and 5, who have not yet developed an intestinal flora. Therefore, an intramuscular injection to a newborn prevents the possibility of hemorrhagic disease of the newborn. Fat malabsorption, broad-spectrum antibiotics, and warfarin are other causes of vitamin K deficiency. Warfarin is an anticoagulant that blocks epoxide reductase, which keeps the vitamin in an active form.

42. The answer is E.   *(Microbiology)*
Actinomyces israelii is an anaerobe that forms part of the normal flora of the oral cavity. Actinomycetes form long, gram-positive branching filaments that resemble the hyphae of fungi, but they are true bacteria and are related to *Corynebacterium* and *Mycobacterium*. After local trauma (e.g., dental extraction), *A. israelii* may invade tissues, forming filaments surrounded by inflammation. "Sulfur granules," composed of a mass of filaments, form in pus, which drains to the outside via a sinus tract. Actinomycosis is not communicable. Treatment consists of prolonged administration of penicillin, coupled with surgical drainage.

43. The answer is B.   *(Behavioral science)*
Latency age children (i.e., children 6–11 years of age) understand the finality of death and may feel guilty and responsible for the death. Children younger than 6 years do not fully understand the finality of death. Children older than 11 years are less likely to feel responsible for the death of a parent than an 8-year-old child.

44. The answer is D.   *(Microbiology)*
Pneumocystis carinii is the classic opportunistic infectious agent associated with AIDS. At least one episode

of *P. carinii* pneumonia occurs in approximately 75% of patients who do not receive prophylactic therapy.

This fungus, which was formerly classified as a protozoan, was the leading cause of AIDS-related deaths before the development of effective drugs. Currently, it is recommended that prophylactic treatment with oral trimethoprim-sulfamethoxazole, aerosolized pentamidine, or isethionate for *P. carinii* pneumonia is initiated when the patient's CD4+ cell count is less than 200/μl.

45. The answer is C.   *(Biochemistry)*
Nearly all of the commonly used restriction endonucleases recognize inverted repeat DNA sequences called palindromes, so the task here is to determine which of these sequences is a palindrome. Only one strand of the DNA is given here; therefore, it is necessary to construct the complementary strand. In order to be a palindrome, the sequence of one strand read in the 5′ to 3′ direction must be the same as the sequence of the complementary strand read in the 5′ to 3′ direction. Answer C is the only sequence with this characteristic:
5′ GTCGAC 3′
3′ CAGCTG 5′

46. The answer is A.   *(Microbiology)*
A cellular oncogene (proto-oncogene) may become activated or overexpressed when a retroviral genome is inserted in the nearby vicinity. Insertion of a strong retroviral transcriptional promoter, or enhancer, sequence close to a cellular oncogene may cause its activation or overexpression. This mechanism of action, known as insertional mutagenesis, or promoter-insertion oncogenesis, was first described for the avian leukosis virus, which activates the expression of the *c-myc* oncogene.

Transduction by a retrovirus (i.e., genetic recombination between the retrovirus and cellular genes) is probably the most potent mechanism by which the viruses induce cellular oncogene expression. If the transduction results in incorporation of an oncogene into the viral genome, the oncogene (now under the control of strong viral promoters) is then expressed together with other viral genes.

The following are characteristics of cellular (proto-) oncogenes:

- They are located in virtually the same positions on the chromosomes of every cell of every individual within a species
- They contain introns
- They are inherited according to classic mendelian genetics
- The nucleotide sequence of each oncogene is similar among different species
- They are normally silent in adults or are transcribed at low levels
- They play key roles in normal cell growth, division, and differentiation during embryogenesis

47. The answer is E. *(Behavioral science)*
Compliance with medical advice increases when the patient is provided with written, in addition to verbal, information. Marital status, race, religion, and educational level are not related to compliance.

48. The answer is C. *(Microbiology)*
The hepatitis B virus is strongly associated with the development of primary hepatocellular carcinoma in humans. Persistent infection with hepatitis B virus can lead to chronic liver disease and increased risk for development of liver cancer. This virus does not carry an oncogene; thus, the mechanism of carcinogens is believed to be indirect. Commonly, there is a 20- to 40-year interval from the time of infection to the development of cancer. Hepatocellular carcinoma is particularly prevalent in Africa, China, and Southeast Asia, where hepatitis B virus is hyperendemic.

The JC virus (Papovaviridae family, polyoma genus) is the cause of progressive multifocal leukoencephalopathy (PML) in individuals with severely depressed cell-mediated immunity, including patients with certain types of cancers (e.g., Hodgkin lymphoma, chronic lymphocytic leukemia). PML is not considered a neoplastic disease.

Feline leukemia virus and simian sarcoma virus are oncogenic retroviruses of animals. They are not associated with human tumors.

Adenoviruses cause generally mild upper respiratory tract and intestinal tract infections in humans. Infected rodent cells, however, can be transformed when early viral proteins are expressed.

49. The answer is B. *(Biochemistry)*
In double-stranded DNA, adenine is always base-paired with thymine. Therefore, the amount of adenine present (22%) must equal the amount of thymine present (22%). The remainder of the DNA molecule consists of guanine–cytosine base pairs. Because the total for all four bases must equal 100% and guanine and cytosine must be present in equal amounts, the cytosine content must be 28%.

50. The answer is C. *(Microbiology)*
All retroviruses, including HIV type 1, carry reverse transcriptase in the mature virion. The enzyme is named because it can use RNA as a template to make new DNA; thus, it is an RNA-dependent DNA polymerase, which is the opposite (i.e., the reverse) of the normal process in cells in which DNA is transcribed into RNA by DNA-dependent RNA polymerases.

The reverse transcriptase uses the single-stranded RNA of the retrovirus to make an RNA:DNA replicative intermediate. It then proceeds to use the new DNA strand in the hybrid to make a second DNA strand, resulting in a double-stranded DNA helix, or a DNA:DNA copy of the viral genome.

The integrase enzyme of retroviruses integrates the newly formed DNA:DNA copy into the genome of the host cell. Thus, it resides as a provirus until it is transcribed by a host cell enzyme (RNA polymerase II) into RNA. Some of the transcripts are spliced, and subgenomic mRNAs are processed and translated into viral proteins. Full-length transcripts are capped at the 5′ end and polyadenylated at the 3′ end. They are then packaged into preformed capsids. After additional maturation, virus particles exit the cell by budding through the cytoplasmic membrane.

Most retroviruses do not kill the cells they infect, and the integrated provirus remains in the genome for the entire life of the cell.

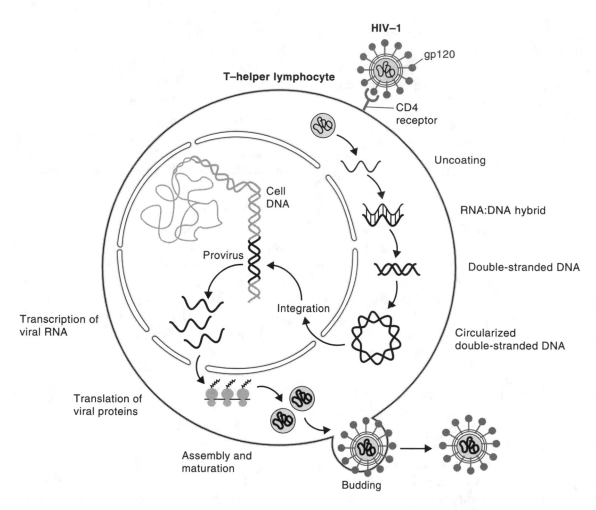

51-52. The answers are: 51-B, 52-B. *(Behavioral science)*

In a normal (Gaussian) distribution, the median is equal to the mean and the mode. Therefore, the median age for contracting disease X is 50 years.

The percentage of people that would be expected to develop disease X between the ages of 38 and 62 years is 68%. This is because age 38 is 1 standard deviation below (34% of the population) and age 62 is one standard deviation above (34% of the population) the mean. In a normal distribution, 68% of the population falls within 1 standard deviation of the mean.

53. The answer is B. *(Behavioral science)*

In this example, the cancer researcher made a type II error because the experimental intervention did make a difference between the treatment and control groups,

but the investigator failed to reject the null hypothesis. A type I error occurs if the investigator rejects the null hypothesis when the experimental intervention did not make a difference between the treatment and control groups.

54. The answer is C. *(Behavioral science)*

According to the DSM-III-R criteria, serious medical illness is considered an extremely severe psychosocial stressor. Divorce and the birth of the first child are considered severe life stressors. Marriage is considered a moderate life stressor, and graduation from school is considered a mild psychosocial stressor.

55. The answer is E. *(Behavioral science)*

Use of aspirin is the independent variable (i.e., the factor that the experimenter can change). The presence of gastric bleeding is the dependent variable in this study (i.e., the outcome that reflects the effects of changing the use of aspirin). Although the age of the patient and the patient's history of cigarette smoking or alcohol consumption may be independent variables, they are not identified as such in this study.

56. The answer is D. *(Behavioral science)*
In negative reinforcement, behavior (e.g., exercising) increases to avoid something bad (e.g., joint pain). Frequently, compliance with medical advice involves negative reinforcement. In positive reinforcement, the patient's exercising behavior would increase to get something good (e.g., a favorite food). Habituation occurs when an individual becomes comfortable with something as a result of repeated exposure. Sensitization results when a person becomes hypersensitive to a stimulus, so that even a weak exposure elicits a response. Extinction is the disappearance of a learned behavior when the reward is withheld.

57. The answer is B. *(Behavioral science)*
The study design is an example of a case-control study. In a case-control study, subjects who have the disorder (breast cancer) and subjects who do not have the disorder are identified and information regarding their prior exposure to the risk factor (relatives with breast cancer) is obtained and compared using the odds ratio.

58. The answer is D. *(Behavioral science)*
In the United States, the prevalence of schizophrenia is approximately 1%. The prevalence is equal among men and women and among all religious and racial groups. The prevalence of schizophrenia is higher in low socioeconomic groups because of the "downward drift" (i.e., schizophrenic individuals move to lower socioeconomic groups because of their handicap).

59. The answer is B. *(Behavioral science)*
For this small sample, the median is a better measure of central tendency than the mean. Range, standard deviation, and standard error are not measures of central tendency.

60. The answer is B. *(Behavioral science)*
The example of a medical student who becomes more comfortable in the gross anatomy lab as the semester progresses is an example of habituation; the student has become accustomed to the anatomy lab because of repeated exposure. Sensitization is the opposite of habituation, in that the person becomes hypersensitive to a stimulus so that even a weak exposure elicits a response. Positive and negative reinforcement are methods of learning using a system of reward and punishment. Extinction is the disappearance of a learned behavior when the reward is withheld.

61. The answer is A. *(Behavioral science)*
Correlation measures the association between pairs of continuous variables such as height and body weight; the correlation coefficient varies from -1 (perfect negative relationship) to +1 (perfect positive relationship). The *t*-test and analysis of variance are used to compare sample means. The chi-squared test tests differences between frequencies in a sample.

62. The answer is E. *(Behavioral science)*
A competent patient may refuse treatment even if her illness is life-threatening. In this case, although the fetus' life is threatened, the pregnant woman is the patient and the physician must respect her wishes.

63. The answer is D. *(Biochemistry)*
The RNA product would have a base sequence complementary to, but in the opposite direction of, the DNA strand used as a template. By convention, all nucleic acid sequences are written in the 5′ to 3′ direction unless specified otherwise. RNA contains uracil (U) instead of the thymine (T) found in DNA. Therefore, as a result of transcription, the product would be:

DNA 5′ AGTACTGC 3′

RNA 3′ UCAUGACG 5′

RNA 5′ GCAGUACU 3′

64–65. The answers are: 64-A, 65-E. *(Behavioral science)*
The standard deviation of these scores is √10/3, or 1.83. Standard deviation is calculated by subtracting each score from the mean, squaring these deviations, and dividing the total by the square root of the number

of scores in the set (n) minus 1. The square root of this result (the variance) is the standard deviation. Therefore:

The mean equals (5+7+4+8)/n, or 6.

$(5-6)^2+(7-6)^2+(4-6)^2+(8-6)^2 = 10$.

The standard deviation is $\sqrt{10/3}$, or 1.83

The standard error is the standard deviation (1.83) divided by the square root of the number of scores in the set (4).

66. The answer is E.   *(Biochemistry)*

The amount and type of proteins produced by a cell are dictated by messenger RNA. Much of this variation is caused by transcription of different genes as a result of cell differentiation. Ribosomal RNA and transfer RNA are the same in all cells, as are nuclear DNA and mitochondrial DNA.

67. The answer is A.   *(Pharmacology)*

Both cyclophosphamide, which is a nitrogen mustard alkylating agent, and cisplatin, an inorganic platinum complex, are believed to act by binding to guanine residues of DNA to cause interstrand crosslinking. Cyclophosphamide is a prodrug that must be activated by hepatic microsomal P-450 enzymes. Both drugs are active throughout the cell cycle (i.e., they are cell cycle–nonspecific agents). Although cisplatin causes relatively little myelosuppresion, nitrogen mustards produce considerable dose-dependent myelosuppression.

68. The answer is D.   *(Behavioral science)*

Women are twice as likely as men to suffer from major depression. Homicide and suicide rates, and the incidence of alcoholism and obsessive-compulsive disorder are higher in men than in women.

69. The answer is B.   *(Pharmacology)*

Rickettsial growth is enhanced in the presence of sulfonamides; therefore, these agents are contraindicated for the treatment of rickettsial infections. The mechanism by which sulfa drugs enhance rickettsial growth is unknown. Tetracycline or chloramphenicol inhibit the growth of rickettsiae; both agents are therapeutically effective.

70. The answer is C.   *(Microbiology)*

In order to determine which antibiotic works best against a specific organism, sensitivity tests are required. The minimal inhibitory concentration (MIC) and minimum bactericidal concentration (MBC) are values obtained during sensitivity testing. Sensitivity can be determined using diffusion (agar plates), dilution (MIC and MBC), or automated processes. The MIC and MBC are determined using an antibiotic dilution assay, which provides quantitative data. In the dilution assay, the antibiotic is carefully diluted and mixed with a standard amount of identified bacteria. Overnight incubation allows growth to occur. Where the antibiotic inhibits growth, the medium remains clear. The antimicrobial will eventually be diluted to a point where the organism can grow, and the medium becomes cloudy.

71. The answer is A.   *(Behavioral science)*

Correlation measures the association between pairs of continuous variables, such as age and blood pressure; the correlation coefficient varies from -1 (perfect negative relationship) to +1 (perfect positive relationship). The t-test and ANOVA are used to compare sample means. The chi-square test tests differences between frequencies in a sample.

72. The answer is B.   *(Biochemistry)*

β-Oxidation occurs entirely within the mitochondrial matrix. The enzymes involved in oxidation of the reduced cofactors produced during β-oxidation of fatty acids are reduced nicotinamide adenine dinucleotide (NADH) dehydrogenase (part of complex I) and succinate dehydrogenase (part of complex II). NADH dehydrogenase oxidizes NADH, and succinate dehydrogenase oxidizes reduced flavin adenine dinucleotide (FADH$_2$). The latter enzyme is the only tricarboxylic acid (TCA) cycle enzyme that is not found in the mitochondial matrix. None of the enzymes associated with the electron transport system are found in the mitochondrial matrix. These enzymes are all located in the inner membrane of the mitochondrion. Approximately 13 of the 100 or so polypeptides associated with oxidative phosphorylation are coded for on mitochondrial DNA. The remaining proteins are coded for by nuclear DNA.

Ornithine transcarbamoylase and carbamoyl phosphate synthetase I are located in the mitochondrial matrix. The other urea cycle enzymes are found in the cytoplasm.

73. The answer is E. *(Microbiology)*
Overexpression of the *c-myc* oncogene is a common finding in patients with African Burkitt lymphoma. Infection of B lymphocytes with the Epstein-Barr virus transforms them into blast-like cells that can multiply indefinitely and secrete antibodies. It is thought that during this inappropriate B-cell proliferation, a distal portion of chromosome 8, which contains the *c-myc* gene, is translocated to a position near an immunoglobulin gene on chromosome 14, which codes for the heavy chains of antibody. Occasionally, the translocation occurs between chromosomes 8 and 22 or 2, close to the genes that code for λ and κ light chains, respectively. The transfer of *c-myc* close to an active promotor of immunoglobulin gene transcription results in the production of large amounts of *c-myc* mRNA.

74. The answer is B. *(Microbiology)*
Azidothymidine (AZT) is an analog of thymidine that blocks the synthesis of proviral DNA by reverse transcriptase (RNA-dependent DNA polymerase). It also inhibits the synthesis of cellular DNA. However, the reverse transcriptase is 100 times more likely than cellular DNA polymerases to incorporate the analog into new DNA. AZT is referred to as reverse transcriptase inhibitor, or DNA chain terminator.

75. The answer is C. *(Microbiology)*
The herpes B virus is prevalent among Old World monkeys (*Macaca* genus, which includes rhesus monkeys). The virus usually does not cause disease in its natural host, but remains latent after infection. However, apparently healthy animals may shed the virus. If disease is present, it tends to resemble human infections with herpes simplex viruses. The virus can be isolated from the saliva, brain, spinal cord, kidney cells, and possibly stool of the monkey.

Individuals at high risk for infection with herpes B virus include animal handlers who work with Macaca monkeys and laboratory technicians who use monkey kidney cells during vaccine development or other purposes. Transmission of the virus to humans can occur through a monkey bite or by direct contact with contaminated animals, their tissues, or cell cultures. Person-to-person transmission of the virus has been recently reported. In this latter case, direct contact with vesicular skin lesions of a patient was believed to be the route of transmission. There are only 20 to 25 documented human cases caused by herpes B virus. In humans, the virus exhibits great neurotropism and has a high mortality rate, approximately 75%. Motor and sensory abnormalities occur about 1 week following infection and progress rapidly. Nystagmus, hyperesthesia, areflexia, flaccid paralysis, decreased consciousness, and seizure have been noted, in addition to the signs and symptoms described in the case history. Paralysis of respiratory function is a common cause of death. The disease is characterized by involvement of the entire brain, in contrast to the herpes simplex viruses, which tend to localize in the temporal lobe.

The herpes simplex viruses can cause a severe form of encephalitis. Cytomegalovirus can affect the central nervous system, especially after congenital or neonatal infection and in the immunocompromised patient. The rabies virus, acquired primarily through a bite from an infected animal, is also neurotropic and highly lethal once symptoms appear.

76. The answer is A. *(Biochemistry)*
The K_m of the enzyme for its substrate is defined as the substrate concentration that gives one half V_{max}. In the table of data, note that the enzyme reaches a maximum velocity of 80 μmol/min at high substrate concentrations. The data also show that one half the maximum velocity (40 μmol/min) is attained with a substrate concentration of 5mmol/L. Thus, the K_m = 5 mmol/L.

77. The answer is D. *(Biochemistry)*
According to the Henderson-Hasselbalch equation for a weak acid,

$$pH = pK_a + \log([A^-]/[HA]),$$

where pK_a is the dissociation constant for the acid, $[A^-]$ is the concentration of the salt form, and [HA] is the concentration of the acid form.

Therefore, pH = 4.8 + log(0.1/0.01) = 4.8 + log(10) = 4.8 + 1.0 = 5.8.

78. The answer is A. *(Biochemistry)*
The mutant enzyme reaches the same maximum velocity, V_{max}, as the normal enzyme. However, the mutant enzyme requires higher substrate concentrations to reach V_{max}. Therefore, the substrate concentration required to reach one-half V_{max} (i.e., K_m) is also higher. The mutant enzyme has a lower affinity for the substrate. The equilibrium constant for the reaction depends on the free energy levels of the substrate and product and is not altered by the presence or absence of any form of an enzyme.

79. The answer is E. *(Pathology)*
Patients with AIDS have hypergammaglobulinemia caused by a nonspecific polyclonal stimulation of B cells by the Epstein-Barr virus and cytomegalovirus. Unfortunately, the immunoglobulins offer no protection against bacterial diseases.

Patients with AIDS usually have a normocytic anemia and a decreased reticulocyte response, indicating ineffective erythropoiesis. Many of the features resemble the anemia of chronic disease (low serum iron, low total iron binding capacity, and increased serum ferritin).

HIV directly inhibits chemotaxis by neutrophils and monocytes.

The p24 core protein is usually increased in active disease.

Macrophage activation of macrophages is decreased, because HIV destroys CD4 T helper cells, which normally release gamma interferon to activate macrophages.

80. The answer is D. *(Physiology)*
This question involves an understanding of the law of diffusion, which states that gases move from high to low concentration. Exposing arterial blood to the atmosphere, where the oxygen tension (P_{O_2}) is 159 mm Hg and the carbon dioxide tension (P_{CO_2}) is 0.3 mm Hg, the oxygen from the atmosphere diffuses into the blood, because the normal arterial oxygen tension (Pa_{O_2}) is 75 to 105 mm Hg. This falsely increases the P_{O_2}, and the CO_2 from the blood would escape into the atmosphere, because the normal arterial carbon dioxide tension (Pa_{CO_2}) is 33 to 44 mm Hg (falsely decreases the Pa_{CO_2}). This underscores the reason for keeping arterial blood in wet ice and capping it by

putting the needle into a cork to prevent any exposure to the atmosphere.

81. The answer is D. *(Pathology)*
The electrocardiogram findings indicate the presence of a U wave, which is indicative of hypokalemia. Primary aldosteronism, which is a mineralocorticoid excess syndrome associated with excess amounts of aldosterone, produces hypokalemia by increasing the exchange of potassium for sodium in the late distal and early collecting ducts.

A pathophysiologic classification for hypokalemia includes decreased intake of potassium, transcellular shift of potassium into the cell, and increased loss of potassium.

The ratio of intracellular to extracellular potassium concentration is the principal determinant of membrane potential in excitable tissue. Hypokalemia increases this ratio, which causes hyperpolarization of the cell membranes—the resting transmembrane electrical potential is lowered and the distance from the threshold potential is increased. This causes the following changes in the electrocardiogram when concentrations less than 3.0 mEq/L are present:

- Low-voltage QRS complexes and widening of the QRS with very low concentrations
- Depressed S-T segments
- Prominent P and U waves
- Prolonged QT and PR intervals

82. The answer is D. *(Pathology)*
Craniotabes, or elastic recoil of the skull on compression (similar to a ping pong ball), is the first sign of rickets in children and is not seen in adults.

Vitamin D deficiency is called rickets in children and osteomalacia in adults. The basic defect in vitamin D deficiency is defective mineralization of osteoid in bone. The main difference between rickets and osteomalacia is that mineralization of osteoid is defective in only the diaphysis in adults, but in both the epiphysis and the diaphysis in growing children. An excess in osteoid widens the osteoid seams beyond normal. The excess osteoid in the epiphyses of children produces the classic rachitic rosary and craniotabes, both of which are not present in adults. The bone is rarefied on radiograph (osteopenia) and cannot be distinguished from osteoporosis, which refers to a decrease in overall bone mass. Because osteoid is soft, the bone is subject to stress and commonly bows outward under pressure to produce bowed legs, which are characteristic of both rickets and osteomalacia.

83. The answer is D. *(Microbiology)*
The pyogenic cocci generally include the genera *Staphylococcus, Streptococcus,* and *Neisseria,* indicating that pus production is a standard feature of their growth in tissue. Isolation of any of these organisms from a wound would not be unexpected. The gram-stain result would be an initial laboratory test that would identify the general group or kind of organism causing the infection.

All streptococci are catalase negative; therefore, *Streptococcus pneumoniae, Streptococcus pyogenes,* and *Enterococcus (Streptococcus) faecalis* would not be possible candidates. *Staphylococcus aureus* is catalase positive, routinely produces β-, or clear-zone, hemolysis on blood agar and, by definition, is *Staphylococcus aureus* if it produces coagulase. The normal flora *Staphylococcus epidermidis* produces hemolysis or coagulase.

Staphylococcus aureus continues to be a significant nosocomial opportunist, with only the gram-negative enteric organisms causing more opportunistic and nosocomial diseases.

84. The answer is E. *(Behavioral science)*
If an individual has a condition that requires treatment, the physician must inform the patient about the diagnosis, the risks, and benefits of the procedure, and the likely outcome if he does not have the procedure. Therefore, under most conditions, you will tell the patient about the diagnosis of prostate cancer. However, if in your medical opinion you feel that his life or health will be compromised if you tell him, you do not have to do so. His wife's opinion concerning this matter is not relevant. It is more appropriate to have the physician, rather than a consultation–liaison psychiatrist, tell the patient about the diagnosis.

85-86. The answers are: 85-D, 86-C. *(Biochemistry)*
Because the ΔF508 mutation is a three-base deletion, the PCR product from this region of the mutant gene is three bases shorter than that from the normal gene. In this example, the normal allele gives a product of

63 bp in length, whereas the mutant allele gives a product 60 bp long. In this family, both parents, I-1 and I-2, and the daughter, II-3, are carriers because they show both the larger and smaller DNA fragments. The son, II-1, is homozygous normal because his DNA produces only the larger band. The daughter, II-2, is affected because her DNA produces only the smaller band, indicating that she has two copies of the mutant allele.

The ΔF508 mutation consists of a three-base deletion. Because codons are three bases long, this mutation effectively represents a deletion of one codon; therefore, one amino acid residue, a phenylalanine at position 508, is missing from the mutant protein. Because exactly one codon is deleted, the reading frame of the ribosome is not thrown off, and the alteration is not a frameshift mutation. Other than the one deleted amino acid, the remainder of the polypeptide product is unchanged.

87-88. The answers are: 87-E, 88-B. *(Physiology)*
The alveolar gas equation can be used to calculate the ideal alveolar P_{O_2}

$$P_{AO_2} = F_{IO_2} (TBP - P_{H_2O}) - P_{ACO_2}/R$$

where the following are given,

- P_{ACO_2} = alveolar P_{CO_2} = 40 mm Hg
- R = Respiratory exchange ratio = 0.8
- TBP = total barometric pressure = 760 mm Hg
- F_{IO_2} = concentration of inspired O_2 = 40%
- P_{H_2O} = partial pressure of H_2O at 37°C = 47 mm Hg

Thus,

$$P_{AO_2} = .40 (760 - 47) - 40/0.8$$

$$P_{AO_2} = 285 - 50$$

$$P_{AO_2} = 235 \text{ mm Hg}$$

Because the arterial P_{O_2} was measured and found to be 60 mm Hg, the alveolar–arterial gradient for O_2 is 175 mm Hg. This measurement is far in excess of normal and implies a V_A/Q_C mismatch. The failure of an enriched O_2 mixture to substantially raise the arterial P_{O_2} suggests the presence of intrapulmonary shunts. This condition is typical of patients with adult respiratory distress syndrome (ARDs) in which lung injury (e.g., aspiration of gastric acids, fat embolus, sepsis) causes an increase in capillary permeability and the exudation of fluid into the alveoli. When this condition occurs locally, a V_A/Q_C mismatch, hypoxemia, and an increase in the A–a gradient results. Although central nervous system depression and obesity can cause hypoxemia, in these instances, the whole lung is hypoventilated and the A–a gradient remains in the normal range (< 10 mm Hg). Anemia does not affect either alveolar or arterial P_{O_2}; hence, the A–a gradient does not change.

89. The answer is D. *(Behavioral science)*
The level of formal education is not related to patient compliance with medical advice. Understanding the instructions, believing the regimen will work, having written as well as verbal instructions, and liking the physician are all factors in compliance.

90. The answer is C. *(Microbiology)*
Mumps is an acute contagious disease characterized by enlargement of the parotid glands. Other organs that may be involved include the pancreas, testes and ovaries, as well as the central nervous system. At least one-third of all mumps infections are subclinical.

Transmission of this paramyxovirus is person to person by airborne droplets. Primary replication occurs in the epithelial cells of the upper respiratory tract and spreads to the salivary glands and other major organ systems. The testes and ovaries may be affected, and the parotid gland is sometimes involved. The virus frequently infects the kidneys and can be isolated from urine. Mumps is a systemic viral disease, with replication occurring in epithelial cells in the various visceral organs. Gastritis, however, is not usually experienced with mumps infection.

Immunity is permanent after a single infection or vaccination with the live, attenuated vaccine. Antibodies against the hemagglutinin–neuraminidase antigen correlate with immunity. Humoral (antibodies) and cell-mediated immunity develop in a normal infection.

91. The answer is A. *(Pathology)*
Both scurvy (vitamin C deficiency) and rickets (vitamin D deficiency in children) have disruption of normal epiphyseal growth. In scurvy, the normal hydroxylation of lysine and proline residues is impaired, producing an abnormal collagen and reduced amounts

of collagen-rich osteoid. Unlike rickets, scurvy has no defect in the mineralization of osteoid. Furthermore, in rickets, there is increased structurally normal but noncalcified osteoid, whereas there is decreased structurally abnormal osteoid in scurvy. In either case, there is disruption of epiphyseal growth. In scurvy, columns of cartilage project into the osteoid in the metaphysis. There is a lateral overgrowth of osteoid at the margins of the epiphyses, which produces a scorbutic rosary in the rib cage. In rickets, there is an overgrowth of structurally normal, unmineralized osteoid in the epiphyses. Distorted masses of osteoid often project into the marrow cavity. Replacement of cartilage by osteoid is disrupted, resulting in overgrowth at the margins and the classic rachitic rosary.

92. The answer is D. *(Microbiology)*
Rubella virus is a togavirus that produces an acute febrile illness and a rash in children and young adults. Rubella can cross the placenta and infect a developing fetus. The earlier in pregnancy this disease occurs, the more serious the permanent damage can be. Control of the disease is best accomplished by use of the live attenuated vaccine.

Hepatitis B can also cross the placenta. The resulting infection is systemic and can lead to a chronic infection. The most effective control is use of the hepatitis B surface antigen vaccine. Hepatitis A is an enterovirus (picornavirus) that is spread by the fecal–oral route. It is endemic in many areas, affecting older children rather than infants and neonates. No chronic carrier situation occurs with hepatitis A infections.

Herpes simplex virus is a significant infection in neonates. This systemic disease can have fatal consequences. For example, the disease can be transmitted to other infants in a neonatal unit because it can be spread by personnel working in that setting. Acyclovir and vidarabine (adenine arabinoside) are effective against neonatal herpes.

Cytomegalovirus causes cytomegalic inclusion disease, the name derived from the massive enlargement of cytomegalovirus-infected cells. This generalized infection is caused by intrauterine or early postnatal infection. The disease causes severe congenital anomalies in about 3000 to 6000 infants in the United States each year.

93. The answer is B. *(Pathology)*
Neither congenital toxoplasmosis nor cytomegalovirus infections are associated with the formation of multinucleated cells.

Multinucleated cells have a varied etiology. Granulomas due to tuberculosis and systemic fungal infections (histoplasmosis) have multinucleated giant cells due to the fusion of activated macrophages. If the nuclei are arranged at the periphery, they are called Langhan cells; if they are scattered throughout the cytoplasm, they are called foreign body giant cells. Many diseases are associated with granulomas and multinucleated giant cells without evidence of caseating necrosis, including Crohn disease, sarcoidosis, and berylliosis. Foreign bodies (e.g., silicone, suture material, glass) also induce a foreign body type of giant cell reaction. In herpes infections, the infected squamous cells frequently fuse together to form a multinucleated cell with eosinophilic (Cowdry A) intranuclear inclusions. The Warthin-Finkeldey giant cell is pathognomonic of rubeola and can be found in the lymphoid organs, lungs, and sputum of infected patients. The nuclei contain glassy, eosinophilic intranuclear inclusions. Subacute encephalitis in AIDS patients (AIDS dementia) has microglial nodules in the brain characterized by the presence of multinucleated giant cells (fusion of microglial cells), tissue necrosis, and reactive gliosis. A characteristic of anaplasia is the presence of tumor giant cells.

94. The answer is E. *(Microbiology)*
Newborn infants may be infected with *Chlamydia trachomatis* by the mother, and 10% to 20% develop a respiratory tract infection that occurs 2 to 12 weeks after birth and culminates in pneumonia. *C. trachomatis* may be the most common cause of neonatal pneumonia. Radiographic examination shows consolidation of lungs and hyperventilation, and *C. trachomatis* should be considered if the newborn also has inclusion conjunctivitis. Erythromycin and tetracyclines (doxycycline) are effective treatments.

Chlamydia pneumoniae (TWAR) is a new species that causes respiratory disease in humans. Whereas most infections are asymptomatic or mild, severe disease has been reported. An atypical pneumonia similar to that caused by *Mycoplasma pneumoniae* is the primary recognized illness. Here, 5% to 20% of community-acquired pneumonia in young persons (but not neonates) is thought to be caused by *C. pneumoniae*. This species also is sensitive to erythromycin and tetracyclines.

The other options (growth in cell culture, reproduction by binary fission within the host cell lysosome, and infective stage as the elementary body) are the same for both *C. trachomatis* and *C. pneumoniae*.

95. The answer is E. *(Pathology)*
Vitamin E deficiency is most commonly caused by malabsorption, because vitamin E is fat soluble. Keratomalacia is softening of the cornea caused by vitamin A deficiency.

Riboflavin (vitamin B_2) is an essential component of flavin mononucleotide (FMN) and flavin adenine dinucleotide (FAD), which catalyze various oxidation–reduction reactions in the body. They can accept two hydrogen atoms, which can be used in oxidative phosphorylation in the mitochondria to generate 2 ATP. Riboflavin is present in meats, dairy products, and green vegetables and can be synthesized by bacteria in the bowel. Deficiency is characterized by

- corneal neovascularization
- a greasy, scaly facial rash in the nasolabial folds resembling a butterfly distribution
- cheilosis (cracking at angle of lips)
- glossitis with a magenta-colored tongue

Niacin is a water-soluble vitamin that is found in meats, fish, vegetables, nuts, and yeast. It is also synthesized by bacteria in the bowel and endogenously from tryptophan, an essential amino acid. Niacin and nicotinamide are required for formation of nicotinamide adenine dinucleotide (NAD) and nicotinamide dinucleotide phosphate (NADP), which are involved in most of the oxidation–reduction reactions in the body. Niacin deficiency, or pellagra, is characterized by

- the 3 Ds—diarrhea, dementia, and dermatitis
- the dermatitis involves increased pigmentation in sun-exposed areas. Cassal necklace is a classic finding
- posterior column degeneration similar to B_{12} deficiency

Tryptophan is also used to synthesize serotonin. Deficiency of tryptophan can occur in the carcinoid syndrome with excess production of serotonin and in Hartnup disease, in which there is an intestinal and renal defect in reabsorbing neutral amino acids. It is also

deficiency in corn, hence leading to pellagra. In either case, this deficiency results in niacin deficiency. Vitamin A maintains the light-sensitive pigment rhodopsin in the rods for night vision and iodopsin in the cones for daytime vision. It is carried by retinol binding protein (RBP) synthesized in the liver. RBP is necessary for the release of the vitamin from the liver. The liver contains large stores of retinyl esters, which can be converted into vitamin A. Vitamin A prevents the keratinization and metaplasia of epithelial cells. It is also important in wound healing and reverses the retardant effect of corticosteroids on wounds. Beta carotene is converted into vitamin A, with the help of thyroxine, and is also an antioxidant that is used along with vitamins E and C for preventing coronary artery disease.

96. The answer is A. *(Microbiology)*
Positive-sense RNA viruses, by definition, contain a single-stranded RNA genome that acts directly as viral messenger RNA. As such, genomic RNA isolated from virions, if introduced within a host cell, is able to initiate the viral life cycle. Picornaviruses (e.g., poliovirus) are the best examples of positive-sense RNA viruses. The released genome associates with host ribosomes and is translated as a large, single polypeptide. This is cleaved by proteases into structural proteins and viral enzymes. This process is called post-translational maturation of proteins. Actinomycin D intercalates at the site of guanine residues and inhibits DNA-dependent RNA synthesis. It has no effect on single-stranded RNA metabolism.

97. The answer is C. *(Biochemistry)*
Riboflavin, not niacin, is an essential component of flavin mononucleotide (FMN) and flavin adenine dinucleotide (FAD), which catalyze various oxidation–reduction reactions in the body. Niacin and nicotinamide are required for formation of nicotinamide adenine dinucleotide (NAD) and nicotinamide dinucleotide phosphate (NADP), which are involved in most of the oxidation–reduction reactions in the body.

Pantothenic acid is a component of coenzyme A (CoA) and fatty acid synthase. Because it is ubiquitous in many different foods, deficiency is rare. Thiamine (B_1) is important in carbohydrate metabolism because it is a cofactor in acetyl CoA production from pyruvate. When it is deficient, there is impaired adenosine triphosphate (ATP) production. It is also involved in

transketolase reactions (2 carbon transfer reactions) in the pentose phosphate shunt in order to provide intermediates for the glycolytic cycle. In Asia, the vitamin is removed from the outer portion of the rice (polished rice), thus resulting in deficiency. In the United States, thiamine deficiency is most often the result of poor diet in patients who are alcoholics. Thiamine deficiency results in beriberi, which affects the nervous system (dry beriberi) and the cardiovascular system (wet beriberi).

98. The answer is C. *(Physiology)*
For water to move by osmosis to or from the extracellular fluid (ECF) compartment into or out of the intracellular fluid (ICF) compartment, a gradient must be established between the two compartments.

The serum osmolality is a measure of the solute concentration in a solution and is expressed in the following formula:

Serum osmolality = 2 (serum sodium) + serum glucose/18 + serum blood urea nitrogen/2.8

Note that sodium is the key component that determines the serum osmolality. Sodium is multiplied by 2 because chloride ions also contribute to the total osmolality. The sodium concentration in the ECF is primarily responsible for the movement of water between the ECF and ICF compartments, because it is limited to the ECF compartment. Either a decrease (hyponatremia) or increase (hypernatremia) in the serum sodium establishes an osmotic gradient between the ECF and ICF compartments, resulting in the movement of water between the two compartments. In hyponatremia, water moves into the ICF (ICF expansion, or edema), whereas in hypernatremia, water moves out of the ICF compartment (ICF contraction). Glucose is limited to the ECF, because it is used in glycolysis immediately on entering a cell. In hyperglycemia, glucose overrides the primary role of sodium as the major osmotic force and draws water out of the ICF compartment. Therefore, water moves out of the ICF compartment into the ECF compartment and initially dilutes serum sodium (dilutional hyponatremia). Eventually, osmotic diuresis causes a loss of sodium, and the patient shows signs of dehydration.

Both glucose and sodium are considered impermeant solutes (i.e., limited to the ECF). Impermeant solutes can establish osmotic gradients in the ECF that alter the overall tonicity of the ECF and are able to affect water movements between the two compartments. Blood urea nitrogen (BUN) diffuses equally between the ECF and ICF; therefore, it does not establish a concentration gradient between the two compartments. Urea is considered a permeant solute. Tonicity of fluid is not the same as osmolality. The tonicity of plasma only refers to those factors (i.e., sodium and glucose) that do affect water movements between the ECF and ICF compartments. The tonicity is calculated the same way that osmolality is calculated, except the BUN is not included. Some clinicians use the term effective osmolality as an alternative for tonicity. It is possible to have an increase in osmolality only from an increase in the BUN without affecting the tonicity of the fluid.

The set of laboratory data that most closely approximates the normal serum osmolality is the set that has the least effect on moving water into the ICF compartment. Because BUN does not affect the establishment of a gradient, it is not considered in the calculations. The calculations are listed below. Note that choice C has an effective osmolality of 285 mOsm/kg, which is normal; therefore, it would have the least effect on causing water to move into the ICF compartment.

	Serum sodium (mEq/L)	Serum glucose (mg/dl)	Effective osmolality (mOsm/kg)
Choice A	120	90	245
Choice B	130	108	266
Choice C	140	90	285
Choice D	145	126	297
Choice E	145	126	297

99. The answer is D. *(Pathology)*

Selenium primarily functions in the metalloenzyme glutathione peroxidase, which is an antioxidant that destroys peroxides in the cytosol. Although glucose-6-phosphate dehydrogenase is in the pentose phosphate shunt, selenium is not present in this enzyme. Selenium coordinates its antioxidant activity with vitamin E, because it neutralizes peroxides in the cytosol, while vitamin E prevents peroxide formation in the membranes of cells. Selenium is also thought to inhibit DNA synthesis and stimulate the immune system. This may explain why low selenium levels are associated with an increase in certain types of cancer. Deficiency of selenium is also associated with muscle pain and cardiomyopathy.

Magnesium activates enzymes, modulates the vasoconstrictive effects of intracellular calcium in vascular smooth muscle, and is a cofactor for adenylate cyclase. When reduced, it will interfere with the proper functioning of parathormone (PTH), because it normally activates adenylate cyclase into cyclic AMP (cAMP).

Reduced PTH results in hypocalcemia. All hospitalized patients with hypocalcemia should have a magnesium level drawn to exclude hypomagnesemia, because it is the most common cause of hypocalcemia in the hospitalized patient. Like calcium, magnesium is partly bound to albumin (35%) and magnesium levels are influenced by the albumin concentration.

Chromium is a component of the glucose tolerance factor, which potentiates insulin. Chromium deficiency is characterized by glucose intolerance. Copper is a component of lysyl oxidase, cytochrome c oxidase, ferroxidase, and superoxide dismutase. Copper deficiency is associated with a microcytic hypochromic anemia, Menke kinky hair syndrome, hypercholesterolemia, and dissecting aortic aneurysms.

Zinc is a cofactor for enzymes in collagen metabolism. It is frequently deficient in the elderly population and in diabetics. Deficiency is characterized by

• acrodermatitis enteropathica
• poor growth and impaired sexual development in children

- poor wound healing
- decreased taste and smell sensations
- diarrhea
- rash around the eyes and mouth

100. The answer is A.   *(Pharmacology)*
Polyvalent crotalid antivenins contain serum globulins from horses immunized with the venoms of pit vipers (i.e., rattlesnakes, copperheads, and cottonmouths). The antivenins do not contain the venom of coral snakes; therefore, they will not effectively neutralize the toxic effects of an eastern coral snake bite. A separate antivenin, known as North American Coral Snake Antivenin, is required for the treatment of coral snake envenomation.

101. The answer is C.   *(Biochemistry)*
Caffeine has not been shown to predispose patients to any cancer. At one time, it was thought to contribute to pancreatic carcinoma.

Control of obesity is important for decreasing the risk for breast and endometrial cancers because of the increased aromatization of androgens into estrogens by the adipose. An increase in unopposed estrogen predisposes patients to the types of cancers previously mentioned.

Diets in which 40% of the total calories are fat predispose patients to colon cancer by increasing the formation of primary bile acids, which increases the formation of secondary bile acids, such as lithocholic acid, a carcinogen. High fat intake has also been implicated in breast cancer, because it increases free estrogen levels. This relationship, however, has now come under attack. The optimal level of fat intake should be less than 30% of the total calories (preferably less than 20%).

An increased intake of dark green, deep yellow, and orange vegetables increases vitamin C and beta carotenes, which are antioxidants that neutralize free radicals (FRs). FRs are able to induce point mutations. Deficiency of vitamin A has been implicated in cancer.

By reducing the intake of salt-cured, smoked, and nitrite-cured foods, there is a decrease in the formation of polycyclic aromatic hydrocarbons and nitrosamines, which have been implicated in cancer.

102. The answer is A.   *(Pathology)*
In endotoxic shock, endotoxins damage endothelial cells and activate macrophages, which cause the release of nitric oxide, a potent vasodilator that contributes to the pathophysiology of shock.

Shock causes the hypoperfusion of tissue with impaired tissue oxygenation. In early endotoxic shock, endotoxin causes vessel dilatation, high-cardiac output failure, and sinus tachycardia.

Endotoxins bind to CD14 receptors on leukocytes, endothelial cells, and other cells. Endotoxins also cause direct injury to cells or initiate the synthesis, release, or activation of chemical mediators derived from plasma or cells. Chemical mediators that are released include:

- Interleukin-1
- Tumor necrosis factor
- Interleukin-6
- Platelet-activating factor
- Nitric oxide
- Complement components C3a and C5a (anaphyla-toxins), which are released from activation of the alternate complement pathway
- Prostaglandins
- Kinins
- Free radicals
- Myocardial depressant factor

103. The answer is A.   *(Biochemistry)*
There is an increased concentration of vitamin A in the elderly, because the liver is not able to clear it out of the blood as quickly. For this reason, it is dangerous for elderly patients to take vitamin A supplements.

The need for calories is also decreased in the elderly. Absorption and utilization of pyridoxine (B_6) is reduced; many aged patients get less than 50% of the recommended daily allowance of B_6 in their diet.

There is a reduction in the need for iron in elderly women, because they are no longer having menses. Increased iron intake is associated with an increased risk for coronary artery disease, because iron increases the formation of FRs, which are capable of forming oxidized low-density lipoprotein (LDL). Oxidized LDL enhances atherogenesis.

Calcium supplementation slows the rate of bone loss in postmenopausal women with average diets. The recommended daily calcium intake for postmenopausal women is 1500 mg of calcium a day and 1000 mg a day for women in their reproductive period of life. The calcium should be taken with vitamin D (400–800 IU), because vitamin D is frequently inadequate in the diet as well.

104. The answer is E. *(Microbiology)*
The nuclear structure (chromosome) of prokaryotic organisms is not bounded by a membrane. Rather, the nuclear material, containing all of the organism's genetic information, is diffused throughout the cytoplasm. Bacteria, such as *Mycoplasma, Chlamydia, Rickettsia,* and *Corynebacterium,* are prokaryotes. Fungi (e.g., *Aspergillus*) and parasites (amoebas, helminths, and flagellates) are eukaryotes; that is, they contain a true nucleus surrounded by a definite membrane.

105. The answer is D. *(Biochemistry)*
Vitamin B_{12} is only found in animal products, so a vegetarian who also consumes eggs and dairy products will obtain enough B_{12} to offset the development of B_{12} deficiency. Pure vegetarians require supplementation of B_{12} in their diets. The liver stores of B_{12} are adequate for 6 to 10 years; therefore, deficiency from diet alone is uncommon.

Biotin deficiency can be caused by an increased consumption of raw egg whites because of the presence of avidin, which binds the vitamin; however, the consumption of approximately 20 raw egg whites a day would be required to produce clinical deficiency.

Folate deficiency is most commonly seen in patients who are alcoholics, because they have a poor dietary intake of vegetables and other nutrients. In addition, alcoholic patients have an increased loss of folate in their stools and urine. Folate deficiency produces megaloblastic anemia, because folate is involved in DNA synthesis and there is a lack of nuclear maturation.

Iron deficiency can occur in a pure vegetarian diet with no iron supplements. Approximately 10 to 20 mg of dietary iron is consumed a day, but only 10% is absorbed. Iron must be in the ferrous (+2) state to be reabsorbed in the duodenum. Heme iron (meats) is already in the ferrous state and is directly absorbed. Nonheme iron (plants) is in the ferric (+3) state and must be reduced by ascorbic acid in the food for reabsorption to occur. Stomach acid is necessary to break up the food in order to release the heme complexes. Women lose approximately 30 ml per period. Because 1 ml of blood contains 0.5 mg of iron, there is a loss of 15 mg of iron per period. A loss of more than 80 ml of blood per period (menorrhagia) on a continual basis is the most common cause of iron deficiency in women.

Pyridoxine (B_6) deficiency is not usually diet induced, but is most commonly related to drugs such as isoniazid (forms an inactive derivative with pyridoxal phosphate), hydralazine, and penicillamine.

106. The answer is E. *(Physiology)*
Ascites in cirrhosis is multifactorial and includes portal hypertension, which is associated with an increase in hydrostatic pressure; hypoalbuminemia (decreased synthesis) with a decreased oncotic pressure; secondary aldosteronism with sodium and water retention; and an increased loss of lymphatic fluid from blockage of lymphatics in the liver.

Edema may be localized or generalized and may represent a transudate or an exudate. Transudates are associated with an alteration in Starling forces, such that the oncotic pressure (serum albumin) is decreased, the intravascular hydrostatic pressure is increased, or both. Exudates imply an increase in vessel permeability and are most commonly associated with an inflammatory condition. The following chart summarizes the laboratory distinctions between transudates and exudates.

	Transudate	Exudate
Definition	Ultrafiltrate of plasma	Extravascular fluid rich in protein and cells
Protein content	<3 g/dl	>3 g/dl
Specific gravity	<1.016	>1.016
Mechanism	Starling forces alterations: low oncotic pressure, increased hydrostatic pressure, or both	Increased vessel permeability
Cells present	Very few cells	Many cells; an inflammatory response

Pulmonary edema in left-sided heart failure is primarily an increase in hydrostatic pressure caused by fluid buildup behind the failed heart. Once hydrostatic pressure overrides the oncotic pressure in the pulmonary capillaries, a transudate leaks into the alveolar space.

Dependent pitting edema in right-sided heart failure is caused by a buildup of venous blood, increasing the hydrostatic pressure, behind the failed right heart.

Pitting edema in kwashiorkor is caused by the decreased intake of protein, which reduces the serum albumin and the oncotic pressure.

Ascites in malabsorption is caused by the loss of protein in the stool with a reduction in the serum albumin and the oncotic pressure.

107. The answer is C. *(Biochemistry)*

Tyrosinemia is an autosomal recessive disease caused by a deficiency of fumarylacetoacetate hydrolase. The deficiency results in an increase in tyrosine, which leads

to severe liver disease (hepatitis, cirrhosis) and kidney disease (aminoaciduria and renal tubular acidosis).

Tyrosine
↓
4-Hydroxyphenylpyruvate
↓
Homogentisate
　↓　Homogentisate oxidase
Maleylacetoacetate
↓
Fumarylacetoacetate
　↓　**Fumarylacetoacetate hydrolase (deficient in hereditary tyrosinemia)**
Fumarate + Acetoacetate

A deficiency of tyrosinase produces the autosomal recessive disease albinism, which results in a lack of melanin pigmentation. Melanin is synthesized in melanocytes, which are derived from neural crest cells that are located in the epidermis. Melanin is formed when the enzyme, tyrosinase, converts tyrosine to 3,4-dihydroxyphenylalanine (DOPA), which, in turn, is polymerized in the Golgi apparatus into membrane-bound organelles called melanosomes.

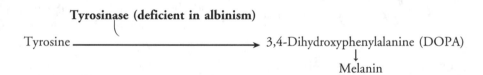

Tyrosinase (deficient in albinism)

Tyrosine ⟶ 3,4-Dihydroxyphenylalanine (DOPA)
　　　　　　　　　　　　　　　　　　↓
　　　　　　　　　　　　　　　　Melanin

Hartnup disease is a defect in the intestinal and renal uptake of neutral and essential amino acids, resulting in a pellagra-like disorder. The loss of the essential amino acid, tryptophan, which can be used to synthesize niacin, is the reason for the pellagra-like findings.

Cystinuria is caused by a defect in the intestinal and renal uptake of cysteine, lysine, ornithine, and arginine, leading to an increase in hexagonal-shaped cystine crystals in the urine and stone formation. Cys-

teine, a sulfur-containing amino acid, is converted into cystine. Cystinuria is the most common genetic error in amino acid transport.

Histidinemia is caused by a deficiency of histidase, which results in an increase in histidine in the blood. Transamination of the excess histidine into imidazolepyruvate results in increased levels of this compound in the urine, which produces a positive ferric chloride reaction. Mental retardation is present in some cases of histidinemia.

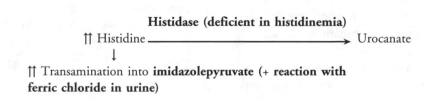

Histidase (deficient in histidinemia)

↑↑ Histidine ⟶ Urocanate
　↓
↑↑ Transamination into **imidazolepyruvate (+ reaction with ferric chloride in urine)**

Maple syrup urine disease is caused by a deficiency of branched chain α-ketoacid dehydrogenase, resulting in elevation of the α-branched chain amino acids and their α-ketoacid analogues. Sweet-smelling urine, neurologic problems, and increased mortality are characteristic of the disease. A diet low in branched chain amino acids (leucine, isoleucine, and valine) can prevent these complications.

108. The answer is B.   *(Behavioral science)*
Up to 65% of medical inpatients have psychiatric problems. Depression is a common psychiatric problem that affects medical inpatients. Psychotherapy and behavioral therapy are useful for treating psychological problems in medical inpatients. People with a history of psychiatric illness are at particular risk for psychological problems when medically ill.

109. The answer is A.   *(Microbiology)*
Viridans (α-hemolytic) streptococci are part of the normal flora, especially in the oral cavity. They can be opportunistic and are most often involved in infective endocarditis (often as a result of dental treatment). Endocarditis is 100% fatal unless recognized and treated with antimicrobial agents. Diagnosis is based on Gram stain examination, hemolysis on blood agar, and resistance to optochin.

Group B streptococci are β-hemolytic and are a significant cause of neonatal infections (e.g., meningitis). These organisms hydrolyze hippurate and are resistant to bacitracin.

Streptococcus faecalis, also a group B streptococcus, is an important cause of urinary tract infections. Group B streptococci are great opportunists outside of the intestinal tract and are capable of growing under more stringent laboratory conditions [e.g., 6.5% sodium chloride (NaCl)] than other streptococci.

Streptococcus pneumoniae may be confused with viridans streptococci because it is α-hemolytic, but it is easily distinguished on the basis of its sensitivity to optochin. Optochin is a quinine derivative that inhibits the growth of pneumococci, but not viridans streptococci.

Streptococcus mutans is often implicated in the formation of dental caries.

110. The answer is A.   *(Biochemistry)*
Histone H1 is bound to the linker DNA between nucleosomes and is not found in the nucleosome core. The basic unit of organization of chromatin is the nucleosome. Each nucleosome consists of a histone octamer with DNA wrapped around the outside. The nucleosome core contains two molecules each of histones H2A, H2B, H3, and H4.

111. The answer is A.   *(Pathology)*
Kaposi sarcoma is the most common type of cancer seen in AIDS patients. The incidence of AIDS-related Kaposi sarcoma has declined from approximately 40% (early in the epidemic when most new AIDS cases were homosexual males) to 20% in the 1990s. The etiology of the neoplasm is not clear, but there is speculation that it may be caused by the virus itself plus certain cofactors, such as cytomegalovirus and other agents. Homosexual AIDS patients have a 6-fold higher incidence of Kaposi sarcoma than heterosexual AIDS patients.

Kaposi's sarcoma is a vascular tumor thought to be of endothelial cell origin. AIDS patients have a 20,000 times greater risk for developing it than the general population. Organ transplant patients also have an increased risk.

Other neoplasms that are part of the AIDS-defining conditions are Burkitt-like lymphomas, primary central nervous system lymphomas, and immunoblastic lymphomas. Approximately 95% of these neoplasms are of B-cell origin. Colon cancer is not an AIDS-defining condition.

To have a diagnosis of AIDS, the patient must meet the criteria as defined by the Centers for Disease Control and Prevention. A CD4+ cell count of less than 200/μl of blood in a person infected with HIV type 1 is diagnostic of AIDS, regardless of whether or not symptoms are present. However, if the patient has an AIDS-defining condition, which includes certain opportunistic infections and types of neoplasms, HIV encephalopathy, and wasting syndrome, a diagnosis of AIDS can be made regardless of the CD4+ cell count.

112. The answer is A.   *(Behavioral science)*
Libido is not affected by menopause because the major female libido hormone is testosterone, produced by

the adrenal glands throughout life. A 55-year-old post-menopausal woman is, however, likely to experience vaginal dryness and thinning of the vaginal walls associated with discomfort during intercourse as a result of estrogen insufficiency. Sexual activity is likely to decrease with aging because of the absence of available partners. This is true particularly for women, because men die approximately 7–8 years sooner than women.

113. The answer is D. *(Microbiology)*

Genital warts are caused by a variety of human papilloma viruses (HPV; Papovaviridae family), none of which have been grown in vitro. HPV are small, double-stranded, DNA-containing viruses without an envelope. They exhibit great tropism for epithelial cells of the skin and mucous membranes. The replicative cycle of the viruses appears to depend on the stage of differentiation of the infected host cells. The late events in the multiplication cycle of HPV (i.e, synthesis of capsid proteins and maturation of virions) occur only in terminally differentiated epithelial cells. In contrast, the JC and BK viruses, which also belong to the Papovaviridae family, can be grown in cultures of human foreskin fibroblasts.

HPV induces a self-limiting cell proliferation, causing skin, genital, and laryngeal warts. Genital warts are among the fastest growing sexually transmitted diseases in the United States.

114. The answer is A. *(Pharmacology)*

Bacterial resistance to antibiotics may involve enzymatic inactivation of drugs, whereas tumor cell resistance does not usually involve drug inactivation. Tumor cell resistance is often mediated by the induction of one or more genes by the antineoplastic agent, and usually involves mechanisms such as decreased affinity or amplification of the target enzyme, increased DNA repair by topoisomerase II, or the efflux of drugs from tumor cells by the P-glycoprotein expressed by the multidrug resistance (MDR)-1 gene.

115. The answer is A. *(Behavioral science)*

Marijuana results in an immediate increase in libido primarily by psychological, rather than physiological, means. Other drugs of abuse increase sexual problems. Cocaine use is associated with priapism, heroin use is associated with premature ejaculation, and long-term

use of alcohol is associated with decreased potency in men.

116. The answer is D. *(Microbiology)*

Tetanus is caused by the anaerobe *Clostridium tetani.* Tetanus spores contaminate a wound where blood flow is decreased and produce an exotoxin. Subsequent necrosis creates an anaerobic environment where the spores germinate into vegetative bacteria. The area of infection remains localized and the tetanus exotoxin (tetanospasmin) is carried via retrograde intra-axonal transport to the central nervous system (CNS) or is delivered into the blood stream. Because the *C. tetani* organisms are seldom released into blood, blood cultures often fail to detect the presence of tetanus infection. The other infections listed in the question (osteomyelitis, brucellosis, typhoid fever, and bacterial pneumonia) all involve bacteremia (bacteria in the blood) or septicemia (bacterial growth in the blood) as part of their dissemination patterns. Although the presence of organisms in the blood may be intermittent in some diseases (e.g., osteomyelitis, brucellosis), blood culture remains the primary diagnostic procedure for confirmation of specific infection.

117. The answer is C. *(Pathology)*

In lung injury, type II pneumocytes are the reserve cell for repair of the alveolar epithelium.

A keloid refers to abnormal wound healing with the production of hypertrophic scar tissue (i.e., thick collagen bands) resembling a tumor. In African Americans, it is a common skin reaction to injury. There is an increased amount of type III collagen instead of the typical type I collagen.

Liver injury has three possible sequelae, mainly regeneration of hepatocytes, scar tissue formation (from the Ito cell), and a combination of regeneration and scar formation.

Central nervous system injury causes gliosis because of a proliferation of astrocytes. In the peripheral nervous system, Wallerian degeneration follows peripheral transection of the axon. The severed nerve exhibits demyelination back to the nearest node of Ranvier, with distal degeneration of the axon and its myelin sheath. Regeneration following peripheral transection of the nerve occurs by the outgrowth of multiple sprouts from the proximal transected nerve stump of the surviving segment of the axon, which reestablishes continuity with the distal nerve sheath.

118. The answer is E.   *(Pathology)*
A patient with a chronic stenosing lesion of the common bile duct would least likely have a problem with a deficiency of B_{12}, because it does not require bile salts for its absorption.

The other choices in the question would all be expected, because bile salts are required for the reabsorption of fats and the fat-soluble vitamins, A, D, E, and K. Follicular hyperkeratosis is a feature of vitamin A deficiency. Bleeding occurs because of vitamin K deficiency and inability to activate factors II (prothrombin), VII, IX, and X, which are synthesized in the liver in an inactive state. Mineralization of bone would be defective because of the lack of vitamin D, which reabsorbs calcium and phosphorus. Lack of mineralization of osteoid in bone is called rickets in children and osteomalacia in adults. Tetany results from the hypocalcemia associated with vitamin D deficiency.

119. The answer is E.   *(Microbiology)*
Chlamydia trachomatis is a gram-negative, obligate intracellular parasite. In the laboratory, cell culture is used to isolate the organisms. Although the elementary bodies are generally too small to be observed under normal Gram stain conditions, immunofluorescent antibody staining is an efficient and sensitive way to observe them. Enzyme-linked immunosorbent assays (ELISA) and DNA probes are also available and will eventually replace the fluorescent antibody technique.

Other organisms listed can be diagnosed with current latex agglutination tests. The group A streptococcus uses latex particles attached to an anti-group A antigen antibody. The *Streptococcus pneumoniae* test uses an antibody against polysaccharide capsules, as does the test for *Neisseria meningitidis*. The latex agglutination test for *Haemophilus influenzae* uses an antibody against the type B capsule.

120-121. The answers are: 120-D, 121-C.   *(Behavioral science)*
This man's educational level, socioeconomic status, intelligence, race, and marital status are not likely to be related to whether he complies with medical advice.

In contrast, a complex treatment regimen, long duration of treatment, presence of symptoms, and long waiting-room time are all associated with decreased compliance.

According to the Health Belief Model, the likelihood of this patient engaging in appropriate healthy behavior increases when he believes that the cost of treatment does not outweigh its benefits. Health behavior increases also when he feels ill, when his usual activities are disrupted by illness, when he thinks that it is practical to obtain health care and that he can overcome impediments to obtain needed care.

122-123. The answers are: 122-C, 123-E.   *(Behavioral science)*
The obese patient's behavior is most typical of a passive-aggressive personality type. She asked for help from the physician and then did not comply with his advice. Her anger with the physician, which she is not even aware of, is the reason for this behavior.

The faculty member's behavior is typical of the paranoid personality type. Paranoid personalities often blame others for their problems.

124-128. The answers are: 124-C, 125-D, 126-B, 127-E, 128-A.   *(Pharmacology)*
Danazol is a partial agonist and competitive antagonist at progesterone and androgen receptors, and it also binds to glucocorticoid receptors.

Mifepristone is a progesterone receptor antagonist and also blocks glucocorticoid receptors.

Clomiphene is a partial agonist and estrogen receptor antagonist.

Cyproterone and flutamide are androgen receptor antagonists.

Spironolactone is a selective androgen and aldosterone antagonist.

129-133. The answers are: 129-D, 130-G, 131-H, 132-A, 133-C.   *(Behavioral science)*
A 56-year-old single man who has voluntarily limited his contact with others during his adult life shows schizoid personality characteristics. Schizoid patients are withdrawn and prefer to be alone rather than with others. A 35-year-old female patient who tells you that she has fallen in love with you and attempts suicide when you recommend that she see another physician

shows borderline personality characteristics. Borderline patients are often inappropriate and impulsive. A 56-year-old female patient who arrives in your office dressed in suggestive clothing and describes her medical symptoms in an emotional, colorful fashion shows histrionic personality characteristics. Histrionic patients are often seductive and dramatic. A 45-year-old male patient who always arrives 15 minutes late for his appointment shows passive–aggressive personality characteristics. Passive–aggressive patients show outward compliance but are inwardly defiant, procrastinate, and often fail to meet deadlines. A 60-year-old male patient who tells you that he has filed numerous lawsuits and complaints shows paranoid personality characteristics. Paranoid patients are often suspicious and litigious and tend to blame others for their problems.

134-138. The answers are: 134-B, 135-E, 136-F, 137-D, 138-G. *(Biochemistry)*

Dolichol is an 80- to 100-carbon lipid onto which an oligosaccharide, containing *N*-acetylglucosamine, mannose, and glucose, is attached. The oligosaccharide is then transferred to an asparagine residue on a specific protein to form a glycoprotein. This process occurs in the lumen of the endoplasmic reticulum. This system of glycoprotein synthesis is in contrast to the way the other oligo- and polysaccharides (including glycogen, the glycosaminoglycans, and the *O*-linked glycoproteins) are synthesized. In the latter process, the sugars are added to a growing chain one at a time, most often as their uridine diphosphate (UDP) derivative.

The A, B, and O blood group antigens are, like many other cell membrane antigens, relatively simple glycoproteins. The non-antigenic O type is a three-

sugar chain consisting of *N*-acetylgalactose bound in a glycosidic link to the base protein, which is then coupled to a galactose and finally bound to a fucose. The group A antigen differs only in having another *N*-acetylgalactosamine bound to the galactose, whereas the group B antigen differs only in having a galactose bound in the same manner to the galactose. That is, the A and B antigens differ only in the presence or absence of an *N*-acetyl group on the galactose.

Niemann-Pick disease, an autosomal recessive disease, is particularly prevalent among Ashkenazi Jews, who have an estimated carrier rate of 1:100. Deficiency of lysosomal sphingomyelinase causes sphingomyelin to accumulate in the liver and spleen. Sphingomyelin is a phospholipid; the alcohol part of the molecule is sphingosine rather than glycerol. Sphingosine is a condensation product of palmitoyl coenzyme A (palmitoyl CoA) and serine:

$$CH_3(CH_2)_{12}-\underset{\underset{O}{|}}{\overset{\overset{H}{|}}{C}}H-\underset{}{\overset{\overset{H}{|}}{C}}H-C-\underset{\underset{\underset{H}{|}}{\overset{|}{N}H_3^+}}{C}-CH_2OH$$

A fatty acid is added to sphingosine, producing a ceremide:

$$CH_3(CH_2)_{12}-CH-CH-C-C-CH_2OH$$

with O, NH$_3^+$, H, C=O, (CH$_2$)$_n$, CH$_3$ — Fatty acid

Finally, a phosphocholine is added to the terminal hydroxyl group to form sphingomyelin:

$$CH_3(CH_2)_{12}-\overset{\displaystyle H}{\underset{\displaystyle O}{C}}H-CH-\overset{\displaystyle H}{C}-\overset{\displaystyle H}{\underset{\displaystyle NH_3^+}{C}}-CH_2-O-P-OCH_2CH_2N^+(CH_3)_3$$

H H
 | |
CH$_3$(CH$_2$)$_{12}$–CH–CH–C–C–CH$_2$–O–P–OCH$_2$CH$_2$N$^+$(CH$_3$)$_3$
     | |
     O NH$_3^+$
     | |
     H C=O   Phosphocholine
        |
     (CH$_2$)$_n$
        |
       CH$_3$

Sphingomyelinase normally cuts the phosphoester bond between the choline and ceramide. In Niemann-Pick disease, this reaction does not occur and sphingomyelin accumulates, resulting in severe mental retardation and death in early childhood.

Tay-Sachs disease, also prevalent among Ashkenazi Jews, is a fatal autosomal recessive disease caused by a deficiency of lysosomal β-hexoseaminidase A, which leads to the accumulation of gangliosides in the neural ganglia. As in Gaucher's disease, Tay Sachs disease is caused by a deficiency of a lysosomal enzyme necessary for the degradation of glycosphingolipids. Glycosphingolipids (gangliosides) differ from sphingomyelins in that they have a polysaccharide chain in place of the phosphocholine. Because they lack a phosphate and are linked to sugars, they are classified as glycolipids rather than phospholipids, despite their structural similarity. In the cell, gangliosides are linked together in a chain-like complex by an *N*-acetylneuraminic acid molecule. Tay-Sachs disease causes mental retardation, blindness characterized by cherry-red maculae, muscular weakness, seizures, and death.

Pompe's disease is an autosomal recessive glycogen storage disease caused by a deficiency of lysosomal α-1,4-glucosidase (acid maltase). This deficiency results in accumulation of glycogen in many tissues, particularly the heart, generally resulting in death from heart failure by the age of 2 years. Pompe's disease is unique among the glycogenoses in that it is caused by an aberrant lysosomal enzyme. This both accounts for the expression of the disease in most tissues and demonstrates the importance of the lysosomal degradative system, even in metabolic schemes that have their own catabolic component (e.g., glycogenolysis).

139-143. The answers are: 139-B, 140-A, 141-A, 142-C, 143-D. *(Pharmacology)*
The vaccine against whooping cough, caused by *Bordetella pertussis*, is derived from killed bacteria.

The vaccine against diphtheria, caused by *Corynebacterium diphtheriae*, is prepared from bacterial toxoid.

The vaccine against tetanus is also derived from bacterial toxoid.

Vaccines against hepatitis B, influenza, and rabies are prepared from killed viruses.

Vaccines against measles, mumps, polio, and rubella are prepared from live attenuated viruses.

144-149. The answers are: 144-E, 145-C, 146-B, 147-A, 148-D, 149-E. *(Behavioral science)*
Because the patient can only get through to the doctor if she finds a gap between the doctor's conversations, she begins dialing the doctor's office very frequently. This is an example of variable interval reinforcement [i.e., her reward or reinforcement (getting through) will occur at unpredictable time intervals].

Studying harder as the final approaches is an example of fixed interval reinforcement (i.e., the student's studying behavior increases in a set time interval to avoid failing the course).

A medical student who allows himself a candy bar after every 50 pages of a physiology text is practicing fixed ratio reinforcement. He receives his reward (candy) after a set number of responses (reading 50 pages).

The office worker who patronizes a vending machine in good working order is receiving continuous reinforcement because a reward (candy) will be obtained after every response (putting in money).

A gambler in Atlantic City will receive reinforcement on a variable ratio schedule, because an unpredictable number of responses (pulling the handle) will produce a reward (the payoff).

As in the first example, catching fish is an example of variable interval reinforcement because the reward (a fish) will occur at unpredictable time intervals.

150-152. The answers are: 150-B, 151-A, 152-C. (Biochemistry)

Alcaptonuria is caused by a deficiency in the enzyme homogentisate oxidase, which is involved in the breakdown of phenylalanine and tyrosine. In this disorder, homogentisate accumulates. Air oxidation of homogentisate causes urine to turn dark when voided.

Phenylketonuria is caused by a deficiency of phenylalanine hydroxylase, the enzyme that converts phenylalanine to tyrosine. Phenylalanine accumulates and is converted to excess amounts of the toxic compounds phenylpyruvate, phenyllactate, and phenylacetate. Unless the patient is placed on a diet low in phenylalanine, this condition will cause mental retardation.

Elevated phenylalanine levels can also occur because of defects in tetrahydrobiopterin metabolism, because this cofactor is required for the conversion of phenylalanine to tyrosine as well as the conversion of tyrosine and tryptophan to catecholamines and serotonin.

Maple syrup urine disease is caused by a deficiency of the branched-chain α-keto acid dehydrogenase, an enzyme involved in the breakdown of the branched-chain amino acids leucine, isoleucine, and valine. The name of the disease is derived from the sweet-smelling compounds that accumulate in the urine. Neurologic problems commonly occur in these patients.

Homocystinuria is due to a deficiency in cystathionine synthetase, an enzyme involved in the metabolism of methionine. Homocysteine and other metabolites of methionine accumulate.

Histidinemia is due to a deficiency in histidase. Elevated levels of histidine occur in the blood and urine.

Defects in amino acid metabolism often lead to mental retardation.

153-154. The answers are: 153-B, 154-C. (Microbiology)

Infection with human papilloma virus (HPV) type 18 or 16 is associated with a high risk for development of cervical cancer. DNA:DNA hybridization techniques have demonstrated that the great majority of cervical carcinoma cells have HPV DNA. The viral DNA tends to be integrated into cell DNA in invasive carcinomas, whereas in dysplasias it is usually episomal. The DNA of HPV types 16 and 18 are most often associated with invasive cervical cancers. Infected squamous cells exhibit a perinuclear halo and wrinkled nuclei, which is called koilocytosis.

DNA hybridization techniques and immunofluorescent antibody assays for viral antigens are used diagnostically for HPV infection. No serological tests are currently available. The viruses do not grow *in vitro* in cell cultures.

The male patient most likely has adult T-cell leukemia (ATL) caused by infection with the human T-cell leukemia virus type I (HTLV-I). ATL is characterized by the presence of pleomorphic cells in the peripheral blood, which have surface markers of mature T lymphocytes and enlargement of lymphoid organs. Skin lesions are present in >50% of cases, and hypercalcemia is common. HTLV-I is expressed at very low levels by infected T lymphocytes (CD4+).

155-158. The answers are: 155-N, 156-H, 157-F, 158-I. (Biochemistry)

The σ factor is a subunit of bacterial RNA polymerase, which helps the enzyme begin transcription. It dissociates from the core polymerase shortly after RNA synthesis begins.

Promoters are binding sites on DNA for RNA polymerase. They help instruct the polymerase what direction to go and where to initiate transcription.

Enhancers are special regulatory sequences in eukaryotes that can be located at various distances upstream or downstream of a gene, oriented in either direction. They are sometimes organ specific. They serve as binding sites for certain transcription factors that affect the rate of gene transcription.

The P site is a binding site on the ribosome for the nascent peptidyl-tRNA during protein synthesis. The A site is a similar location for the attachment of the new aminoacyl-tRNA specified by the latest codon encountered by the ribosome. An aminoacyl-tRNA only enters the P site directly during the binding of fMet-tRNA in the initiation of protein synthesis.

Ribosomes bind to the Shine-Delgarno sequence on prokaryotic mRNA molecules. The anticodon region of a tRNA molecule binds to its corresponding codon by the formation of complementary base pairs. Elongation factors aid in the process of protein synthesis as the ribosome moves down the messenger RNA molecule synthesizing the polypeptide strand. Release factor assists in the termination of protein synthesis when the ribosome encounters a nonsense (chain termination) codon.

The repressor protein binds to the operator region of DNA to regulate gene transcription in prokaryotes. Rho factor is a protein subunit of bacterial RNA polymerase involved in the termination of transcription at rho-dependent termination sequences. The attenuator is a special terminator of transcription used in the regulation of certain bacterial operons.

159-163. The answers are: 159-E, 160-B, 161-C, 162-D, 163-A. *(Pharmacology)*

Busulfan, an alkylsulfonate alkylating agent, is used to treat chronic myelogenous leukemia. It is slowly reactive and administered orally.

Mechlorethamine, a nitrogen mustard alkylating agent, is used to treat Hodgkin disease. It is highly reactive and must be administered intravenously. Prednisone is also used to treat Hodgkin disease; however, mechlorethamine is the first-choice agent for this disease.

Prednisone, a glucocorticoid with lymphotoxic effects, is used to treat acute lymphocytic leukemia.

Cytarabine, a pyrmidine analog with S-phase specificity, is used to treat acute myelocytic leukemia.

Chlorambucil, a nitrogen mustard alkylating agent, is used to treat chronic lymphocytic leukemia. It is slowly reactive and administered orally. Prednisone is also used to treat chronic lymphocytic leukemia; however, chlorambucil is the first-choice agent for this disease.

164-169. The answers are: 164-K, 165-L, 166-H, 167-H, 168-M, 169-E. *(Biochemistry)*

All water-soluble vitamins, except vitamin B_{12}, are rapidly excreted in the urine and need to be replaced daily. However, once saturated, the liver has a 5- to 7-year supply of vitamin B_{12}.

Vitamin B_6 is a collective term for pyridoxine, pyridoxal, and pyridoxamine. All three forms are phosphorylated and are used as the cofactor pyridoxal phosphate. This cofactor forms Schiff bases with the α-amino groups of the amino acids and helps catalyzation, transamination, deamination, decarboxylation, and condensation reactions. In addition to its role in amino acid metabolism, vitamin B_6 is an essential part of glycogen phosphorylase.

Niacin, or nicotinic acid, and nicotinamide are substituted pyridine derivatives, which are coupled in the body to an adenosine via a pyrophosphate bridge to form the adenine dinucleotides, NAD^+ and $NADP^+$. A deficiency of niacin results in pellagra, which is characterized by the four Ds: dermatitis, diarrhea, dementia, and if untreated, death.

Tryptophan can be converted to niacin in the body. However, the conversion is inefficient, because about 60 mg of tryptophan is transformed into only 1 mg of niacin. The conversion only occurs if there is excess tryptophan following protein synthesis. Serotonin is also formed from tryptophan.

Pantothenic acid is a component of coenzyme A, which functions in the transfer of acyl groups. Coenzyme A plays a central role in metabolism cofactor for pyruvate and α-ketodehydrogenases, fatty acid β-oxidation, and the fatty acid synthetase complex.

Ascorbic acid (vitamin C) is a required cofactor for the posttranslational hydroxylation of proline and lysine during collagen synthesis. Ascorbic acid deficiency causes weak collagen, resulting in a condition called scurvy that is characterized by perifollicular hemorrhages, glossitis, and gum and hematologic diseases. The latter is caused by a secondary iron deficiency caused by the inability to maintain iron in the ferrous state during digestion and absorption. Scurvy is prevented with a daily intake of 10 to 15 mg of ascorbic acid. The antioxidant function of ascorbic acid requires a 100-fold higher intake. Ascorbic acid is also used to treat methemoglobinemia, because it also reduces ferric to ferrous iron in the heme molecule.

170-171. The answers are: 170-A, 171-C. *(Physiology)*

According to the Henderson-Hasselbach equation, the arterial pH is proportional to the ratio of bicarbonate (HCO_3^-) to carbon dioxide tension (P_{CO_2}), which is approximately 20:1. Because the relationship is a ratio, an increase or decrease in either the HCO_3^- or P_{CO_2} concentration automatically alters the arterial pH. Compensation is for acid–base disorders in an attempt to bring the ratio back to 20:1, which should bring the pH back to the normal range (full compensation).

If the HCO_3^- concentration is increased and the arterial pH is decreased, the patient must have a primary respiratory acidosis. In this case, metabolic alkalosis is the compensation.

If the HCO_3^- concentration is decreased and the arterial pH is decreased, the patient must have a primary metabolic acidosis. In this case, respiratory alkalosis is the compensation.

172-175. The answers are: 172-G, 173-J, 174-A, 175-D. *(Biochemistry)*

Magnesium is a critical element in energy metabolism. It is chelated by adenosine triphosphate (ATP) and adenosine diphosphate (ADP), thereby neutralizing negative charges on the phosphates and altering their conformation. All ATP and ADP requiring reactions use magnesium ion as a cofactor. It also forms bridges between negative charges on some enzymes and their substrates. Magnesium deficiency is common among the elderly, alcoholics, and with individuals taking certain medications (e.g., aminoglycosides, cisplatin).

Zinc is an essential cofactor for a large number of enzymes, including collagenases involved in collagen remodeling, carbonic anhydrase, carboxypeptidases, alkaline phosphatases, lactate dehydrogenases, and for RNA and DNA polymerases (which bind to "zinc fingers" on the DNA).

Loss of acuity in distinguishing taste, smell, or both may accompany the aging process and also appears to be associated with a decreased ability to absorb zinc. Gustin, a 27 K molecular weight polypeptide, is necessary for the development and maintenance of taste buds. This peptide is a close relative of nerve growth factor and has two atoms of zinc per molecule bound to it.

Chromium is a constituent of glucose tolerance factor. A deficiency of chromium, which may be induced by parenteral nutrition, decreases a person's ability to lower blood glucose levels and may be a contributing factor to type II diabetes.

Iodine is used by the thyroid gland to synthesize thyroxine and triiodothyronine. It is stored in the thyroid gland on thyroglobulin. To compensate for an iodine deficiency, the thyroid gland enlarges, causing goiter. Iodine is found naturally in seafood, and goiter was endemic in areas in which seafood was unavailable. In the United States, most individuals obtain the required amount of iodine from iodized table salt.

176-180. The answers are: 176-G, 177-D, 178-C, 179-A, 180-B. *(Behavioral science)*

Nausea on seeing the needle (even before the medication has begun to flow) in a woman who has received five previous intravenous chemotherapy treatments is an example of a conditioned response. A conditioned response is one that is learned by an association, such as nausea that has occurred in the past in conjunction with exposure to the needle. Now, just seeing the injection needle causes nausea. Receipt of candy each time a child prints a letter more clearly is an example of the learning technique of shaping (i.e., rewarding closer and closer approximations of a desired behavior). The medical student who observes a surgeon doing a procedure on a patient before attempting it herself is using the learning technique of modeling (i.e., observational learning). After 4 weeks of Gross Anatomy lab, the medical student who no longer notices the smell of formaldehyde is showing habituation; she has become "used to" the noxious stimulus. The reverse phenomenon, sensitization, is exemplified by the medical student who is more bothered by the smell of formaldehyde after 4 weeks of Gross Anatomy lab than she was on the first day of lab.

SUBJECT ITEM INDEX

Test 3 : 1, 3, 5, 7, 9, 20, 35, 47, 53, 57, 63, 65, 66, 67, 68, 69, 70, 75, 76, 77, 81, 91, 92, 94, 107, 117, 119, 125, 126, 132, 133, 134, 144, 145, 146, 147, 148.

Test 4 : 1, 2, 28, 43, 47, 51, 52, 53, 54, 55, 56, 57, 58, 59, 60, 61, 62, 64, 65, 68, 71, 84, 89, 108, 112, 115, 120, 121, 122, 123, 129, 130, 131, 132, 133, 144, 145, 146, 147, 148, 149, 176, 177, 178, 179, 180.

MICROBIOLOGY

Dx Test : 8, 11, 12, 17, 18, 20, 24, 26, 29, 33, 35, 37.

Test 1 : 2, 8, 15, 22, 26, 28, 30, 32, 34, 35, 37, 39, 41, 43, 45, 47, 48, 50, 52, 54, 56, 58, 60, 62, 64, 66, 68, 70, 85, 90, 91, 94, 101, 106, 110, 112, 114, 115, 116 121, 127, 130.

Test 2 : 2, 5, 7, 11, 13, 15, 17, 20, 29, 37, 43, 46, 48, 50, 52, 54, 56, 58, 60, 61, 64, 66, 77, 87, 89, 94, 96, 100, 106, 109, 111, 113, 115, 118, 121, 124, 148, 149, 150, 156, 157, 176, 177, 178, 179, 180.

Test 3 : 2, 6, 10, 14, 25, 33, 37, 41, 45, 49, 52, 54, 56, 58, 60, 62, 64, 80, 82, 83, 89, 90, 97, 103, 108, 111, 115, 120, 122, 163, 164, 165, 177, 178, 179, 180.

Test 4 : 3, 8, 12, 16, 20, 24, 32, 36, 38, 42, 44, 46, 48, 50, 70, 73, 74, 75, 83, 90, 92, 94, 96, 104, 109, 113, 116, 119, 153, 154.

BIOCHEMISTRY

Dx Test : 2, 14, 15, 28, 39, 40, 41, 45, 46, 47.

Test 1 : 3, 4, 5, 7, 9, 11, 13, 14, 16, 17, 19, 21, 24, 29, 31, 36, 38, 40, 53, 59, 63, 69, 72, 74, 78, 86, 93, 100, 103, 105, 107, 119, 123, 125, 129, 134, 144, 145, 146, 147, 148, 149, 155, 156, 157, 158, 159, 160, 169, 170, 171, 172, 178, 179, 180.

Test 2 : 3, 4, 8, 12, 18, 27, 31, 35, 39, 49, 69, 70, 71, 72, 78, 79, 80, 84, 88, 91, 92, 93, 97, 99, 101, 103, 114, 123, 135, 136, 137, 141, 142, 151, 152, 153, 154, 155, 163, 164, 165, 166, 174, 175.

Test 3 : 11, 13, 15, 17, 19, 21, 23, 27, 31, 39, 51, 55, 59, 71, 73, 79, 84, 85, 86, 88, 93, 96, 98, 100, 104, 110, 113, 116, 121, 124, 127, 128, 129, 130, 131, 135, 136, 142, 143, 171, 172, 173, 174.

Test 4 : 6, 10, 14, 18, 22, 26, 30, 34, 37, 39, 41, 45, 49, 63, 66, 72, 76, 77, 78, 85, 86, 97, 101, 103, 105, 107, 110, 134, 135, 136, 137, 138, 150, 151, 152, 155, 156, 157, 158, 164, 165, 166, 167, 168, 169, 172, 173, 174, 175.